S0-EKO-387

BALLET TECHNIQUE
FOR THE
MALE DANCER

BALLET TECHNIQUE FOR THE MALE DANCER

BY

NIKOLAI I. TARASOV

ADAPTED BY MARIAN HOROSKO
TRANSLATED BY ELIZABETH KRAFT
EDITED BY N. T. FINOGENOVA
ILLUSTRATED BY N. M. VOVNOBOY

DOUBLEDAY & COMPANY, INC.
GARDEN CITY, NEW YORK
1985

The author of this book was a famous teacher of classical dance, formerly a soloist of the Bolshoi Ballet. The first edition of the book received the State Prize of the USSR in 1975. In preparing the second edition, the author enlarged the book with new exercises and illustrations. A foreword by Tarasov's pupil Maris Liepa, Lenin Prize Laureate, has been added. The text is addressed to teachers, ballet masters, and students of the choreographic schools.

Photographs of M. Lavrovsky, A. Vetrov, I. Mukhammedov with L. Semenyaka, and Andris Liepa are by Vladimir Pcholkin.

Photograph of Irek Mukhammedov in class is by Shigeo Yamamoto.

BOOK DESIGN BY BEVERLEY VAWTER GALLEGOS

Originally published as Klassicheskiy tanets by
"Art" Publishing House, 1971, 1981
Sobinovskiy per. 3
103009 Moscow

LIBRARY OF CONGRESS CATALOGING IN PUBLICATION DATA
Tarasov, Nikolai Ivanovich, 1902–1975.
Ballet technique for the male dancer.
Translation of: Klassicheskiĭ tanets.
Includes index.
1. Ballet dancing for men.   I. Horosko, Marian.
II. Title.
GV1788.2.M46T3513   1984   792.8'2'088041   82-46042
ISBN 0-385-18448-4

Copyright © 1985 by Marian Horosko
All rights reserved
Printed in the United States of America
First Edition

CONTENTS

PART ONE: THE SCHOOL

PART TWO:
ELEMENTARY MOVEMENTS OF CLASSICAL DANCE

(Plié, relevé, battements and ronds de jambes; forms of port de bras.
Descriptions are given with movements of the legs; arms, torso, head;
rhythm of the step and suggested accompaniment for given levels.)

PART THREE: POSES AND DANCE STEPS
(The poses of classical dance. Positions of the arms for poses;
description of rounded and elongated positions.)

PART FOUR: JUMPS AND BEATS
(Small jumps, beats and large jumps.)

PART FIVE: TURNS AND TURNING

(Turns and spins par terre—on the floor—and en l'air—in the air—are described as changes in direction and as a virtuoso element added to basic vocabulary. Tours—turns—are further divided into small pirouettes, big pirouettes—grandes pirouettes—and tours in big poses. Tours move en dehors—outward— or en dedans—inward.)

FOREWORD

BY

MARIS LIEPA

A WORD ABOUT A TEACHER

The small library of textbooks for teaching ballet has been enriched by this book, *Ballet Technique for the Male Dancer*. Its author, Nikolai Ivanovich Tarasov, represented Moscow's ballet. He was a Muscovite by birth as well as in his character and artistic ideals. His entire life was bound to Moscow and he rarely left his beloved city. During those rare absences, his life still flowed with the rhythm of the city, its interests which he felt everywhere, its breath and life-giving character. The author of this book is no longer with us, but if death is ever wise, it was so with Tarasov. He worked up to the end of his life. He taught and discussed the teaching of ballet, maintained an unvaried interest in new ballet premieres and did not bother anyone with his physical troubles. He demanded neither care nor compassion and passed on as quietly, bravely and beautifully as he had lived.

The work of the ballet teacher is passed from generation to generation, becomes perfected, acquires new traits and lives not only in the classes of the ballet school but also on stage, where the complexities of the art of dance come alive. In the choreographic schools of Moscow, Riga, Kiev, Berlin, Prague, Budapest, Sofia and many other cities, Tarasov's pupils are teaching and preserving the precepts of their famous teacher.

Tarasov became eloquent and animated only when he talked about ballet, artistic news or new books. He seldom spoke about himself even in intimate moments of talk with his pupils at his home. All that can be told here is what has been learned from brief lines in his autobiography, from my personal work with him and from impressions during study with him, talks, and reports from those who knew him in his youth and mature years.

Nikolai Ivanovich Tarasov was born on December 19, 1902, in Moscow into a family of dancers of the Bolshoi Ballet. There are indications that his father recognized his abilities and decided his future by placing him, in 1913, into the Moscow Choreographic School. His teachers were N. Domashev and N. Legat.

The future dancer stepped through the doorway of the Choreographic School during a complex and contradictory period in Russian ballet. Gorsky and Fokine were creating new works. Pavlova, Karsavina, Geltser, Fedorova and Nijinsky, in guest appearances all over the world, extolled Russian art.

Domashev was one of the outstanding dancers of his time. His views on art were realistic, consistent, wide in scope. All who saw him dance were amazed at his brilliant virtuoso technique, his noble manner and amazing elevation. One could compare him only with St. Petersburg's Nijinsky.

Legat, Tarasov's second teacher, studied at the St. Petersburg School. He knew the pedagogical system of Christian Johansson and Petipa. Legat learned to dance from Gerdt, another outstanding teacher and artist, a stylist and master of the art of partnering. Lopukhov, a connoisseur of classical choreography, characterized Legat's method: "Intuitively he understood the need of each pupil in the class. He gave the same movement to all, but for each made corrections relating to his given possibilities. This individual approach to each student was the superiority of Legat over other teachers. He tried, with additional exercises, to strengthen and develop musculature where he saw weakness."

Many years have passed since Tarasov left the stage. For that reason, we recount the appraisal of his contemporaries: "Tarasov had a brilliant ballon. In big jumps, the size of his figure was not felt. In Leningrad, he brought glory to the Bolshoi Ballet when he performed sixteen entrechats-six in a row in Basil's final variation." "He was an ideal cavalier. All the ladies loved to dance with him," recalls A. Tsarman.

It is probable that none of his contemporary ballerinas was as exacting a partner as Marina Semenova. She demanded not only exactness and adroitness, but also the ability to feel inner rhythms of dance, momentarily changing nuances. She called Tarasov a brilliant partner. Ballerinas always felt secure with him and portrayed their roles well against his acting. A. Radunsky refers to his beautiful plastique and a special importance he imparted to the role of Apollon in *Esmeralda*. Appearances with such famous ballerinas as Geltser, Semenova, Krieger, Podgoretskaya, Abramova and others helped to perfect his mastery and gain the ability to work with a variety of stage temperaments.

In the 1920s excited discussions were in progress on whether ballet should live, whether it was needed by the Soviet audience or if it was only a part of bourgeois culture. The young and older artists of the ballet defended their art with passion and action. In spite of the difficult living conditions in the early years in Soviet society, they continued tirelessly to pursue perfection. They appeared in numerous concerts for the military and in the schools. They learned to know their new audience through the performances and by talking freely with them afterward in clubs and barracks. This exchange was of enormous value to form a new outlook and to widen their horizons of understanding.

Curious and observant, Tarasov gained a great deal from these meetings. During this period he read history books, books on the problems of the revolutionary movement and art books to seek answers to troubling questions. His last years at school, so important to the forming of the intellect, were linked to the Civil War and destruction. So much was lost, general education was superficial, but as a young artist he caught up with the rest by enriching his education by going to the Tretyakov Gallery, the Pushkin Museum, and the Moscow Philharmonic.

Tarasov loved nature. He waited impatiently for the two-month vacation at the end of the school year in the outskirts of Moscow. Later he chose a village near Lake Seliger, where he would always spend his vacation with classmates: Ulanova, Vecheslova, Gusev, Lopukhov and Chekrygin, with whom Tarasov shared a long working friendship throughout the years.

Tarasov, in the theater, survived the discussion on whether ballet was to be or not to be. In spite of enormous material difficulties, the Bolshoi was saved, its school, its traditions of the performing art, and, even more important, the ballet masters were able to maintain these traditions and to perfect them under the new conditions. Gorsky created, in a very short time, two stage versions of *Swan Lake,* and *The Nutcracker,* and Tikhomirov restored and lightly retouched *The Sleeping Beauty.*

Within the ballet company itself, there were discussions on the future development of the art. The lexicon of dance was the object of the most heated discussions. The question was if it should remain academic and strict, gradually being renewed through union with new themes, new stage methods, or if it should be rebuilt as fast as possible, assimilating elements of nonclassic dance. For the most part, the company favored the gradual and normal inner rebuilding. Before the first heroic-romantic Soviet ballet, *The Red Poppy,* to the music of Glière, in which Tarasov performed, there was a new treatment of *Esmeralda,* with emphasis on folk themes and nonclassical motifs. These two works defined the future development of ballet and its school.

The artists of Moscow were not alone. The outstanding teacher, Agrippina Vaganova, while not deviating from the fight for classical choreography, recognized the need for the art to renew itself and gain further perfection.

Tarasov firmly joined those who believed in the classical school as the basic beginning of the balletic art and who, following its strict laws, accepted the need for development and renewal.

A large number of artists began to teach in the middle or at the end of their performing career. Rarely did a teaching career start at the same time as the artistic career, but Tarasov began teaching almost from the first years of his career on stage. In 1920, he became an artist of the Bolshoi, in 1923, a teacher. His teaching activity started in the rehearsal studios of the Bolshoi when he led company classes for the leading soloists. This he did until 1936.

In his daily class, artists such as A. Messerer, Yermolayev and Gabovich, as well as others, maintained their mastery and developed their technique. In addition to those classes, Tarasov taught from 1923 to 1960, without interruption, in the Moscow Choreographic School.

His fate was to be an artistic leader and director of a school during the hardest years during and after World War II. Tarasov repeated the feat of Glushkowski, who, in the Patriotic War of 1812, evacuated the Moscow School under dire conditions and thus saved it from destruction. The task of saving the school during the years of the Great War—World War II—was placed directly on Tarasov's shoulders. In Vasilsursk, where the school was moved and which was filled with the evacuated, Tarasov found room for studios, hostels for the students, living quarters for the teachers. He was always known as an exact man, contained, softhearted and kind, but no one realized he possessed remarkable organizational talent and had the ability to find solutions to the most difficult problems and to overcome hopeless conditions. Because of his efforts, the school did not close during the war, and Tarasov became to the students not only their teacher-director, but also a loving, caring father. That was extremely important to the children who had been torn away from home and family.

"We lived in the club of people working in water supplies," reminisces People's Artist R. Struchkova. "We studied there, and had a studio for lessons with all the other rooms used as bedrooms. We were cold, hungry, depressed and without a parent's caress. Sometimes we would wake and see Nikolai Ivanovich near the stove, seeing to it, so that the pupils would be warm for the day's studies. His care for the youngest was amazing and touching. No matter what age the child, Nikolai Ivanovich saw the future person in him. Although he was strict and demanding in class, at other times he was a caressing, kind person to each of us. He received letters from Moscow and from the front, thanking him for his care of the children. In the studio, there was a small stove. The pianist, Potanov, in felt boots and gloves, like a magician, produced sounds from an old, broken instrument.

"It was 1942 and we studied, rehearsed for concerts for the patients—wounded soldiers. We gave more than forty concerts in the hospital and performed a children's ballet, *Son Dremovich,* staged by Kasyan Goleizovsky."

While giving his professional energy and the warmth of his heart to the school, Tarasov thought of the future of ballet. He had, by this time, already composed a pedagogical system and methodology. Doubtless Tarasov in creatively reforming his view used much of his experience with Domashev, Tikhomirov and Legat. But it would be a mistake to consider his pedagogy a synthesis of his predecessors. Tarasov's methods have his unique character and rest basically on his own enormous experience. But this personal experience has the blood of theater life, that relatively novel something that stage adds to the vocabulary of dance and to the professional image of the actor.

He participated directly in the ballets of Petipa, Ivanov and Gorsky, Tikhomirov and Goleizovsky. Before his very eyes, he saw the emergence of young choreographers like Vainonen, Zakharov, Lavrovsky, Chabukiani and Grigorovich. While building his daily lessons, creating methods and programs for teachers, he knew what was going on in the theater and knew how to combine strict academic laws with the demands of the times.

During the years of study, his pupils acquired the ability not only to master the technique of classical dance, but to add a sense of plastique, insight and imaginative interpretations. He himself said: "Classical dance as a subject of study does not place as its goal the mastery of the study of the basics of acting. Nonetheless, from the first to the last lesson in classical dance, the learning of a means of expression is indivisibly connected to the ballet artist as a basis of his mastery. As the technique strengthens, the student's knowledge of the expressive gesture strengthens as well."

Whenever anyone came for the first time to Tarasov's class they were amazed by the even, quiet academic pace. And indeed, academic strictness in the combination, musicality, a correct and polite manner toward the students and inner constraint created this atmosphere of quiet and balance. Beneath this understanding by both the pupils and the teacher was hidden a creatively active and total dedication to the work. There were no pointless tasks in Tarasov's lessons. They all contributed in some way to the goal of the lesson. An attentive eye could discern what he intended to introduce next as new material.

In working with the future teacher, Tarasov always demanded exact knowledge of the elements in each exercise already learned and knowledge of what must be prepared before new movements were studied. This principle was applied equally to separate elements as well as to an entire section of the study.

In this way, Nikolai Ivanovich considered that turning, as a unit, should be taught at the barre and not in the center. The dancer's entire mechanism should be prepared in this way for turning. In the center, he required that the pupil already be spinning—that is, dancing freely, using the technique of spinning as a part of the ballet artist's mastery.

Tarasov's lessons had a strict general composition: barre with the adagio dominant; a center consisting of adagios and allegro movements; and the finale. Each section of the center work had its own culmination, the highest point of effort.

Tarasov, like every teacher, had his characteristic methods and combinations, which makes it easy to recognize Tarasov's training in his pupil's teaching. With their inner structure and artistic finish, Tarasov's lessons were like a performance. The lessons at times ended in an etude danced to classical or modern music. It was, for the most part, a heroic theme. The etude served as a link between class combinations and future roles.

Tarasov attributed great importance to the musical structure of the lesson and forbade the accompanist to play bits from operas, ballets, or improvisations on popular songs. Lessons were accompanied by new and improvised music. It, as a rule, had a clear rhythm which did not follow the pupils but led them.

When I studied with him, he was already ill and rarely demonstrated a movement himself. One of his strong pupils showed us the movement, but for the most part, Tarasov explained the combination with his hands. He did this clearly and it seemed to us that we saw the contours of the overall form. We also got used to having our task explained verbally. His descriptions were full of images and rhythms. In the higher levels, we had no difficulty in translating the verbal instructions into the speech of movement.

Tarasov remembered that the creative life of many artists ends in teaching. For this reason, in the senior classes he analyzed combinations and entire lessons, teaching us to think like a teacher.

Tarasov led his class sitting down. He had to see us all. Not one fault escaped his attentive eye. His concentration was unbroken. Work with him was easy and joyful. I don't remember ever waiting impatiently for the end of a lesson. Although his manner was not assertive, the student willingly fell under his influence and our trust in him was limitless. His authority at school and in GITIS (the State Institute of Theatrical Art) was unquestioned.

The pupils of this talented teacher and fine psychologist not only performed in full detail all their given movements and combinations, but also became co-workers in the creative process. This developed analytical thinking and imagination. Tarasov studied his pupils attentively. He knew the physical abilities, the creative possibilities, the endurance and temperament of each, as well as his psychological traits, interests and living habits. Everything interested him. To a wise tutor, this was necessary for the harmonious forming of the future actor/dancer. It helped overcome faults sensibly and with understanding. In the forming of the dancer, a man and citizen was formed as well. The actor and citizen—an indivisible idea in Tarasov's teaching—was rightly considered one of the most important principles of the Soviet Choreographic School.

His students were always open with him. They shared their innermost thoughts and fears and their ideas about their future profession. And in turning to their beloved teacher, they knew they would always receive a useful answer.

Nikolai Ivanovich respected his young but not yet strong brothers in art. He respected them with a sense of human dignity and, even when punishing them for serious faults, he always remembered that before him was an unformed character, vulnerable, easily hurt and in need of special attention. We who were fortunate to study with him never heard an irritable voice, a peremptory remark, a derisive or biting comment. His control, inner restraint, politeness and good will forever remain an example. As a teacher, Nikolai Ivanovich had another interesting ability. He taught us to think about the performances we saw in the theaters of the city, the guest appearances by foreign groups, the film premieres and exhibitions. Each time he would ask, with a kind smile, "Well, from what you have seen, what have you put into your actor's briefcase?"

The problems in methods of classical dance training and aesthetic education always concerned him. I especially understood and felt this when I became a ballet artist and talked with him on questions of teaching. Tarasov was among those who gave choreographic pedagogy a truly scientific basis and systematic organization. In 1940, together with A. I. Chekrygin and V. E. Moritz he created his *Methods of Classical Training,* which was issued in large numbers and at once became a rarity.

In 1945, GITIS, in the name of Lunacharsky, was opened with a faculty of ballet masters. A few years later, there was also a faculty of pedagogues of choreography. For the first time in the history of ballet, higher education was established for the education of choreographers. As an organizer of the faculty, the great Soviet choreographer Zakharov was able to find co-workers and helpers able to author a program in the separate sciences of the entire teaching plan. Colleagues of Zakharov were strongly associated with the Bolshoi and its school: Tarasov, Vasilieva-Rozhdestvenskaya, Tkachenko, Tseitlin and, soon, Lavrovsky.

In GITIS, a new and very important page in Tarasov's biography was begun. Officially, he was the head of the course in the composition of classical dance. In reality, he headed the various branches associated with classical dance. Tarasov saw to it that the daily study of classical dance turned into a creative laboratory enriching the palette of the future choreographer.

In creating a new branch, Professor Tarasov added his own extremely rich experience of style and theatrical knowledge, and also included contemporary theater—what life asks of the art of dance.

As a talented and experienced master of methods, Tarasov created the program for a course called "Composition of Classical Dance," defining exactly the problems of the subject and the method for its teaching. He seemed to have a premonition that this subject would soon take a respected place in the teaching plan of the choreographic institutes. This program is still in existence today.

Life presents new demands to art, and it is possible that, in time, there will be changes and additions to the program created by Tarasov, but the foundation of this complex subject will always be that which he created.

Tarasov understood new harmonious movements, new stylistic characteristics, and contemporary themes. At the same time, he constantly reminded his pupils of the limits of genre and the specifics of ballet art, the disregarding of which, he predicted, would lead the artist to catastrophe.

The creation of GITIS and of a faculty of choreographic pedagogues was proper. Many new schools opened throughout the country, and they demanded qualified teachers. Tarasov worked out a general plan and program of methods in teaching classical dance. Graduates of the pedagogic faculty of GITIS and pupils of Tarasov are teaching in almost all the schools in our country and in many abroad. Tarasov lives today in his students and they preserve his teachings and are, as he was, true to the art.

The faculty has grown. It prepares teachers for the choreographic school and teaches répétiteurs, which are necessary for our theater. Tarasov's pupils and followers are in both professions.

The first printing of the book *Ballet Technique for the Male Dancer* was in 1971. It was Tarasov's gift to his art while he was still alive. The book is unique. The works on Classical dance, up to that point, had been mainly concerned with female dance. Tarasov devoted his work to male dance.

The Soviet theater is a theater of high aesthetics. Heroic, revolutionary and contemporary themes are the pivot of the repertoire. In this repertoire, a special place is occupied by the male heroic figure—flying, large and expressive. In many ballets of classical heritage, newly restaged, the male roles have become expanded. All this makes the study of dance for males more complex and includes much that is new in the technique. But the uniqueness of this book lies not only here. Tarasov begins with a chapter on the school and its divisions, which formulate the main line of Soviet choreographic art. This line is the traditional realistic direction in the art of Russian and Soviet ballets. It defines the character of the creative activity of the theater and of the ballet schools and their teaching.

In 1975, for his book *Ballet Technique for the Male Dancer,* Nikolai Ivanovich Tarasov was awarded the State Prize of the USSR.

He dedicated his book to those who maintain the great traditions of the Russian School of dance, who nurture in ballet artists not only virtuoso professionalism but also citizenship and patriotic strivings.

A NOTE FROM THE AUTHOR

Nikolai Ivanovich Tarasov

This book is dedicated to the training principles of the Russian and Soviet School of classical dance. It is written for future teachers on choreographic faculties of theatrical institutions and in choreographic* schools.

This work may also be of use to future choreographers[†] and performing artists who must possess an excellent knowledge of the school[‡] in order to make full use of its means of expression in their creative activities.

The material in this book is divided into two parts. The first part discusses the goals and tasks of the school of classical dance, the planning of the teacher's work and the grading of the pupils' progress. The second part includes the system of exercises—educational material—accepted in the school of classical dance and examples and methods of studying these exercises. Sketches illustrate the rules of executing these exercises.

The book as a whole discusses the school of classical dance as a method, a system of educating and training the future dancer of the professional ballet stage. However, I would like to emphasize that no book, even the most useful, can substitute for practice, as only with the aid of practice can a teacher's mastery be forged and his experience accumulated. At the same time, a book can extend, make more precise, and deepen the teacher's knowledge of the theory and the method, and bring purposefulness and regard for system and principles, into his work.

In this book I have endeavored to answer as fully and in as much detail as possible the following questions: Why, how, and what does the school of classical dance study? What is the essence of technical mastery from the point of view of the teacher? How I have succeeded in these objectives only the reader and time will tell. I myself will be entirely satisfied if my work is of some use to the beginning teacher, if only in a small degree. It would please me especially if the book were to prove of use to choreographers of folk theaters, institutes of culture, and amateur groups.

Finally, I would like to heartily thank all those who in word or deed helped me prepare this work for publication.

---

* The word "choreography" is used in the USSR to describe the art and technique of dance as well as to describe the arrangement of steps into a dance or larger work.
[†] A ballet master is the Soviet term for a choreographer.
[‡] The "school" refers to the artists and the art of classical ballet as taught and performed in the USSR. It has a common teaching and a similarity of execution.

BIOGRAPHY

OF
NIKOLAI IVANOVICH TARASOV

Born December 6, 1902, in Moscow
Died February 8, 1975, in Moscow

Soviet artist and teacher (pedagogue), Tarasov became an Honored Artist of the USSR in 1937. He studied at the Moscow Choreographic School, under N. G. Legat, and graduated in 1920. From 1920 to 1935, he danced in the Bolshoi Ballet in the following roles: Colin, Siegfried, Albrecht, Basil, Désiré, Jean de Brienne, and many others.

Tarasov is considered a very important teacher and methodologist of classical ballet. From 1923 to 1960 he taught at the Moscow Choreographic School (the official school of the Bolshoi Ballet). From 1942 to 1945 he was its general director and its artistic director and, from 1953 to 1954, its artistic director once more.

From 1929 to 1930, Tarasov taught the "Classe de perfection" at the Bolshoi Theater and at the Moscow Artistic Ballet Company led by Victorina V. Krieger. From 1933 to 1937, Tarasov was the artistic director of the Technicum (Institute) Lunacharsky. From 1946 he worked as a teacher and artistic director of the department for pedagogues and choreographers at GITIS (State Institute of Theatrical Arts), and was given the rank of professor in 1962.

Among his pupils were the dancers Yuri T. Zhdanov, Alexander A. Lapauri, Mikhail L. Lavrovsky, Maris E. Liepa and Yaroslav D. Sekh.

Choreographers and teachers who studied with Tarasov included A. Chichinadze, P. A. Pestov, A. A. Prokofiev, E. P. Valukin and A. A. Khercul.

Tarasov was the author of *Metodika klassicheskogo trenazha* (Methodology of Classical Training), with co-authors A. I. Chekrygin and V. E. Moritz (1940).

In 1971 he wrote *Klassicheski tanets* (Classical Dance, School of Male Technique), which won the State Prize of the USSR in 1975.

Tarasov also wrote a scenario with Agrippina Y. Vaganova for the teaching film *Methodology of Classical Dance* (1947).

—From *Ballet Encyclopedia,* page 509
Moscow: Soviet Encyclopedia, 1981

PREFACE TO THE AMERICAN EDITION

The days in America when anyone with a foreign-sounding name could open a studio and teach ballet are almost over. The requirements now are a professional background, administrative ability and a board of directors!

This development, along with tremendous audience response, has stimulated creativity and given opportunity to dancers and choreographers on an unprecedented scale. Increased career security has attracted male dancers, with the result that they are almost equal in number to female dancers in professional companies.

Although the larger centers of dance provide some separate study for male students, many boys begin their classes wedged between girls of greater size and more advanced technique, imitating each step except for those minutes when they are taken aside and shown a "boy's step" or two. In some schools, there is a schedule of classes for older boys. But by the time that level of study is reached, a good deal of imitation has passed through the reflexes.

In his book, Tarasov describes the vocabulary of the male dancer, not in the form of a syllabus, but taking each step from its generic foundation through its embellishments and additions that lead, through mastery of each part, to virtuoso performance. He defines basic structures, outlines the elements necessary for their correct execution, and takes each to a tasteful, artistic goal.

While a preference for the *style* of Leningrad's Kirov or Moscow's Bolshoi Ballet is a matter of choice, technique is not. The principles of dance are more or less the same throughout the world. The overall Soviet syllabus, followed by Soviet teachers, who are taught to teach, is standard, although modified from time to time. Yet the Soviets have produced great male dancers, notably in the classes of Tarasov, Pushkin and Messerer. What is the difference in the teaching?

Naturally, being able to choose the most talented youngsters with no concern for the economics involved in giving each a nine-year course is no small advantage. In his book, however, Tarasov is not speaking only to his peers in the State schools. He hopes to reach teachers of "folk theatres, institutes of culture, and amateur groups"! While folk theatres and institutes of culture may be a bit removed from the American scene, Tarasov has valuable advice to give every dancer, teacher, régisseur, ballet master/choreographer, and, I might add, critic, whatever the circumstance. It is to rethink the teaching of the male dancer on the basis of mastery of each new element before progressing to the next, and beginning in that approach in separate male groups, from the very first to the very last class.

For example, the grand jeté en tournant and the tour en l'air would not be taught as a whole until the graduating class, when the elements of jumping, landing and turning have been thoroughly mastered.

Like American students, some Soviet students begin the study of dance later than at the recommended eight or ten years of age, and they are just as pressed for time as their American counterparts. There is some comfort in knowing that they make the same errors as all students everywhere. But Tarasov, in pointing out the errors, continues to admonish the teacher to continue in the tradition of teaching each new element with stops or pauses throughout the learning process, even into the last year. This gives the student exactness in each portion of the new step, a sense of security in its performance and a final, correct rhythm in its execution.

Tarasov emphasizes a *masculine* style with a dignified respect for the female counterpart. From the first, he makes us aware of the physical characteristics. He is wise in the guidance of the psychological differences and gives us, as his aim, the development of the male dancer's artistic potential and versatility on stage.

He provides a frame of reference which is not based upon pyrotechnical display and he clearly states what "feminine" qualities should be eliminated from stage work.

He encourages *general culture*—the need to develop slowly in technique while adding knowledge of music, acting and art to enhance the artistry of the student. The expansion of technique includes classes in character dance, pas de deux and historical dance.

No less important, Tarasov, for all his discipline, exhorts us to show love. Love for dance and love for one's pupils. In return, he received love.

Maris Liepa, one of his famous pupils, who is now ballet master in Sofia, Bulgaria, writes at length in his autobiography about his teacher's pedagogy, but remembers him in this way: "I doubt that any one of us who has gone through his classes does not cherish within himself a feeling of deep gratitude and warmth toward this remarkable man."

What more can a teacher ask than to be given talent, to nurture it, and to be loved for guiding it.

MARIAN HOROSKO

PART ONE

THE SCHOOL

The art of ballet originated in folk dance. The vital, inexhaustible source provided by folk choreography permitted ballet to acquire and create the richness and the multifaceted means of expression it now has at its command.

In striving to embody on the stage the most varied themes derived from real life, ballet, as it grew and developed, evolved a specific means of expression. It is due to this that one can differentiate character dance from historical dance, and classical dance from grotesque dance or from mime.

In time, books will be written on when and how these dance genres evolved. Here, we need only note that classical dance possesses a highly ordered, clearly developed system of stage movement. Its range of technique is very great—a characteristic that enables the choreographer to create a wide variety of compositions, much as the composer, on a given scale, is able to create a wide variety of musical combinations. In other words, classical dance has the means of expression to allow the choreographer to create works of varied content and in various forms from small concert works to full-length ballets; from corps de ballet ensembles to leading solo roles such as Odette/Odile, Giselle, Raymonda, Juliet, Maria, Esmeralda, Paquita, Kitri, Laurencia, Swanilda, and Aurora, or Danila, Romeo, Philippe, Vaslav, Spartacus and so forth.

In short, classical dance possessed the richest means of creating drama in ballet spectacles as well as the character traits of heroes and heroines. All this does not mean, however, that classical dance is the *main* component of theatrical choreography. Indeed not. All varieties of stage dance are an equally valuable means of expression in and of themselves and also as components of the ballet performance as a whole.

The path of development for classical dance has been complex and difficult. There was a time when modernists and other would-be innovators insisted that the vocabulary of classical dance was so outmoded that it could not interpret the content of modern life or portray a contemporary person. Therefore, classical dance, together with its academic school, it was thought, should be immediately and forever relegated to the archives.

It is well known that modernisn and decadence, with its advocacy of pessimism, unhealthy symbolism, mysticism, sex, etc., is rightly doomed in Soviet art. But classical dance has withstood the test of time perfectly and continues to develop successfully along the path of realism. The work of Soviet choreographers has fully proved that through works created for classical dance, the content of life can be vividly represented. This is confirmed by a series of new concert works and ballets such as *Fly, Doves! The Lady and the Hooligan, Leningrad Symphony, Shore of Happiness, Goryanka, Asel, Jacqueline* and many others. In these works, the means of expression of classical dance were used to their fullest extent. Retained in these works was the perfection of choreographic form, an elevated, poetic style of movement and faultlessly refined performing technique. The compositional language, the personality and the actions of the heroes has changed, but the perfect choreographic foundation remains immovable.

It is true that, in the past, classical dance was used to portray princes, princesses, their friends, slaves (male and female), fantastic creatures and fairy-tale characters. But the basis on which the vocabulary of classical dance arose was life-like and natural. It was based upon the very nature of man, the mechanics of his movements, his creative imagination, his emotions, his love and his striving for beauty, nobility and high ideals, which was used first by the common people and later in ballet. For example, it would hardly be possible to use movements of character dance to portray the characters of Juliet and Romeo or Parasha or Yevgenii. Incorrect use of the means of expression of a genre proves the weakness of the choreographer, not choreography itself. Classical dancing may be perfected along the lines of choreography, performance, teaching methods and theory, but, I repeat, the choreographic foundation, its school, must be as unchangeable as a scale of music. Those remarkable Russian choreographers of the past—Petipa, Ivanov, Fokine, Gorsky—knew classical dance and its school to perfection. And on this basis they created choreographic works of high artistic quality, harmonious with the trends and style of their time. That is the reason why the work of these masters is considered innovative. The same may be said of our contemporaries: Fedor Lopukhov, Goleizovsky, Lavrovsky, Zakharov, Vainonen, Sergeyev, Burmeister, Grigorovich, Belsky, Jacobson, Vinogradov, and many others.

Finally, for vivid and true reflection of life, not only a knowledge of the school is required, but also a deep understanding of contemporary life and mastery of the arts of stagecraft and dance as well as an understanding of music and theater. Therefore, the teacher of classical dance must be firmly aware that he is called upon to form not only high technical standards but also the moral and aesthetic awareness of the future artist. How his pupils will portray his contemporaries in new ballets depends upon this awareness.

THE STYLE AND REPERTOIRE OF SOVIET BALLET

The repertoire of Soviet ballet is acquiring an ever-deepening ideological content. The drama of contemporary ballets demands not only excellent technique, but also a more perfect mastery of drama, music and general culture.

The education and training of the future Soviet dancer in a large measure defines the school—its traditions, trends, and the mastery of its teachers. The oldest professional schools of classical dance, French, Russian and Italian, have their own deep national traditions, but the choreographic basics, the composition of movements is the same for all three schools. At the same time, the performing style, manner of movement, ideological and national peculiarities in the dancing of the artist are different.

THE FRENCH SCHOOL

It is customary to consider the French School as possessing a high level of technical performance; an elegant style; a soft, light and graceful manner of movement, at times overly refined, which is the nature of French art in general.

THE ITALIAN SCHOOL

The Italian School possesses virtuoso technique; a strict style leaning somewhat to the grotesque; a manner of movement that is impetuous, somewhat strained and at times angular.

THE RUSSIAN SCHOOL

The Russian School has perfect technique; a strictly academic style; simple, restrained, and soft movements free of superficial effects. In addition, the so-called "modern dance" style is totally foreign to it.

Some foreign choreographers believe that the Russian School is an amalgamation of the French and Italian traditions. Of course, the movements and terminology of classical dance were established in France, not in Russia. However, the ideological, artistic, and national peculiarities evident in the creations of the Russian dancer are completely independent.

Similarly, it was not in Russia that the musical scale became established, but the Russian school of music possesses its own profoundly national traditions of performance and ideological and artistic trends.

Undoubtedly, a mutual influence among the schools existed. In the past, Russian and foreign masters of ballet borrowed, during guest appearances abroad, one another's most perfect examples of dance technique. Foreign choreographers also trained Russian dancers. In pre-revolutionary Russia the style and manner of the French and Italian schools were propagated. At the same time, the creative work of outstanding Russian choreographers—Yevgenia Kolosova, Avdotia Istomina, Yekaterina Sankovskaya, Timofei Bublikov, Andrei Nesterov, Adam Glushkovsky, Sergei Sokolov, Didelot, and many others—shows that they struggled for the development of the Russian School of classical dance, which always adopted the finest achievements of the technique of foreign schools without changing, however, their own national traditions.

The Great October Revolution finally freed the Russian School of classical dance from foreign influences.

Agrippina Vaganova wrote, "Beginning in the first decades of the twentieth century neither the French nor the Italian School in its pure form could be encountered on our stage." Thus, as early as the 1920s the Russian School gained complete independence in performance practice.

About the mid 1920s, professional choreographic schools began to appear throughout the Union republics. The Russian School gave wide and friendly support. Russian teachers and choreographers work in the various republics, in schools and in theaters. In Leningrad and Moscow, dancers, choreographers and teachers are trained for them.

Some of the choreographic schools in the national republics are very new and are still in the process of establishing themselves in regard to both technical training and professional artistry. But in the matter of developing their own national creative traditions, all the schools of the republics are absolutely independent.

At the present time a strict academic style is characteristic of all the schools of classical dance in the Soviet Union. But this includes the most varied manner of performing the movements. The strictness of style does not limit or constrain the dancer's individuality but, on the contrary, allows for the fullest and deepest opportunity to reveal creative abilities and national characteristics.

The art of the Soviet dancer is seen in creative individuality, not in manner of movement learned from his teacher or favorite artist. One of the prime traits of the Russian School of classical dance is the development of independent artists.

At first pupils inevitably imitate the performing manner of the teacher. But as they gain confidence in their strength and a certain independence of movement, the teacher must gradually encourage each pupil to bring his *own* feelings, his *own* approach, to every classroom combination in order to develop his *own* manner of movement without breaking the rules of strict academic style.

During this transitional period, it is necessary to watch attentively that the pupil shows sincerity and freedom from affectation, for a manner of movement must not be "acted out" but must be natural and not forced. This teaching approach will allow the pupil to "find himself," his individuality, which is important to the future dancer.

The teacher must avoid a monotonous "cold" and unchanging manner as well as false emotion, false temperament, a self-satisfied air and other examples of tastelessness.

The manner of movement of the dancer is determined by his level of culture as a performing artist and as a person which, of course, cannot be taught without precise training, just as perfect technique cannot be imparted without a corresponding level of culture. The dancer's manner of movement is his own means of expressing his individuality through movement; it is his own art and no one else's; it is a true art, not a means to imitate another dancer, even a beloved and famous artist.

One cannot imagine the performance style of Smoltsov, Shavrov, Sergeyev, Chabukiani, Yermolayev, Gabovich, Messerer or Fadeyechev as a copy of their remarkable teachers. There is, of course, the influence of the teacher, the succession of the tradition, a high level of technique and a reflection of the times, but no imitation.

One would wish, in the new generation of teachers, that in affirming their contemporary and individual manner of movement, they will not forget the traditions of the beautiful, inspired mastery of the generation that has now left the stage, that the new generation will never accept formalistic interpretations, insufficient stagecraft or musicality, or careless or imprecise technique.

A realistic trend is traditional in Russian and Soviet ballet.★ It determines the character of the creative activity not only of the theater, but also of the school and its teachers. If, during the lesson, there is life and creativity, then the dancer is being educated in this realistic trend. If the pupil understands that technique is the means by which he can express his thoughts and feeling, then the teacher is teaching the pupil within the realistic trend. Not even the highest level of technique, if it is dead or mechanical, can serve an art that glorifies life and creation. During the lesson, even a simple battement must be done artistically, intelligently, musically and with understanding and feeling for the technical and performing aspects of the combination.

Any theatrical dance, including classical dance, will only influence the spectator when the dancer's art is based upon an expressive, not mechanical, gesture; a realistic, not abstract, action.

The talented young generation of Soviet dancers—Vasiliev, Soloviev, Liepa, Lavrovsky, Vladimirov and many others—were educated first at school and now in the theater, in just such a realistic, not formal manner.

The Russian and Soviet School of classical dance is proud of its distinguished teachers: Gerdt, Domashev, Tikhomirov, Nikolai Legat, Leontiev, Semenov, Ponomaryov, Shavrov, Pisarev, Pushkin, Messerer, Rudenko and many others. Each of them had his own method of teaching but each fought for the purity of classical style and the realistic trend in choreography, which helped to create onstage such diverse works as the classical ballets, *Coppélia*, *Giselle*, and *Swan Lake*, and the newer ones, *Shore of Hope*, *Leili and Medzhnun*, *Legend of Love* and *Spartacus*.

THE VOCABULARY OF DANCE: POSES, MIME AND THEIR CHARACTERISTICS

To master classical dance, it is necessary to learn and grasp its nature, its means of expression, and its school. While the movements in classical dance are very numerous and varied, its basic unit is the pose (position) with all its artistic and compositional variety.

The characteristic of the pose, in classical dance, is its freedom from resemblance to everyday life. Stage action—and its emotional content—is presented poetically, not in a prosaic, everyday manner.

Of course, the pose in classical dance is conventional. In it, all is subject to the rules of space and time of theatrical choreography, which sculpturally strengthens, expands and elevates it, bringing extraordinary virtuosity to the natural body

★ The term "Russian" is used to describe pre-revolutionary art. "Soviet" describes post-revolutionary art.

movements of man. But this conventional nature is fully realistic. It gives the art of classical dance an exceptionally full and flexible means of expression.

For instance, in performing just one pose, the arabesque, while not violating its technical correctness, one may express a diversity of stage actions, from subtle, glowing lyricism to profound drama.

The pose may enter as a basic or auxiliary component within movements accepted in the school of classical dance. It may be performed slowly or quickly, be held for a long or short duration, or increase or weaken in dynamics. A pose may be small, medium or large; executed on the floor (par terre) or in the air (en l'air); incorporate a turn (en tournant) or not; be performed en promenade (a walk or tour lent); with beats, as a cabriole, and so forth. Poses may be joined to form an entire choreographic composition with the help of the most varied connecting movements.

And if this composition is performed with interpretation, inspiration, musicality and technical perfection, then the pose is transformed into a live, expressive gesture of dance, and is able to portray the characters, genre, style and era of the ballet as well as the feelings, aspirations and experiences of man.

However, when the pose or composition as a whole is executed in a formal manner, with no feeling or interpretation, it remains no more than a conventional choreographic scheme of movement.

Thus, the pose is a sort of gesture flowing from interpretative and expressive movement, but a gesture in which the entire body of the dancer takes part, not only the arms, which usually accompany our speech to give it greater expressiveness.

The choreographer in creating his compositions chooses the poses in his choreography that best enable the dancer to portray character and express the idea behind the theatrical action most fully and with greatest artistic truth. And if both choreographer and dancer perform their work with talent, then feelings, aspirations and unexpected shadings can be brought into the gesture of classical dance.

In our time, the pose of classical dance has become changeable and multifaceted. Its classroom rules can be sculpturally transformed by the choreographer in a great many ways. It is naïve to believe that only the classroom pose is purely classical and that everything else is a violation of historically established form, style or expressive possibilities.

It would be wrong to think that classical dance itself is conservative, closed or aloof from other forms of theatrical dance. On the contrary, it is tied closely to them.

For instance, classical dance may be enriched by stylistic suggestions of folk dance—Russian, Ukrainian, Byelorussian, Georgian, and so forth—stylized imitations of a bird—swan, eagle or dove—a fantastic lizard, a flower or a jewel. Certain sport movements—fencing or tennis, and so forth—may be included if the choreographer needs such movements for the stage action.

Movements of folk or character dance, fortified by classical technique, achieve greater virtuosity, plasticity, force, nobility, imagery, and artistic expression. In short, all forms of theatrical dance are used in one measure or another, even in such sports as skating and gymnastics, to acquire a higher, more perfect level of performance.

In the choreographic schools, beginning with the first stages of the study of classical dance, a professional bearing is developed. The entire moving apparatus of the student is strengthened and further developed, and the pupil's sense of pose and musicality is cultivated. That is, a basis of performance and technical mastery is laid, without which the pupil cannot establish himself firmly in his chosen genre of theatrical dance. Modern dance, so widely performed in capitalist countries in the West, cannot do without the professional school of classical dance, for without it this form cannot reach the necessary height of technical preparation and dramatic expressiveness.

Stage experience has convincingly shown that classical dance, possessing an enormous range of technical and expressive means, can serve as a basis for performers of all forms of theatrical dance. But this refers only to the school, to dance technique, as the future dancer must have the ability to create a psychological image of his hero, to work on a role as an actor does.

It must be remembered in connection with this that, in classical ballets of the past, leading dancers used to perform the most dramatic scenes with the help of mime. Contemporary ballet, having overcome the constraints of so-called narrative gesture in classical dance, its illustrative quality, is capable of resolving the most complex dramatic tasks by means of dance, without the help of mime.

For example, in Romeo's monologue in the scene "In Mantua" from Prokofiev's *Romeo and Juliet*, choreographer Lavrovsky expressed with great clarity the drama of the action and the depth of what the hero was experiencing psychologically, without the use of mime.

In the scene between Maria and Vaslav at the ball in *The Fountain of Bakhchisarai* by Asafiev, staged by Zakharov, it is confirmed that classical dance has enormous resources of expressiveness and that mime is not always needed.

The best example of the art of performing classical dance is in the art of Galina Ulanova. Consummate technique, poetry, simplicity, elegance, truth, naturalness, freedom and inspiration were always the mark of this exceptional actress. Her pose was always alive with the plasticity of dance and the choreographic, not mimed, composition of the movement. Without effort, Ulanova's pose always joined into the whole with the music, and she brought the finest nuances into the sense of the action. She always created an especially clear and psychologically refined interpretation graphically and intensely rendered by means of dance, not mime, which, incidentally, she performed with mastery and talent. Ulanova achieved her mastery of classical dance not only because of her rare talent, diligence and experience, but first of all because of the best traditions of the Russian and Soviet choreographic school, which has educated many remarkable masters of dance by giving the most critical attention to the development of a high level of technique.

It would be wrong to say that contemporary classical ballet acquired its true psychology and depth of expressiveness on stage because it borrowed the methods of mime. Today, our performers of classical dance derive their living, dramatic truth and inspiration from life itself.

In short, one cannot say that mime in ballet is always an expression of life, while classical dance is an artificially conceived system of stage movements which the choreographer or dancer can fill out with one or another acting method of mime where necessary.

It would be wrong to believe that mime should never be present in contemporary ballet, that all scenes should be realized exclusively by means of dance. I personally would find it difficult to imagine Khan Girei (*The Fountain of Bakhchisarai*) dancing during the course of the entire ballet.

Without going into detail in assessing mime, one only needs to say that it is a very ancient fine art, stemming from daily life, with a rich variety of forms. In ballet, mime performs independent and very important artistic functions. The art of classical dance and mime are very different by nature, in acting requirements and technique of movement, just as in opera singing parts are different from recitative. The differences are even more sharply defined since the contemporary performer of theatrical dance, and especially of classical dance, relies on the art of reliving experience rather than the art of acting out scenes.

Naturally, the choreographer knows best where, when and how to use mime in a ballet. But truthfulness, imagery, psychological subtlety and depth of dance action depend not only upon the skillful use of mime but upon the content of the libretto, the musical ideas of the composer, on the professional and creative maturity, knowledge and talent of the choreographer and, on the theatrical mastery, experience and gifts of the performer. In order to master the expressive gestures of the ballet actor, one must penetrate the essence, character and interdependence of the performing elements of the art, which will be presented in the following pages.

Classical dance as an academic discipline does not set out to teach the basic principles of acting. Nevertheless, lessons in classical dance from the first to the last year of study are insolubly linked with the assimilation of the expressive means on which the mastery of the ballet dancer depends.

And the more solid the pupil's technique, the more closely he will come to understand the expressive gesture of the ballet actor.

MUSICALITY IN THE PERFORMER

Ballet is an art of musical theater. How obedient, flexible and responsive and finely tuned the art of the dancer must be to truthfully reflect and reveal the sense of the music!

To be able to "dance" the content of the music creatively and with inspiration and with virtuosity, is to possess one of the main elements of technique. For this reason, it is very important that the future teacher know how to develop this ability. The problem of teaching musicality is both simple and complex. It is impossible to establish a single approach to this delicate problem. The ballet stage creates new dance works, striving to profoundly reveal the content of the music. However, not all performers always possess a sufficient degree of musical and theatrical culture, which is established in school, in classes of dancing and acting.

If the pupil is educated to consider music a conscious creative element, to exploit its inner feeling of movement, then the school is adequately preparing him for the stage. The theater will gratefully and more successfully complete this education because the theater is a second school for the young artist, one that will give final form to his musical and theatrical culture. True dancers must not only know how to listen to music and penetrate its inner content, they must love, understand, feel and be carried away by it. Therefore, both the teacher and the pupils must pay special attention not only to the development of a feeling for rhythm but to the emotional and dramatic link between music and dance. And, of course, it is well to be aware that music is an art in which ideas, emotions and experiences are expressed rhythmically and intonationally by organized sounds; by the same token, dance is an art in which ideas, feelings and experiences are also expressed rhythmically and intonationally by means of organized stage movements, or, in other words, with the aid of choreographic composition, the pose and theatrical gesture.

Musicality is an aptitude for music and a subtle understanding of it; dance talent (or dance ability) is an aptitude for dance and, likewise, a subtle understanding of it. Theatrical dance is not simply a component which visually recreates the contents of the music. It is an independent art form possessing its own means of expression with the assistance of which (music) a sense of stage action is revealed. Finally, without true musicality, one cannot have true dance ability, for musical content and stage action are one indivisible entity. A musical and choreographic image is a synthesis of artistry in the performing art of theatrical dance. Therefore, in classroom work, the teacher must encourage the pupil to strive to perform each combination not only with technical correctness and physical self-assurance, but also with creative enthusiasm and with musicality.

DEVELOPING MUSICALITY

The musicality of the future dancers consists of developing three interdependent elements.

The first component is the ability to correctly coordinate movements with the rhythm of the music.

Every musical composition has, as we know, its own rhythm which is measured and sensed by meter (the structure of a bar of music) and tempo,* the degree of speed of its performance and the character of movement of the musical work.

---

* The tempo—that is, the degree of speed and the character of the performance of the dance exercise— is analogous to the tempo and character of a musical work. The tempo may be largo (very slow), adagio (slow), andante (calm and flowing), allegro (fast) or presto (very fast).

Every dance creation should strictly follow the rhythm of the musical work, and this, in great measure, defines the dynamics of the development and the character of the stage action.

The smallest violation of musical rhythm robs dance of dramatic and artistic precision of expression.

Special attention must be given that the pupil perceive musical rhythm not as a simple, mechanically exact beat, but as an expressive component of dance.

At first, naturally, the pupil must assimilate the most simple music and dance rhythms: 2/4 and 4/4. Then the more complex rhythms: 3/4 and 6/8, and so on, advancing gradually from slow to faster tempos and to increased dynamics in the performance of the exercises. This will aid in teaching a more sensitive and artistically true connection between music and dance.

The dynamics of the performance of the dance exercise may also be analogous to the force of intensity of sound of a musical work. It may be basically forte (strong), or piano (weak); increasing in force, as a crescendo may be indicated, or, likewise, decreasing in force, diminuendo.

The second component of musicality is the ability to consciously and with creative enthusiasm perceive the melodic theme and embody it artistically in dance.

As we know, the content of every musical work is recognized in its themes, which, through expressive sonority, can evoke various images and moods possessing qualities of intonation, rhythm, dynamics and timbre. Every dance attempts to reveal the theme of the musical work, defining at the same time the character, image and essence of the stage action. This theme must be perceived by the pupil not in the abstract, but artistically. The music and movements must not be felt as parallel entities, but as a unified whole.

In the art of dance, emotion and a truly lively imagination may arise and be revealed only if the performer is captivated by the musical theme, which always has a tremendous influence upon the creativity of the artist. Without this inner creative excitement, dance cannot become the living expression of the stage action. Emotional perception of the musical theme always arouses in the student the desire to act not only with technical physical perfection but with sensitivity and animation—that is, with creativity and without formality or falseness.

In other words, the dancing pose and gesture, on stage as well as in class, must reflect the live feelings of the theme, not merely an abstract scheme of movement: It must be an active means of expressing the content of the music.

CHOICE OF MUSIC FOR CLASS

No one in the teaching profession has any doubt that technique must develop together with a feeling for musical rhythm, an ability to coordinate movements with absolute precision with sequences and combinations of musical time values and accents.

At the same time, there are differences of opinion concerning whether emotions and imagination as well as meter in classroom music should be perceived by the pupils simultaneously, as an integral whole, with equal clarity; or whether this distracts them from developing a strong and precise technique. For this reason, the music in class must always be very exact and clear, mainly in 2/4 or 4/4, and the musical theme must be as abstract in character as possible; it should not arouse the pupil's imagination and lead him to active emotional interpretations.

An interpretive and enthusiastic perception of a musical theme does not at all impede the development of a strong technique; on the contrary, it activates it in a suitable measure and with suitable taste, in accordance with the classroom goals and the age and professional ability of the pupils.

It is therefore very important that at the basis of the course of instruction in classical dance, in every class and every combination, even the most elementary, there be a lively and intelligent perception of the music. This is an immutable rule of theatrical dance, without which it cannot exist.

While the future dancer is still in school, it is necessary to cultivate a striving for conscious rather than intuitive creativity. The music must not merely be a musical "support" for the movement but also an inner stimulus for emotional enthusiasm, which is expressed in a lively, technically perfect and inspired plastique of the dance pose. The musical theme or melody must not be perceived by the pupils superficially or approximately, but as the emotional beginning of imagination and action.

The future dancer, if he loves music, is drawn internally to its theme. Like a musician, he brings to his daily exercises, even the most elementary ones, traits of his own enthusiasm, from which his creative individuality as an artist is formed. As a result, the musical theme must always manifest itself as the pupil's artistic, emotional, conscious feeling for dance, as a vital, fully conscious choreographic cantilena. However, there should be no dramatic plot or elements of acting—that is the task of the acting class.

The relationship to the musical theme must be manifested in the pupil's motions naturally, simply and freely, without excessive deliberacy, emphasis or force. *The smallest attempt of the student to portray, act or mime his relationship to the musical content, must be immediately stopped.* This only confirms falseness, affectation and tastelessness and it destroys the creative individuality of the future dancer-actor.

The ability to comprehend music attentively and truly, and to be excited by its contents, must be expected from the first year of study, as soon as the pupils are standing firmly on their own two feet and have begun to assimilate the movements of exercises at the barre as well as in the center. This work must be developed and furthered gradually—not indiscriminately, but in the closest connection with the assimilation of dance technique.

The ability to listen to a musical theme under the strongest physical and nervous tension is proof of true mastery on the part of the dancer. To interrupt the inner link with the musical theme is to depart from interpretive movement into mere technique.

If pupils at the point of extreme psychological and physical exhaustion attempt to listen to the music actively, maintain aplomb and precision of movement and execute complex big jumps, beats and various turns strongly, freely and with elasticity, this means that they are acquiring a genuine mastery of theatrical dance.

Likewise, it is not proper to depart from a precise and clear perception of the musical theme in class—this is professionally incorrect.

The performing dancer knows the musical theme before going out on stage and has the opportunity to familiarize himself with the content. The pupil acquaints himself with it only during class.

However, both the performing dancer and the pupil, when at the point of extreme tenseness of all forces, experience enormous difficulty connected with the task of maintaining musical and creative enthusiasm. The teacher must train his pupils in this art, and not only at rehearsals but also in ordinary classes of classical dance.

As the pupil leaves class he must precisely remember not only the combinations given by the teacher, but also the musical tempos, which gave him an inner excitement and sense of movement (even if only in a slight degree) and also helped to develop his dance technique.

Therefore, it is worthwhile to repeat a combination—for example, an adagio or allegro combination—two successive days—not only to develop a more precise technique but also for the sake of a better, more artistic interpretation of an already familiar musical theme. However, themes of melodies, especially favorite ones, must not be played too much, since overexposure dulls the emotional sharpness of the pupil's understanding. Melodies of popular songs and themes known to pupils from current ballet repertoire to my mind ought not to be used during lessons of classical dance, because they are always associated with a definite literal content or the portrayal of a specific character. Work on those aspects does not belong in the structure of a class.

The musical content, in summation, must not only be correctly understood but must be correctly reflected in the pupil's movements. It should not be acted out or mimed, thus turning the lesson in classical dance into an acting class. The face and the entire body of the pupil must respond freely and with animation, but in full harmony with the rules of classical dance, not those of mime. This should constitute the principal difference in the education of the dancer from the education of the mime.

The third component of musicality is the ability to listen attentively to the intonations of the musical theme while striving to embody them in dance with technical correctness and creative enthusiasm. Thus music and choreography become a single object for the pupil's attention in all respects.

The experience of Soviet ballet confirms that the ability to truthfully feel and freely express intonations of music must be cultivated in the pupil just as the ability to sense the rhythm and theme of music must be cultivated. A performer may be able to dance rhythmically, to perceive a musical theme subtly and correctly and yet not be able to express the music's intonations sufficiently in his movements. Consequently, the pupil must understand not only what a musical theme says, but how it speaks and it is during the lessons of classical dance that he must understand this. There is no need for fear when the pupil introduces intonational nuances into his movements or his musicality, for in so doing he is not breaking teaching traditions or choreographic rules but rather surmounting

what might otherwise become a cold technique, a robotlike manner and monotony.

The pupil may clearly express musical intonations by changing the plasticity
of movements in an exercise (of course, only to the extent that this is useful) or
by intensifying or weakening rhythmic accents—for example, by making a
movement strong and energetic, soft and restrained, fluid and with a "singing"
quality, or firm and brisk. These changes are not exercises in acting, but work
on the musical plasticity of dance. The surmounting of a "cold" technique requires
an intelligent and purposeful gaze, not a blank stare, and puppetlike movements
of the head, arms, torso and legs even in the performance of the most elementary
battements. Therefore, I repeat, to fear that musical intonations in class may destroy technique or interfere with its logical development, is the same as to fear
life itself. On the contrary, the ability to perceive musical nuances will make the
student learn combinations as living, creatively effective plasticity in dance and
not as an abstract, mechanical, rhythmic scheme of movement.

The future musician, as well, learns the method of playing his chosen instrument
not in an abstract fashion, but with the specific intent to achieve in addition to
rhythmic precision, a pure, supple, soft and deep tone capable of expressive intonations. The composer Asafiev once said, "When people say of a violinist that
his violin sings, this is the highest compliment for him. It means they are not
only listening to him, but striving to hear of what his violin sings."

Of course, the ability to hear music as a whole, its rhythms, themes and intonations, must be taught gradually, step by step from the simple to the complex
over the entire course of the study, taking into account the age of the student,
his knowledge and the character of the given exercises. In the early classes, especially the first year, very simple, clear and even naïve music, understandable
and accessible to the psychology of pupils nine to eleven years old should be
chosen. For students between the ages of twelve and fifteen, music may be more
complex; in senior classes the music must be suitable for pupils between the ages
of sixteen and eighteen. Beginning in the very first year, the content of the music
must be closer in character to the psychology of boys than that of girls. Although
this aspect of the music does not have such great importance in the earlier classes,
it should be anticipated for intermediate and especially senior classes. It is self-
evident that the music selected for exercises in all classes and groups must be
considerably simpler at the barre than for center, adagio and allegro portions of
the class.

USE OF IMPROVISATION AS MUSICAL ACCOMPANIMENT

In teaching classical dance, the music for classical dance and the music for class
may be improvised or selected from music literature. Improvisation is used quite
widely as accompaniment, just as the teacher himself improvises when he gives
combinations, without reproducing actual examples of stage choreography. The
accompanist is the teacher's immediate assistant in these choices. By knowing
the character, rhythms and components of dance exercises, the accompanist can

choose proper theme, tonality, dynamics, meter and accents suitable to the exercise. True, some people believe that improvised music for class cannot be of the highest artistic merit because it is created not by great composers, only accompanists. But it is also true that class exercises are composed not by great choreographers, only teachers.

The work involved in classes of classical ballet is unusually difficult and complicated, full of endlessly and scrupulously repeated exercises, some already learned and others new to the student. In regard to music, such work must take form in strict correspondence with the true essence of dance. It is very good when the music's rhythm easily and exactly corresponds with the teaching exercise, and very bad when the musical theme and its intonations do not correspond with the character of the exercise; the pupils develop no true creative enthusiasm, no desire to correlate the combinations with the music and their own inner reactions. It is also bad if the music is abstract and monotonous in character. Therefore, the accompanist who improvises must not be apathetic when giving musical form to the idea or goal behind the teacher's combinations; he must do this creatively and with interest, avoiding, however, extremes of primitiveness and complexity in his music.

The outstanding Russian teacher Nikolai Legat improvised on the piano when giving his own classes. After giving us the combination, he would hum a theme, then play and properly harmonize it on the piano as we danced. These themes were, of course, not remarkable by artistic standards, but, first of all, they were always perfectly easy to understand, and we hummed them to ourselves, of course, as we danced. Secondly, each theme corresponded exactly in character to the choreographic composition of the exercise, whether in the adagio or allegro portions of the class. And thirdly, the themes were exactly suited to the individual qualities of the pupils, the girls and the boys.

In the late nineteenth century in Russia and abroad, teachers accompanied their classes on the violin. It seems to me that this was not accidental and not only because the bow was handy to punish a pupil, but because the violin "sings" better than any other instrument, intones the theme with especial clarity, and it is nearer to the orchestra in sound than a piano. Ballet pupils of the time were taught to play the violin instead of the piano and were also taught solfeggio (sight singing). Those studies helped them understand, hear and become inspired by the intonation of the musical theme, as well as to develop a musical ear, taste and knowledge. This does not mean, of course, that we should return to the old system of educating a dancer. Not at all. Today's pupils are given excellent training in playing the piano and understanding music. But one must be moved by the respectful and careful attention teachers of the past gave in training the dancer to feeling the inner music of dance.

The methods of training the artist of the contemporary ballet stage deepen the inner ties of music and dance in all choreographic disciplines. The contemporary stage demands it. The ability to hear and dance the music must be entered into the teaching program as an obligatory element and be learned creatively, not formally nor superficially.

USE OF THE LITERATURE OF MUSIC FOR ACCOMPANIMENT

The use in the classical dance lesson of works from the literature of music, like improvisation, has received wide application. The literature of music must be included in ballet exercises as an organic element in the art of theatrical dance, and this is a very difficult task. The accompanist must have a fine sense of meter, artistic taste and judgment in offering compositions suited to the teaching goals. Selections from the literature of music are used in the lesson somewhat differently from the use of improvisations. Using a musical work as a basis, the teacher creates a classroom choreographic étude; it is not the music that is selected or adapted to suit the combination, but the opposite—the choreography must express the content of the music. This is already more than an ordinary combination— it is a classroom dance phrase. The teacher, in creating these études, must include only those movements that the students have learned sufficiently. The étude should not be composed indiscriminately, but in strict accordance with upcoming work on specific aspects of dance technique, just as specific aspects of piano technique can be worked on with the aid of études by Czerny and other composers. What would a music teacher say if it were suggested that he teach his pupils using musical masterpieces that were not intended for classroom use? Only purposeful work on these études can properly shape the technique of the future dancer. That is the reason for choosing good music for them—that is, music that is suited to the goals of the classroom. The ballet master creates compositions for stage, while the teacher creates études for the classroom. To substitute one for the other is a gross professional error. The creative aims of the choreographer and those of the teacher are quite different in content even though both compose on the basis of musical content and know to perfection the school as the basis of theatrical choreography. As mentioned above, the character of the music must correspond strictly to classroom goals. Pessimism, loneliness and false temperament must not be taught through music. Sentimental lyrics, overemotional themes or salon or jazz music must be totally excluded. Music of emotional imagery, dance action, optimism and resolution with clearly expressed and finished melody, is the most acceptable for teaching. A high level of musical taste in both teacher and accompanist enriches classroom work and increases the diligence and creative activity of the students. The absence of musical taste in the teacher creates a negligent and superficial attitude toward music in the student.

It must be underscored once again that the primary task is the teaching of a precise, uncompromisingly finished technique; not a mechanical technique but one capable of responding to the emotional and intellectual content of the music. That is why the music of the lesson must be recognized and comprehended as a means of educating the future dancer, not as an accompaniment that pleasantly eases physical labor.

As the pupil's range of dance technique increases, he will himself begin gradually and actively, without prompting from the teacher, to perceive the emotional content of the music. Although this striving is natural, it demands from the teacher unfailing and strict control: first of all, the teacher must demand, without deviation, that each exercise as a whole, and in the smallest detail, be performed with technical precision. Second, he must demand that the pupil relate freely and naturally to the content of the music. Forcing the pupil into an adult interpretation of the music leads to formal imitation, the portrayal of feelings invented by others not the student's own feelings.

Pupils must be guided to truthful and independent perceptions of music, since forcing will rob the pupil of the creative activity so necessary to the future dancer-actor. A sense of meter, strictness, simplicity, naturalness, and a fine taste for form and music must become the immovable qualities of the pupil's musical culture. Displays of false temperament, affectation or attempt at acting must be immediately stopped.

In summary, the teacher must strive for the pupil to be able to perceive the character of a theme; its tonality; its living rhythmic beat; and to be able to "sing" the music through the plasticity of dance, that is the movements of the entire body. It is for this reason that the combinations and the music of each lesson must harmonize.

The creation of musicality does not need a new or special training system. It requires only that each lesson be kept to an unswerving commitment to instill in the pupil the ability to overcome difficulties of dance technique and to creatively perceive musical content. This will prevent a showoff technique. At the same time, a creative penetration into the character of the music alone cannot substitute for technique. The technique of dance is, first of all, the teaching of the entire organism of man—muscles, psyche, nervous system—which is impossible without systematically repeated physical demands and the acquisition of movement skills necessary for the execution of theatrical dance. But for inspiration, the future artist needs a creative impulse, a dream, which is born by music, and not only on stage, but also in the daily class.

Therefore, the teacher should be reminded to be bolder in allowing the pupil to dream freely of that most important, essential goal, even though it is distant and not always clear or concrete: the acting gesture; the vital breath of musicality; and plasticity in dance which later will become transformed on stage into a powerful and active means of expression.

How can one forget that bare technique always leads the performer to inner lifelessness, robs the scenic action of the imagery and force of artistic expression, and that subjugation of the performing technique to intellectual and emotional content, is an irrevocable condition of the true art of theatrical choreography.

The dream is the basis of every creation. The preference of technique over all else as a rule leads the dancer to mechanization, not imagination, and to action that destroys his individuality. Insufficient or limited musical culture does not allow the artist to achieve true creative heights. The performances of such a dancer, even if he is richly gifted as an actor, may be technically effective, brilliantly virtuosic, filled with temperament, and may coincide with the stage portrayal of the role, but they will not be profoundly artistic—that is, musical and emotionally and psychologically truthful, and this is the difference between true realistic art of theatrical dance and its imitation.

If the future ballet artist is unable to perceive musical content as an artistic component of dance, as the imaginative world of human dreams, as a high, noble poetry of emotions, as a living, creative basis of dramatic inspiration, then he cannot or is not ready to become a true artist.

ALIGNMENT OF THE BODY

It is known that the body's support is its skeleton and the system of joints that enable man to move in space. If the body of the dancer is not sufficiently supple, the movement will be constrained and inexpressive. If the spine bends with difficulty and only to a limited extent, it cannot give the deep resilient and elastic arch necessary in certain forms of port de bras, arabesque, renversé and so forth. Tense shoulders, elbows, wrists and fingers also constrain the movements. Hips that are tight (not "open" enough) rob the body of turn-out and freedom of movement. Poor flexibility in the knees and ankles make the movement of the legs in plié and especially in jumps more difficult.

A lack of suppleness of the body will cause coarseness, stiffness, rigidity in performance and will not harmonize with the concept of classicism.

The suppleness of the future dancer depends in large measure on innate gifts which, of course, must be developed, strengthened and perfected as a basis of technique. Acrobatic flexibility, splits, the turnout of the "lying frog" position (a stretch on the floor that resembles a frog lying with inner thighs touching the floor), overstretching the wrists, fingers, knees or ankles cannot be allowed as a means of fortifying technique. Grotesque and eccentric movements in classical dance are *stage elements* and are introduced by the choreographer.

The true image of the art of classical dance must be firmly established in the pupil's consciousness; its strictness of style, precision of choreographic composition and artistic essence. Consequently, developing flexibility in the body must not resort to artificial "breaking" of the hip, spine, foot, and other parts of the line of the body. This habit will only lead to a mechanical and formal feeling of movement and eventually will do violence to the natural organism. Classical dance needs flexibility born of a natural sense of movement. It is senseless to stretch an ungifted pupil to the point that he cannot maintain the extension actively, freely and musically while dancing. The ballet has excellent performers of classical dance with low extension but great dramatic gifts and fine musical taste. It also has performers with high extension and a lack of feeling for dance.

Of course, before the start of the lesson, the pupil may do stretches at the barre, but making up in this way for what is not an innate gift should not be allowed. The classical school possesses all means necessary for the development of elastic, soft, free and stable movements, harmonious with the character of the stage action and its musical content. Flexibility in the performance of classical dance is a means of musical and dramatic expressiveness. It is flexibility that lends the necessary nuances and color to movement. Ordinary flexibility does not give the necessary character and style to dance. Just as in singing, for instance, one must sing with flexibility and musicality and not merely shout, so in classical dance one must move with artistic flexibility.

Therefore, the physical flexibility of the future dancer should be developed along with musicality and plasticity. Flexibility may be great and elastic but ordinary—that is, inexpressive and unmusical; on the other hand it may reflect exactly and subtly the character and content of the stage action.

CHOOSING STUDENTS FOR THE CHOREOGRAPHIC SCHOOL

If the children chosen to study in the choreographic schools are sufficiently flexible, there will be no need to stretch the joints of the body artificially. While exercising for flexibility of the shoulders, elbows, wrists and fingers, the dancer must be kept strictly within the normal bounds of bending and stretching without exhibiting extremely angular or stick-straight lines.

ARMS AND FINGERS

The straightening and rounding of the arms from the shoulder to fingertips must be free and supple. Changing arms from one position to another must be natural, without excessive stretching of the wrists or turning of the hands. Fingers should retain their natural grouping, bending and unbending without opening out for "effect."

NECK AND SPINE

When working on the flexibility of the neck and spine, it must be remembered that the naturally most mobile sections are the vertebrae of the neck and small of the back, and the least mobile section is the upper-back and upper-chest portion of the body.

But in teaching, one must require that the pupil use all vertebrae while bending backward or to the side. This imparts perfect, finished lines—rounded, rather than angular—to movements of the torso, for example in arabesque. The forward inclination of the torso is done most often using the vertebrae of the small of the back and to some degree those of the neck; otherwise the back will become stooped (or rounded).

HIPS AND LEGS

When working on extension it must always be taken into account that the height of the extension must not be increased at the expense of the placement of the hip. A high but turned-in extension does not perfect technique or enhance the leg's plasticity. Extension and turnout, in classical dance, must be viewed together as a whole. A pupil's attempt to raise a turned-in leg as high as possible always destroys the harmonious proportion and the aplomb of movements especially of large poses.

The development of the extension is not achieved by kicking (or yanking) the leg upward but by relying upon the natural abilities of the pupil—that is, by raising a turned-out leg to a comfortable height, increasing over the years from 45 degrees to 90 degrees and higher, once again depending on the pupil's abilities. If the leg is kicked or yanked instead of raised with control, slackness and roughness of movement will result. Turnout in its own way supports the leg, leads it to its necessary point in space; it disciplines the body's movements and perfects its plasticity. Therefore, the development of extension begins with turnout, not with the height of the raised leg.

KNEES AND ANKLES

In working for flexibility of the knees and ankles, the pupil must strive for light, free and, at the same time, sufficiently strong movements, depending upon the tempo, character and form of the movement, in the bending and straightening of the knee while maintaining the proper turnout.

An insufficiently flexible knee, and, even more an insufficiently flexible ankle, Achilles tendon, instep and toes, interfere with free movement of the legs and imparts laxness and an unfinished look to the movements.

Therefore, I repeat, it is necessary for the choreographic school to accept only children with good body flexibility. Otherwise, their progress will always be tortured, mediocre and little suited for professional art. Of course, perfect knowledge of the school and the skill of the teacher may work wonders but cannot substitute for innate gifts. A pupil with too much flexibility, on the other hand, must be restrained to avoid acrobatic looseness and disconnected movements. During the lesson, it is necessary to develop flexibility that will perfect not only the correctness of the execution of the movement but also the musical and sculptural variety of rhythm and tempo. In working on flexibility in dance, attention must be devoted to everything related to the dance "palette," especially precision, plasticity, and intonational musicality (phrasing) in the movements of the head and the gaze, hands and torso.

LEGS

The use of the legs in classical dance includes their progressive formation and firming, making proper movement simpler to achieve. Still, much depends upon the flexibility of the extension, the turnout and the ability to maneuver their movement in full harmony with the movements of the head, arms and torso. The coordination of these movements contains enormous possibilities of expressiveness which may be used by the ballet master and performer in infinite variety. Flexibility that is used artistically can become part of the art without which classical dance cannot be truly alive and musical.

APLOMB

The ability of the dancer to move on stage with assurance and precision is referred to as aplomb. Literally, aplomb means the maintenance of perpendicularity, and in dance, this means the stability that allows the artist to perform not only with perfect technique, but with artistic integrity and musicality. Insufficient aplomb (stability) disrupts and distorts imagery and the content of the stage action and introduces an element of haphazardness and amateurishness.

If the performer does not possess sufficient aplomb, the true artistic process will prove beyond his grasp, and he will find it impossible to perfect his tasks as an actor.

For instance, the roles of Kitri (*Don Quixote*) and the Dying Swan are direct opposites. Kitri is life itself; the Dying Swan, doom. The first role requires resolute, energetic movements reflecting joy and the affirmation of life. The second role reflects extinction, death. But both roles demand excellent aplomb. The fluttering frailness of the swan is achieved not by means of a loss of balance, but by a sensitive, virtuosic aplomb, through which the dancer projects the idea behind her roles.

In other words, aplomb must become so organic, constant and pliable an element in the technique of the female dancer, that it may be used as a means of dramatic expressiveness. While mastering aplomb (or stability), all the rules of technique in movements of the legs, torso, arms and head, as they apply to the school, must be strictly observed.

Obviously, highly developed aplomb must not be *unnecessarily stressed* lest it upset the characterization and content of the stage action. An unnecessary pirouette or a prolonged pose on demi-pointe opposes the dancer's dramatic tasks. Aplomb to some degree is emphasized in all dance lessons. During the lesson, it is subject to the most meticulous work, beginning with the study of the positions of the feet. The pupil is taught first to stand firmly and correctly on turned-out feet. Turnout is obligatory in the performing technique of classical dance. As is well known, it allows for freer movement in the pelvic area and more finished leg movements, enlarges the area of support and therefore increases aplomb.

The largest area of support on turned-out legs is in First Position. In Second Position and especially in Fourth Position, the area of support is still greater.

ESTABLISHING STABILITY OR APLOMB

Aplomb is successfully achieved by strictly observing the following rules:

The foot should always be placed on the floor firmly and evenly. The toes, like clinging tentacles, should forcefully keep the balance of the body, not allowing the slightest faltering during the movements. The heel is also placed on the floor, providing a supple support.

It is necessary to avoid rolling over onto the big toe, since this would diminish the area of support and weaken aplomb. If the weight of the body is equally and firmly distributed on the entire foot, including the heel (only the arch remains off the floor), the dancer will be able to maintain stability. If this rule is not observed, the legs will usually quickly lose the turnout and the foot will weaken as it rolls from one side to the other or slides from its position on the floor, especially during the landing from a jump. In general, in classical dance, the foot must press against the floor very softly and flexibly from the tips of the toes, noiselessly, but with a strongly placed heel. Otherwise the stability will be uncertain and insufficient.

The ankle also plays a part in preserving the stability, since it is able to return the off-kilter body to proper balance through supple movements invisible to the spectator's eye.

It is easier to keep the body stable while standing on the whole foot than on demi-pointe, where the area of support is lessened. At the same time, when on demi-pointe, the ankle becomes more tense and mobile, allowing for free and active correction of the balance. These movements of the ankle must be as invisible as possible in order not to introduce an element of instability into the movement.

No less essential is the work of the knee and hips in developing stability. Knees and hips must be kept turned-out with flexible coordination to the foot. During a plié, it is necessary that *the knee remain in a vertical line over the foot.* This gives direct support in relation to the foot. If the knee falls *inside* the vertical line over the foot, the turnout of the hips will be disrupted and the foot will roll over onto the big toe for support, which will be weak and unstable.

Stability of the body does not permit an outward thrust of the pelvic region (as seen from the back), or a dropping of the pelvic girdle (as seen from the front of the torso), which must always be lowered or dropped (from the back view) or pulled up (from the front view) in order not to destroy the dancer's entire line. This placement must not be misunderstood as tucking the buttocks under or leaning backward, but simply a lowering or dropping of the lower spine and a maintenance of the hips and pelvic region in an uplifted and supportive position at all times.

It is just as necessary to maintain aplomb according to the same rules while standing on one leg. However, it is practically impossible to keep a total turnout of the supporting leg when the working leg is at 90 degrees only at the barre. Therefore, in center work, in big poses in Second Position and especially in Fourth Position back, the supporting leg is not completely turned out.

The rules for the turnout of the working leg at 22 degrees, 45 degrees or 90 degrees off the floor are the same as the rules for the standing leg. Otherwise, the dancer loses more than his line—he loses aplomb as well. The working leg must observe all rules of movement just as strictly as the standing leg. (See description of battements.)

If the working leg is moved incorrectly or holds its position in space weakly, if it is lowered, even mechanically, or if the pelvic region, the instep or the toes weaken, the turnout is lost and the movement becomes unstable.

Classical dance can change weight from one leg to another by means of a variety of steps. The slightest loss of stability during these changes introduces the element of uncertainty and technical error. Therefore, the ability to transfer the center of gravity from the standing leg to the working leg in a firm and sure manner must be scrupulously developed, in a progressive variety of rhythms, tempos and in the character of the movement.

The transfer from one leg to another must be done in place, or while traveling slowly or quickly, with simple or complex movements, but the center of gravity must always be correctly transferred to the new point of support with stability.

The ability of the student to keep his torso pulled up helps the development of aplomb. One knows that all movements of the torso are related to the spine, the vertebrae. This physically strong and flexible rod from the small of the back to the head allows for the preservation of balance of the body during the performance of any movement accepted in classical dance.

The center of gravity must always be over the standing leg, which is a principle of balance. The necessity of keeping the balance arises especially during the performance of multiple or fast turns, complex jumps, etc., when any weakening of the torso is totally inadmissible.

The expressions used in the teaching profession—"Pull up the torso (body)," "Hold the back," "Open and lower the shoulders freely," "Don't sit, *stand* on the leg,"—all indicate that several parts of the body must be used in unison for the development of stability. Movements of the torso, just as movements of the entire body of the dancer, may reflect different actions on stage, but the body, nonetheless, must not lose its sense of wholeness and consequently break that very elementary principle of the law of stability so necessary for the art of expressive dance.

Correct positions and movements of the arms, like those of the legs and torso, actively help in preserving the physical balance of the body. If the dancer cannot precisely control his arms in coordination with the movement of the body, it means that he cannot move with aplomb. The arms of the dancer can portray a vast array of characters and actions, but always on the basis of a precisely worked-out system of movement.

While assimilating the positions of the arms, the student already acquires performing aplomb, that is, the ability to fix them firmly in specific positions in space. Port de bras teaches the student to change arms from one position to another with equal plasticity. Poses teach the student to fix exactly the many positions of the arms in dance. (See port de bras section.) In this way, a finely proportioned and stable system of arm movements is established in the pupil's consciousness.

Aplomb, in addition, demands that arm movements be active and sure. The entire arm must sense the specific plastic quality of every dance gesture. Therefore, it is unacceptable for elbows and hands to hang lifelessly or acquire weak, angular or passive movements. It is likewise unacceptable for the arms to be excessively tense, to jerk in a reflexlike manner, or to move in response to the motion of the legs. The movements of the legs and arms must always display plasticity and rhythmic coordination, as this perfects aplomb, but each must retain independence and freedom from the other. No less important for acquiring aplomb are correct movements of the head. It must turn and incline in strict coordination with the rhythm, force and character of the movement of the dancer's entire body. The slightest inexactness in plasticity or rhythm in the use of the head may sharply weaken balance, especially in the performance of multiple turns, pirouettes, tours chaînés, and tours en l'air. Movements of the head in classical dance are extremely varied and they complete in their way the sculptural pattern of ports de bras, poses, etc. This requires free yet calculated movements including the direction of the dancer's gaze. It is therefore very important to develop in the student the ability to move the neck precisely and without excess force, as it is the neck, that effects all turns and inclinations of the head.

While developing the stability of the entire body, the pupil must be taught at the same time how to firmly fix and perform every movement and pose. The smallest break in a movement or pose or in rhythmic coordination always creates an impression of instability, unsureness in performance. The same is true of an interrupted or rhythmically imprecise connecting motion from one movement to the next. The flow of one pose into the next must also be worked on as a form of stable cantilena (a graceful, flowing quality).

For the same reasons, every exercise, from the simplest to the most complicated, must have a clearly fixed finish or ending. It is well known that the inexperienced dancer expending his strength inefficiently usually gets excessively tired and limp by the end of his variation and is unable convincingly—that is with stability—to perform a finish (end in a fixed pose that is stable). For this reason, the pupil must always finish each class exercise with aplomb, in the same character in regard to the music and plasticity in which it began and continued.

It was mentioned earlier that while developing aplomb, it is essential to build the strength and endurance of the entire body. If, for instance, the student's legs are insufficiently developed, they cannot sustain a pirouette or change the weight of the body with lightness in a complex big jump, much less finish that jump softly and with stability. Similarly, the same will happen if the student does not have a strong, properly aligned back, even if his legs are excellently developed and the movements of his arms and head correct. To develop strength for support in movements, the teacher must introduce into the barre and center work a sufficient number of demi-pliés and relevés on demi-pointe. These should be especially included into forceful movements like battement developpé, and grand rond de jambe en l'air, grand battement jeté, etc. With the same aim in mind, it is useful to perform battement developpé tombé in the exercise to develop the pupil's ability to correctly and stably transfer the center of gravity to the supporting leg.

Into the execution of battements developpés, it is useful to introduce various ports de bras and inclinations and turns of the torso. Turns, pirouettes and fouettés at 90 degrees, jumps such as sissonne simple, temps levé simple, pas ballonné, rond de jambe en l'air sauté, and jeté passé, should also be introduced. These jumps must be done in small measure and singly as a connecting movement and small forceful addition confirming that the development of virtuoso aplomb begins with elementary movements.

Exercises in the center floor work must be done en tournant* (turning), which develops endurance and stability of the supporting leg and the ability to orient oneself in space. All these abilities are used later in pirouettes† and other forms of turns. The ability to maintain stability in exercises en tournant must be exercised as well as the mechanics and form of the pirouette itself.

Especially useful in each lesson, and in the center floor work, are battements divisés en quarts (a battement performed while turning one quarter of a complete turn). This exercise is excellent for developing all parts of the body necessary for the stable execution of grande pirouette and all forms of fouetté at 90 degrees.

The older the pupil, the more compact and full the exercises should be. The demands on strength and coordination must clearly be present in the execution of these exercises for stability, otherwise the pupil will be insufficiently prepared to move on to the more complicated part of the lesson, the adagio; he would, as it were, be skipping a very useful stage of learning that must provide a firm foundation for strengthening elementary stability in the legs and the entire body.

DEVELOPMENT OF STABILITY IN ADAGIO MOVEMENTS

In composing adagios for class, the teacher must remember that stability develops not only in the simple or complex and slow and fast transfer of weight from one leg to another, but mainly in connecting several different movements with the weight of the body *on the same supporting leg.*

Only exercises of sufficient duration, tenseness and complexity in developing the standing leg in the adagio portion of the lesson will aid in the development of virtuoso stability. Of course, the demands on the standing leg must be increased gradually, in regard to complexity and physical difficulty, in sensible balance with the entire syllabus and in correspondence with the abilities of the pupil.

DEVELOPMENT OF STABILITY IN PIROUETTES

A special exercise for correct and stable turning during grandes pirouettes is four pirouettes executed on the same leg. The pupil begins with a tour lent (slow turn) à la seconde en dehors (away from the body) followed by an uninterrupted transition into grande pirouette en dehors still à la seconde. There follows a small pirouette en dehors, with a final transition into à la seconde. The entire exercise is repeated four times, then repeated on the other leg, then reversed (turning en dedans, toward the body). The exercise may also be done in different poses, varied or made more complex.

---

* En tournant refers to turning slowly or quickly once or several times.
† Pirouettes refer to spinning movements or multiple turns.

This exercise is technically difficult and very tiring, especially if a great number of pirouettes are performed. But it develops endurance and strength of the supporting leg and assures the turning coordination of the entire body. It also proves the determination and character of the pupil—no less important in the development of stability.

Of course, the supporting leg must not be overworked, especially in the lower classes, since it leads to overtiring the muscles and various injuries. Therefore, the difficulties in the composed adagio in each class must be suited to the teaching program and the pupil's progress. It must not be forgotten that stability is developed by hard work demanding the pupil's strength. But difficult adagios will prepare the pupil to be sufficiently prepared for jumps in the next part of the lesson, the allegro. Consequently, big jumps may be introduced into the adagio portion in a limited number and singly, with the same aim. For instance: grande sissonne ouverte, grand jeté from an open position of the leg, grand fouetté, jeté entrelacé or any beaten step.

DEVELOPMENT OF STABILITY IN JUMPS

Jumps require well-developed strength in the legs, stability of the torso, exact movements of the arms and head. All these qualities are executed first in a simple, elementary way at the barre, then in a more complex manner in adagio and finally in allegro, where it is ultimately perfected.

Stability in jumps largely depends upon a strong turnout and supple demi-plié, which allows the student to push his weight away from the floor lightly and freely, and to accept the weight once more at the completion of the jump. Short, weak, poorly stretched Achilles tendons and weak calf and thigh muscles are faults in the development of a good stable jump. These are overcome by sufficient work for the legs in demi-plié at the barre and in adagio movements.

To achieve a jump marked by aplomb, it is very important to be able to hold the torso correctly. During the push from the floor, in flight and in landing a lax back is unacceptable. If the torso is not lifted, supported and gathered into proper alignment, it cannot actively sustain the work of the legs and take part in maintaining the stability of the entire body.

It is necessary to be able to propel the body with sufficient force during the jump along a vertical line as well as along the trajectory of the jump. If the body is pushed off with insufficient force, the finish of the jump will be haphazard and unstable.

Arms also aid in the stability of a jump. They cannot remain passively uninvolved or reflexlike or jerky in movement; this would give the plasticity of the movement an unsure and constrained character. If the arms maintain a position motionlessly during the flight of the jump, they must be free but actively support the force of the pushoff from the floor. If they move they must do so energetically, increasing the propelling action of the whole body from the push off the floor. The term for this arm movement is "catching up." (The arms catch up with the body and legs, to assume a strong and fixed pose in flight.) The higher and more complicated the jump, the more strong and exact the "catching up" required.

Special attention is given to this matter in the section on jumps executed en tournant and in complex turns, where clearness and correctness of performance demand the exact use of this force. Here the expression "taking needed force" is used—that is, to give to the arms a propelling force of sufficient precision and strength to allow the pupil to execute a given combination with aplomb.

These methods must not be practiced in an indiscriminate way but with thorough calculation of all details of this "catching up" and "taking force" in each jump. Arms thus become a component in maintaining aplomb in jumps.

Head movements also aid in the stability of the jump as well. The head, like the arms, during flight must be motionless or move, but in either case must be part of the general tempo of the force of the whole jump. Active and precise use of the head plays a decisive role in the execution of such steps as tours en l'air and double saut de basque with aplomb. Weak and inexact movement of the head cannot give reliable stability and self-assured character to the jump.

The work of the legs, torso, arms and head as a whole, constitutes a factor of considerable force capable of assuring good stability in a jump. This force may be useful only if the three phases of the jump-pushoff, flight and finish are performed with coordination, calculation, at the same tempo and in accordance with all the rules of technique of classical dance.

The ability to perform a series of jumps with elasticity and lightness while retaining the plasticity and rhythm of the movement with aplomb is called "elevation."

But it is a mistake to think one may have good elevation with insufficient mastery of stability in jumps or the ability to foresee in the push off from the floor the necessary height and length of the jump in the correct tempo and rhythm. That is to say, mastery of elevation begins with the logical study of the elementary principles of aplomb in jumps and the smallest details of classical technique.

In the development of aplomb in jumps, special attention must be given to movements executed on one leg, which will develop the pushing force of the legs; stable movements of the torso, arms and head, as well as all movement discussed in the "en tournant" section must be done a sufficient number of times at every lesson. All these exercises develop stability, elevation and ballon. (Ballon is the light, supple quality in jumping in which the dancer bounds from the floor, pauses a moment in the air and descends lightly and softly, only to rebound in the air like the smooth bouncing of a ball.)

With the same purpose in mind, combinations devised by the teacher must be physically difficult and technically complicated. Jumps will acquire aplomb if all technical skills of the pupils are developed just as fully as their knowledge. It sometimes happens that pupils know and understand more than they can do. This does not aid in the development of stability.

In addition, it is extremely important not only that the pupils be able to move strongly and precisely but that they be equally good at seeing the space in which their movement takes place.

The dancer who can orient himself on stage is better able to carry through the pattern of the dance composition, to cope with his tasks as an actor, and to relate to the other dancers. Therefore, pupils must be taught to maintain firmly not only the structure of the movements and poses but the positions en face, épaulement croisé and effacé; lines of direction (straight, diagonal, curved); and single and multiple turns par terre and en l'air (en dehors and en dedans).

It is also important to teach the pupils to judge the space of the classroom floor, to strictly keep distance from one another, and to do all exercises in the reverse direction.

---

1   Numbers of the room. At left, Stepanov system; at right, Vaganova system in current use; a: dancer

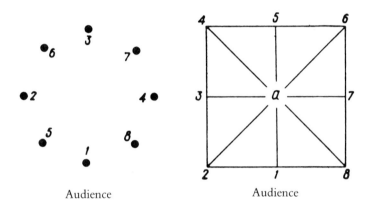

Audience   Audience

It is necessary to compose combinations in strict correspondence with the dimensions of the classroom in order not to impede or limit the spatial movements of the pupils. It is possible to acquaint them with the divisions of the classroom by the aid of the special scheme devised for dance notation by V. I. Stepanov and perfected by A. Vaganova (see diagrams). But it is rather conventional and abstract to acquire knowledge of stage space in the classroom with the use of numbered points. For this reason it is best of all to explain concisely and precisely the dimensions and spacial divisions of the stage. (The rake of the stage—slant downward toward the orchestra pit—is part of the European construction and is not frequently found in America. The degree of the rake affects the alignment of the body, the tempo of the movements and relationships in patterns.) The relationship must be an awareness of the width, depth and height of the stage as well as the pupil's relationship to the spectator. It is very important that the future dancer not only know all this, but that he feel it. Then, on a real stage, he will act with more assurance and stability. In short, classwork must be conducted on the basis of real stage conditions, not an abstract numbered system.

The development of aplomb also depends on how work on coordination is conducted. Excessive complexity in combinations does not aid the pupil's concentration, does not develop precision or harmony of movement, and does not sharpen his sense of rhythm and space. In short, it does not help the development of his aplomb, but hinders it. Combinations that are too "comfortable" likewise are not suitable for this goal. It is important to review steps already mastered, but this must not become an endless repetition of monotonous combinations over the course of weeks, months or even years. This one-sided approach does not enhance work on the development of aplomb as such work requires, especially for virtuoso performance, sufficiently intense complex and diverse use of the musculature.

Finally, the development of aplomb largely determines the degree to which the pupil is able to hear the rhythm and character of music; to remember combinations; and to strive ceaselessly toward the perfection of his knowledge and skills.

Additionally, another kind of stability, psychological aplomb, will give the pupil an inner desire for movement, faith in his own capacities, and a performing temperament as well as resoluteness and boldness in his creativity. Without all these qualities, the art of theatrical dance cannot exist on an artistic level.

DEVELOPMENT OF PRECISION IN MOVEMENTS

The content and depth of a choreographic work can be revealed exactly and fully only through precise technique. Precision is not simple professional pedantry, not a cliché, not a goal in itself, but first of all living, poetic inspiration which is determined by maturity and mastery in performance. Precision permits the dancer to acquire harmony of form, clear phrasing, confidence in his strength and creativity. Where there is no technique developed with precision, there cannot be true art. No high artistic concept or exciting plot can substitute for precision in technique.

The words "approximately," "about," "nearly," are all incompatible with professional dance technique. The smallest error in rhythm or form or digression from the character and phrasing of the music, or an unpersuasive gesture, all point to the fact that the dancer has not mastered his technique.

The discovery of all the "secrets" of precise technique begins with the first steps, based on the strictest of principles: Start with the simple and then go to the complex. That is why one may go to the next more complex task only after the previous principle has been assimilated and worked out completely. Great care must be taken that all the elements comprising a new movement are scrupulously prepared. The study of a new movement in the syllabus without adequate preparation prevents the proper development of exact technique.

As a rule, when imprecision becomes a habit, it is reversed with great difficulty and sometimes does not allow for correction at all. *The causes of small and large imprecision: carelessness and an undemanding teacher!*

It is no less important to make the student accurately coordinate the rhythm of his movements and the music and correctly recognize the character and tonality of the music—that is making an orientation in time as well as in space within classical dance. The experience of the Soviet ballet theater has proved conclusively that the language of classical dance is extraordinarily rich, able to reveal the artistic essence of real life, from romantic passions to depths of the psyche. But this is possible only with the thorough mastery of a precise technique.

With this in mind, I should like to warn the beginning teacher against the so-called method of "dancing out" pupils, that is, imparting musicality only very late in their studies. As a result of that method, the pupils commit technical inaccuracies or portray musical content superficially. Therefore, exactness must be part of the work from the pupil's ABC's which have their own artistic basis; and if there is no such basis, it really will become necessary to "dance them out"—settle for an unwelcome compromise. Of course, in teaching, one must establish the choreographic and rhythmic basis of movements studied, and then the musicality. But this must be done without delay and at the proper time, so there will be no need to "dance out" one's own or another's pupils, but to conduct work normally along a clearly conceived plan.

DEVELOPMENT OF LIGHTNESS

To move lightly, freely, without excess physical effort, means to hide from the spectator all the difficulties of technique, and the enormous expenditures of strength and energy it requires. The slightest constraint in the movement of the head, torso, arms or legs, lack of physical strength, energy or resoluteness, make the dancer's movements encumbered and heavy, and prevent him from fully realizing his gifts. However, lightness of movement in technique is not a mere "elegant weightlessness." It is first a means of expressiveness in acting that may be used in all its variety of plasticity. Lightness imparts a loftily graceful "winged" plastique, especially in poses, big jumps and turns.

In classwork, lightness is based upon flexibility, aplomb, precise movements, and flawless musicality. The pupil's performance must always be sufficiently strong, clear, determined, enthusiastic and varied in character, but always light—never impeded and consequently heavy.

DEVELOPMENT OF SOFTNESS IN THE MOVEMENT

It is also very important to make students, especially in the intermediate and senior classes, realize that softness of movement is not only the ability to move with elasticity, turnout, suppleness and rhythm, but is one of the most expressive means of the ballet artist. In teaching, it is most important to develop a supple demi-plié, especially in jumps, that the pupil can control softly in slow to fast tempos, with a small or greater degree of plié, in simple to complex rhythms.

In working on all battements, too, elasticity and clarity of movement must be developed along with the soft resiliency. All port de bras forms must be exact but softly flexible in the use of the hands, wrists, elbows, torso, neck and head. In poses, even the most complex, there must be a masculine softness, not a coarse, forced form.

In developing musicality, one must teach the pupil to strive always for clear, but sufficiently soft linked phrasing in the performance of combinations. In this way, softness in technique will acquire variety of plasticity and a volume of expressive means particular to classical dance.

DEVELOPMENT OF INDIVIDUALITY

Movement brought to its highest form of development in accordance with the rules of natural human motion is essential for the future actor-dancer as a vital creative basis; without this, he cannot create realistic dance image. Young, inexperienced dancers often make use of excessive displays of emotion and form and add general pomposity to their movements which renders their characterizations primitive rather than profound.

The ability to express dramatically the subtlest logical shadings in a role, can only be developed out of a natural sense of movement; it cannot be achieved with superficial posturing, even with technical virtuosity.

The education of the future dancer follows a highly complex, and at times contradictory, path. The pupil must do all exercises clearly and convincingly, but with a clearly expressed feeling of his own attitude to the art of dance and music. A teaching tradition that allows the pupil to remain himself throughout, leads to naturalness, depth and simplicity of movement.

This approach allows the pupil to fully discover his individuality, his inner world, his imagination and steers him away from formal emulation and programmed emotions. In the performing arts, simplicity is the supreme degree of brevity. It does not tolerate anything superfluous or alien, although it does not exclude the continuing traditions of realism. The art of Anna Pavlova, Ekaterina Geltser, Mikhail Mordkin, Galina Ulanova, Konstantin Sergeyev, are clear examples of this simplicity and individuality.

In teaching, one must inculcate the love of simplicity in dance. Pretentiousness, superficial prettiness, and self-admiration are unacceptable. Masculine modesty, willful resoluteness, and firmness—these are the qualities to develop for simplicity in performance of the future dancer. At the same time, simplicity of movement in classical dance cannot be total without strictness. Strictness denotes not only academic perfection and subtlety of form, it indicates above all a healthy and high artistic taste, a thoughtful attitude toward the musical content and the movement. But the desire of a dancer or pupil to turn strictness into cold elegance or asceticism, thus hiding his inner emptiness of feeling and thought, would show lack of integrity. Strictness is truly a professional quality that allows the dancer to find that measure of generalization and precision of characterization without which he might start on the path toward naturalistic verisimilitude, brilliant in form but cold in regard to thought and feeling. Some say that this strict performing style in classical dance has become obsolete as a means of expression, because contemporary style demands sharper, more contrasted, angular movements and dissonant forms of expression and that rounded lines, a cantilena style developed to a full, logical, and sculptural form, cannot reveal the essence of the contemporary stage—that "old," strict classicism is now archaic.

I am not in agreement with this statement because I feel that future dancers must be trained and developed on the basis of strict academic style and healthy artistic taste. Future dancers must be prepared to portray psychological action within the strict rules of the classical genre, not the passing fashion of modern dance. This strict performing style is an integral trait and traditional trend of the Russian and Soviet school of classical dance.

DEVELOPMENT OF MUSCULATURE WITHOUT STRESS

One of the most important elements of technique in classical dance is freedom in performance. We know that man's actions are governed by his intellect and emotions. No less active are the functions of his muscles in the performance of physical actions. A dancer's muscles must possess sufficient strength, endurance, elasticity and mobility to do his work efficiently and to achieve the purpose with no excessive stress, which would lead to constraint rather than freedom of physical action. The more developed the muscles, the more freedom of action on stage.

If, for instance, during the lesson, the muscles of the face, neck, arms or torso are extremely tensed, the student will not be able to do various poses and ports de bras freely. To preserve the proper position of the legs (position, turnout, extention), it is necessary to have sufficient but not excessive tension in the muscles. Too much tension interferes with the performance of various forms of plié, relevé, battements, ronds de jambe, simple jumps, tours lents, and turns, which later are used in the most complex movements of classical dance.

From the first year of study, the student must be taught to move energetically and confidently but always efficiently, avoiding excessive muscular tension before it becomes a habit. This habit will interfere with the development of coordination, restrict and limit the free expression of the pupil's individuality and produce a mechanical performance.

Special lessons are not needed for the proper development of muscular freedom. In the ordinary class, the teacher must *constantly* create a desire in the pupil to move economically and with integrity, with no excessive muscular tension. Otherwise, even the most excellent acting lessons will not help the pupil acquire true freedom of movement.

If the muscles are to acquire sufficient strength, endurance and mobility, they must be exercised regularly for two class hours every day, except for the weekly day of rest and vacations.

The interruption of the class schedule, for even the shortest time, does not permit the muscles to maintain the firmness required by classical dance, but will develop them irregularly, with sharp setbacks and overtenseness. Professional dancers know very well that if they miss a few lessons separately or consecutively, it will show in their performance technique. The muscles become weak and insufficiently obedient. It demands more than a little effort and time to reacquire necessary elasticity, endurance, precision and freedom of movement. Only in regular and sufficient work adequate in amount, complexity, and intensity can the future dancer acquire a high level of technique—that is, make use of the strength and endurance of his muscles freely and efficiently, without stress and in the proper degree.

In the more advanced classes, especially the graduating class and with the permission of the school doctor and teacher, the student may be given additional and vacation time to work the muscles with the aim of developing more mastery for stage appearances. The most remarkable Russian and Soviet dancers, while students in the more advanced classes, perfected their performing technique with uncommon enthusiasm, love and sensitivity, at special times in addition to the regular schedule. This additional work must, of course, be coordinated with the teacher's general schedule and workload, and planned with regard to the state of the pupil's health.

The study of new movements in classical dance must be strictly progressive and systematic and consist of thoroughly assimilated elements to which have been added one or more choreographic details. This allows the muscles to work more actively, precisely, efficiently and freely, without excessive tension. Gaps in learning the technique usually destroy cohesiveness and the logical use of the muscles. The quality of cantilena in movement can be developed only if the pupil knows well and in full measure the extent of his own muscular tension and its fluctuations. For this reason, a strict, progressive and accumulative approach in the study of the elements of classical dance is necessary.

The pupil must not care only about the "what" and "how much" of his performance, but also the "how" and "why" of it. Then he will be in control of the form and rhythm of the combinations and also learn to care about the work of his muscles.

Overstressed muscles result when separate steps, combinations, or even the entire lesson, are given at too fast a tempo. Each movement of classical dance has a definite spatial pattern and duration of performance, which may be made faster or slower, depending upon the stage of study, on technical preparedness and on its coordination with the general rhythm of given combinations. If, at the beginning of the study of a movement or pose, the tempo is too fast, the result will usually be overexertion and strained muscles.

First, the student must learn to tense his muscles, not to the limit, but slowly, with due restraint in each composite movement. This allows the student to better understand and feel the rational measure of effort required by the muscles in relation to performing difficult technical movements.

The tempo should not be slowed too much, but still it is important to "make haste slowly" for the slow comprehension of the normal energy required to work the muscles. Learning to combine separate movements into combinations must also, at first, be done in a somewhat slower tempo. When all the elements and connecting steps have acquired a certain steadiness, precision, and elasticity, the teacher may proceed to the normal tempo.

Periods of rest between the execution of the exercises must be sufficient so that the muscles may rest without cooling off, and the whole musculature does not lose its working condition. If the period is too short, the muscles will not have time to rest and become resilient once more and the next exercise will require fruitless overexertion.

DEGREE OF ENERGY REQUIRED

Each movement of classical dance demands from the performer a specific degree of muscular tension. One cannot execute a grand jeté and a petit jeté with the same amount of muscular effort, despite the fact that both must be executed with sufficient strength, clarity, lightness and elasticity.

On the other hand, the execution of that same grand jeté or petit jeté on stage, in a scenic action, changes the effort required. If, for instance, the character of the movement is lyrical, the muscles will contract softly for a protracted length of time. If the character of the movement is heroic, it will demand more energetic and perhaps very sharp tension in the muscles. Therefore, the performing technique of classical dance consists not only in the force and tempo of muscular contraction, but in the plasticity required to portray the musical, ideological and psychological content of the stage action truthfully. This work of the muscles may be compared to the touch of a pianist who placing a determined amount of weight on the keys influences the force and color of the sound. The inability of the dancer to hear and feel music or penetrate its content can result in ordinary muscular stress which, under certain conditions on stage, cause the movements to become too forceful or insufficiently energetic. Intense joy or sharp heartache may be expressed by the dancer with the same degree of muscular tension but only if this tension is related to musical character and plasticity. The development of "dance touch" must be begun not only on stage and in acting classes, but in daily class, while the pupil gains precision in movements developed with confidence in combinations. In this way first, stability of classroom muscular tension is established and a certain variety may be introduced gradually in musical character and plasticity. The exercise will be performed not only with physical strength, precision and economy, but in the character that the music suggests. This usually occurs freely and naturally, as if by itself. If a gifted, diligent and well-trained pupil senses confidence in his abilities and if his muscles have achieved the necessary mobility and elasticity, then he cannot remain indifferent to the content of the music which seems to define the character of his physical actions.

If the teacher hurries, and allows the student to become excited by the music too early in his development, before his muscles have acquired the necessary strength, endurance and precision of movement, then the teacher is guilty of a gross professional error.

If, on the other hand, the muscles *have* achieved the necessary development and the teacher has not allowed his student to impart diversity corresponding to the character of the music, he also is in error, but in the opposite extreme.

Excessive emotional and nervous excitement in the pupil can interfere with the normal work of the muscles. If the pupil, as a result of an unbalanced and overly enthusiastic character, begins to force his movements and does not keep the musical-rhythmic order and plasticity, he loses control over his muscles, which have begun to tense too strongly and unrhythmically, that is, without freedom of movement.

PHYSICAL FREEDOM

If the teacher uses an excessive amount of drill, this will usually result in blind obedience and inner constriction, which will be reflected in the work of the muscles. Physical freedom of movement must be exercised not only through the development of muscular strength, endurance and mobility, but also the development of the pupil's confidence in himself and in his creative abilities.

Excessive labor and drill are always reflected in the work of the muscles. One must develop not only a standard of physical obedience, but the inner discipline that will aid the development of creative individuality in the future dancer. It is especially important to remember that the development of freedom of movement must be based on the moral, ethical and aesthetic principles of Soviet art. Each teacher is obliged to develop this freedom. Of course, it must be done according to the psychological age of the pupil and in an accessible and understandable form.

Work on physical freedom in exercises at the *barre and center* must always be done with the accent on stable muscular tension—that is, diversity in musicality and plasticity must be introduced in small, careful amounts in strict accordance with the teaching tasks of various parts of the lesson.

In doing the adagio portion of the class, the pupil must not slacken the work of his muscles begun at the barre but add to it—not only through the increased complexity of various combined movements, but also by striving to penetrate, comprehend and become enthusiastic over the more complex exercise characterized by the adagio. This enables him to add stability of muscular tension to an already worked-through exercise, a clearer and more definite sense of the music stemming from its content and the creative individuality of the pupil. Of course, this too must be in strict harmony with the age, capability and professional preparedness of the student.

Allegro combinations, which demand the utmost effort and complex work from the muscles, must be approached just like the barre and adagio. If the jumps are done as an elementary exercise, attention can be concentrated on muscular stability, which can guarantee the development of good aplomb, exactness, freedom, cantilena and softness of movement. In allegro combinations, more attention can be given to nuances in plasticity and musicality—that is, to the development of the ability to find a suitable "tonality" and muscular tension in each individual case on the basis of the stability already achieved. This proposed method of work may, of course, be changed to suit the individual method used by the teacher in the education and training of the pupil. But one thing must not be forgotten: classical dance is the art of musical theater. The language of this art is a means of expressing live, human feelings, not an abstract choreographic scheme of movement.

ADDITIONAL EXERCISES TO GAIN STRENGTH

In working on muscular strength, one must always try to develop the dancer's body in strict, elongated proportions, not in bulk. This also has a direct relationship to the body's beauty and its freedom of movement. The basic work in creating muscular strength, depends on the legs, which carry the weight of the body and perform the complex progressions of movements, especially in grand adagios and big jumps. Because of this, the lesson must be constructed so that the capacity of the muscles is developed without enlarging the shape of the legs in relation to the upper portion of the body.

Some young dancers are criticized because their upper body is weakly developed and does not harmonize with the powerful muscles of their legs. But in reality, one must not be concerned with the development of the size of the muscles of the torso, arms or neck, but work so that the muscles of the legs retain their normal size and shapeliness in proportion to the upper figure and correspond to the proportions of a dancer's figure, not a weightlifter's body.

Development of the muscles of the upper body must be done additionally by means of a special system of gymnastic exercises and partnering classes. These additional gymnastic exercises must be approved by sports specialists and choreographers with respect to the individual needs of each pupil. In the end result, musculature in the classical dancer should be of minimal size and must possess maximum strength. In choosing future students, one must prefer the asthenic figure over the athletic or pyknic.

For the pupil's muscles, especially calf and thigh muscles, to preserve their harmonious proportions and not become bulky, one must avoid excessive, long, repetitious and monotonous, forceful effort. Without destroying the composition of the lesson and individual combinations, it is necessary to alternate exercises demanding much muscular tension with easier ones, giving the muscles suitable variety and rest. Repetition is the mother of learning, as the saying has it, but repetition must be moderated and reasonable, not excessive or monotonous.

STUDY OF ANATOMY

Teachers of classical dance are often reproached for rarely or never directing the pupil's attention to the functional work of muscles—criticized that not doing so leads to "blind" and intuitive technique and that one must care about the pupil's more basic knowledge of the anatomy of the human form.

This reproach is fair, since this knowledge helps the future dancer understand and, consequently, feel the work of his muscles. But one must not forget that if the student does not grasp the feeling of a live pose, or its musical breath, he will not be able to master his art and the most comprehensive theoretical knowledge of anatomy and physiology will not help him.

Anatomy is studied in the choreographic schools, but the teaching of anatomy has little to do with the teaching methods of the art of dance. It seems to me that choreographic schools should offer not a general anatomy course, but a specialized one, developed according to a program established by specialists in anatomy and choreography. The students should study this course not during classical dance lessons, but as a special subject which might be called the Anatomical Principles of Choreography (technique). Then, during the dance lesson, the teacher might incidentally show the pupil which group of muscles should be given special attention and how that group works. The muscles then would make the proper effort and in the proper measure, freely performing their functions in regard to movement as well as artistry and plasticity.

As for developing creative freedom, that begins the moment when the student correctly regulates the work of his muscles, can hear music attentively and with interest, and is able to use his imagination, emotions and desire for an elevated style of performance in dance.

BREATHING

Any dancer, and especially the performer of solo and leading roles, must have strong and controlled breathing. The rhythm of breathing on stage is an expression of the emotional life of the artist, linked with the content and character of the stage action. Therefore, one cannot establish unchangeable performing formulas of breathing for each separate movement, since their compositional possibilities are limitless in their variety of plasticity and musicality.

Consequently, the breathing of the dancer must not only uninterruptedly support his work capacity but also serve as a means of dramatic expressiveness. During the most intense and complex physical work, the dancer's organism always unconsciously finds the most rational and artistic rhythm of breathing. It may be quiet, deep and even, or the opposite, very intense, impetuous, accelerated, reflecting the dramatic force of the stage action. This does not mean, however, that the dancer's breath submits only to emotional situations; it should support and replenish the physical and nervous forces of the dancer. Therefore, the technique of breathing must be well placed and developed.

The dancer must be able to breathe uninterruptedly, evenly and deeply. Abdominal and chest breathing may be freely combined. This process will give the performer great force and capacity, qualities that allow for the greatest intake of oxygen, and to receive the needed amount of life-giving energy. Such breathing should be developed in school, during the execution of the simplest combinations and later in longer and more complex ones; it should be further developed in student performances and finally in the theater, in rehearsal and performance.

A dancer's body cannot be strong and have stamina if the breathing mechanism is poorly placed or underdeveloped. Just how can a dancer hear the music clearly, orient himself properly in space, have a feeling for his partners and the ensemble, as well as the imagery and style of the stage action, if he is exhausted—that is, if his muscles and will have weakened? It is impossible to maintain correct and even breathing always, for in classical dance there are extremely complex and virtuoso movements that demand maximum effort of all forces on the part of the dancer. This makes the dancer hold his breath temporarily—for example, when doing jumps à grand ballon, or multiple turns on the floor or in the air. Technically complex and lengthy stage compositions require the dancer, especially the principal dancer, to accelerate and shorten his breaths.

In classwork an even rhythm of breathing can be maintained only in the simplest exercises. Complex and demanding movements naturally require intensity and a certain acceleration of breathing.

In the adagio and especially in hard allegro combinations, the pupil breathes with greater intensity and in an accelerated rhythm in accordance with the demands of each combination. But no matter how physically hard or complex the combination, it is necessary always to make sure that the pupils inhale and exhale—despite any acceleration—as uninterruptedly, deeply, and evenly as possible, and that they not become unnecessarily upset or tighten their muscles—especially those of the face, neck and shoulders.

Future dancers must be able to breathe freely, with no outward signs of exhaustion or loss of nerve. From the beginning of the study of dance, the pupil must be taught to breathe through the nose, not through the mouth. In difficult exercises, which cause faster breathing, it is recommended to inhale through the mouth and exhale through the nose. This allows a short span of time for freer and deeper breaths, thus regulating the rhythm of the breathing. (Most American dancers are taught to inhale through the nose and exhale through a slightly opened mouth.)

Special attention must be given to the ability of the future dancer to overcome the "dead point" or extreme level of physical exhaustion through willpower. After that "dead point" of tiredness, there appears to be a kind of second wind, which restores the organism's workability for those periods of greatest physical strain. Having overcome this barrier of utmost fatigue, the dancer is able to tolerate further muscular and nervous tension.

In the beginning classes—the first, second and third years—combinations must be constructed and executed in a tempo that allows for the first wind to pass smoothly to the second wind.

In the intermediate classes—the fourth, fifth and sixth years, the heart muscles and lungs are considerably stronger, which allows the student to overcome the heavier class load. At this point, combinations may be composed in a manner to give the student skills to work on his second wind and give him the understanding of its significance to him as a professional dancer.

In the senior classes—seventh and eighth years and especially in the graduating class, the ninth year—the second wind must receive a greater degree of development. The best way to work on the second wind is in repeated demanding exercises—adagio and allegro—taking into account the more intense pace of the whole class.

Pupils in the intermediate and senior classes may work on variations and excerpts from ballets which enter the syllabus at this time as additional stage material.

It must be emphasized once more that insufficient strength and stamina in breathing as a rule limits the technical and acting capabilities of the dancer. Theatrical experience has revealed that such dancers are unable to reach the artistic heights of dramatic expressiveness and acquire true freedom of physical movements.

Errors in the development of correct breathing may occur for the following reasons: (1) The teacher may not be competent in composing and conducting the lesson. (2) The teacher may not be working on an individual basis with each pupil. (3) The classroom may not be sufficiently ventilated. If such conditions are not taken care of, even the most perfect system of breathing will not aid the pupil to master classical technique.

It is good that some schools teach the basics of breathing, but this factor of the performing technique is not as yet sufficiently incorporated into the teaching methods and practices.

It is therefore to be desired that choreographic schools incorporate a specially designed course, which might be called a dancer's course in breathing. Such a course should be put together by choreographers and medical specialists. It should be taught separate from dance lessons, where the pupil's attention may be focused on general principles of breathing only in an incidental and elementary way.

The teacher need not give special directions to those pupils who naturally possess correct and strong breathing.

Some of our most outstanding dancers, without giving much attention to the anatomy and physiology of breathing have acquired this facility simply by having gone through the School of classical dance. It is, of course, unfortunate that those dancers know less than they should about this mechanism, but since they are able to practice free and organic breathing, they are able to give their attention to musicality, imagination and acting.

Of course, the school doctor and teacher of the course in breathing would have to give certain pupils special attention to aid their breathing capacity, bearing in mind that not all pupils will require the strength and endurance needed by the soloist or principal dancer.

IMPORTANCE OF DEVELOPING ATTENTION

Much of the dancer's mastery depends on a highly developed and well-trained attention. The attention of the dancer should be understood to mean his ability to gather and direct his psychic activity to performing creatively. As with any other artist, the attention of the dancer must have professional qualities bound to clearly stated objectives, without which it is impossible to become truly carried away by movement and to reach artistic results in class or on the stage. If the dancer works in an organized manner, thoughtfully and with no major technical or creative flaws, then his attention is working in a totally concentrated manner. The ability to grasp at one and the same time, all sides of the performing mastery—the intentions of the dramatist, composer, and choreographer—means that the dancer's attention is working to its full capacity. The ability to expend rationally, all of one's forces—change quickly from one rhythm to another; change the character of the role according to the stage action—means that the dancer's attention is able and working with flexibility.

All these qualities of a dancer's attention work in every facet of his performing mastery, but in the process of characterization they work in a deeper and more complex way than in technique. The more psychologically complex and subtle the character to be created, the deeper the dancer must enter into the inner world of his hero and the more he must concentrate his attention on the expressiveness of his acting rather than his technique.

One cannot, nonetheless, artificially divide the dancer's attention into mechanical and creative aspects. Technique of movement is not a purely automatic process. There is always a certain amount of creativity involved, although it is impossible to compare it with the work involved in creating a character. In the creation of a character, the dancer's attention is concerned with many very complicated, profound, and at times, imperceptible psychic processes which give the role imagination, musicality, truth and poetic emotion.

The dancer's performing technique is always in a stable and definite form. The process of characterization is always a search, an inner improvisation. Therefore, the ability of the dancer to overcome the most difficult technical and physical burdens with the least expenditure of attention will help him act more creatively, freely and truthfully on stage. Enthusiastic acting overshadows all physical difficulties of the performance. Creative inspiration is assured the dancer who has paid the price of heavy physical labor, which will bring, all the same, enormous joy of mastery, if the desired goal is reached with success.

A totally developed attention allows the dancer to master a perfect technique and musicality, and acting as well as the means of finding himself, his individuality, and of determining his capabilities as a performer.

The cultivation of attention is the strongest attribute of the contemporary actor-dancer. It frees his thoughts, arouses his creativity and perfects and ennobles his technique. The development of the pupil's attention is an integral part of the development of his will. A weak-willed and unstable pupil cannot properly direct his attention. Whatever sort of will the pupil has, it is always expressed in his attention and ultimately in his actions.

The basis of developing the pupil's will and attention is conscious discipline, this is precisely what will form the pupil's strength of character, his diligence, and a demanding, unwavering ability to withstand a high level of physical and nervous tension. A toughened will aids the pupil in directing and retaining his attention in all performing activities. If the pupil's attention is insufficiently developed or one sided, the teacher is remiss.

If a healthy pupil is absentminded in class, this means he is being lazy, which signifies a lack of discipline—the opposite of will. The future dancer must be taught to respect and love his work, his art, to believe in his own strengths, and to honestly and fully strive to achieve the highest results.

In developing the pupil's attention, the following rules should be observed:

1. *Upon entering the room, the teacher should find the pupils standing quietly in place at the barre.* This allows the pupil normally, with no special remarks from the teacher, to begin the class after the traditional greeting to the teacher and accompanist, in the form of a stage bow.

This beginning is not a tribute to tradition or just a formality, but a useful approach to the work on the pupil's attention.

If the students, especially those in the elementary classes, upon appearance of the teacher, continue to be distracted and can be quieted down and made to take their places only with great difficulty, then they are not ready for the lesson, since their attention is elsewhere.

The beginning of the lesson is a teaching upon which the future success of the pupils' work depends. It must be organized very clearly, bearing in mind that the big is created from the small and the ability to collect oneself before going on stage is extremely important to the future dancer. Such an approach to the beginning of the lesson must be established in all classes, from the first to the last.

All exercises begin with various preparations, each of which give the rhythm and character of the music; the preparatory position from which the exercise is begun; and directs the attention of the pupil to the coming movements. If the preparation is done in correct form, but in an abstract manner, it means the pupil has not concentrated his attention on the exercise.

2. *All combinations must be given without repeated explanations, except for new movements.* The teacher must clearly and thoroughly but briefly give the combinations, incorporating demonstration and explanation, especially when new elements are worked on. Thus, the pupils' visual and aural perception will allow them to work

better on their attention and better understand all the details of the combinations—especially in elementary classes.

In composing a combination, the teacher must see that the pupils' attention span is not overtaxed. True, such overloading develops mental acuity and the pupil immediately can grasp the structure of the combinations without confusing the order of the steps and can orient themselves in space and in the rhythms required. But very often the sense of the music, the plasticity of dance, the artistic completeness and the refinement of the choreographic pattern will receive almost no attention.

Complexity of composition is necessary in every combination, but it must not take all of the pupil's attention. Each difficulty must be overcome thoughtfully and artistically, not mechanically. The difficulties must be increased gradually from simple to complex, from small to large, with no sharp increases or decreases in complexity. The line of development of the pupil's attention must rise evenly and gradually, with consideration for the meaning and development of each lesson and for every part of it, every combination.

The barre, and also exercises at the beginning and at the end of the center, call for less attention than the adagio and allegro portions, since these sections contain less complicated elements. But whatever the combination, excessive complexity will force the pupil to fix his attention on *what* to do instead of *how* to do it. Of course, a pupil sometimes will devote more attention, and sometimes all his attention, to technique when studying new steps. But once the step is learned, the pupil's attention again strives for fullness and flexibility. Then he is again able to perceive the movement as dance and to become aware once again, of the plasticity of dance and the musical content—that is, to deal with the art of dance rather than gymnastics.

An unduly light, primitive composition of a combination or an excessively fast or slow tempo also will not do, since they do not develop the needed sharpness of attention.

The teacher should make comments at the proper time, supporting, not distracting, the attention of the class and all the while demanding that while doing one step they prepare in detail for the next one, linking them as a single whole. This teaches the future dancer to anticipate all his actions while considering the pattern, character, and musicality of the combination. The art of cantilena in dance can only be learned in this manner.

Stopping the student during the performance of an exercise must be done as rarely as possible and only at the appearance of a gross error caused by a lapse of attention. Each teacher, of course, arrives at an individual approach in correcting mistakes. But it must be stressed again that the development of the art of dance requires active and concentrated attention. Therefore, frequent interruptions for insufficient reason or constant prompting are of little use as a means of developing attention.

Naturally, new movements must be totally explained, demonstrated and observed for correctness, then corrected if there are errors. But, when a pupil still makes elementary errors after a time, it means his attention cannot act inde-pendently and long enough because it has become dependent upon prompting. One must request less and demand more independence and personal responsibility from each pupil.

3. *When the exercise has been completed, the pupils must not immediately "turn off" their attention.* The end of each exercise must be clearly fixed as the teacher at this point makes corrections. The pupils are then permitted to rest a bit and relax their attention in order to be able to begin afresh the next exercise.

For the normal development of the pupil's attention, the previous material must have been learned properly; it is also necessary neither to oversimplify nor to complicate the lessons, but to develop an artistic relationship to technique and music. This will permit the pupil to gradually acquire necessary attention, without which the creative work on characterization will, as a rule, be superficial.

IMPORTANCE OF MEMORY

If the dancer is able to recreate impressions and experiences in his consciousness, and clearly remember all facets of the role's characteristics and stage action, then his memory is well developed, which allows him to reach a high level of technique as well as mastery of acting. A well-developed memory illuminates the actions of the dancer, leading him directly to the goal he sets. A weak memory limits his actions, causing unexpected lapses in performance. In projecting the depth and subtlety of the inner life of a hero, an excellently developed memory is re-quired. The shortest lapse of even one moment, lowers the performance into an unclear, inconsistent, unmusical and false characterization. Memory for classical dance is divided into aural, visual and motor responses. The aural memory fixes in the artist's mind all he has heard and hears from his teachers, the répétiteur (ballet master or ballet mistress, rehearsal person or captain), and choreographer, and all that the music, accompanist, and conductor "tell" him.

The visual memory fixes in the dancer's consciousness all that has been and is shown to him by his teachers, répétiteur, choreographer, and stage and costume designers, and the entire pageant of stage action in which he takes part.

The motor memory (or reflexes) fixes in the dancer's mind and body all the performing methods of technique acquired at school, in rehearsals and on stage.

These forms of memory are indivisibly meshed to form the entire store of memory. This store allows the dancer to act freely in his technique and char-acterizations. If one of the forms of memory is not functioning precisely—for instance, the motor memory—the form of the dancer's movements and, con-sequently, their content can suffer. Figuratively speaking, the dancer's memory is the musical score from which he projects all his stage actions. If he cannot remember the content and sense of his role, his character and image, his world of feelings, desires and psychological traits, then the dancer is not able to create a free, whole, deep, truthful and inspired image.

The memory of the artist is based upon well-developed attention. Sometimes it is not the memory that fails a dancer but his attention. Inattention does the greatest harm to memory, for only attention can remove the reason for a lapse in memory.

WAYS OF DEVELOPING MEMORY

The dancer must perfect his memory in a regular, systematic way, and only through consciously repeated actions. No matter what his innate capacity may be, his ability to remember cannot become stronger or develop any other way. Purposeful action leaves the most enduring traces in the memory. Therefore, the dancer must strive for conscious and indelible actions and precise, well-worked-out skills. Then his memory will acquire the necessary clarity, stability, depth and strength.

THE AURAL MEMORY

The professional memory of the dancer is developed and perfected from the first steps at the school just as methodically and systematically as his attention is developed. Aural memory is developed through the spoken word and music. The teacher must speak to the pupil purposefully, concisely and exactly. Vague, verbose remarks are ineffective. The teacher's speech must always be vivid and alive and express his thoughts exactly. If the speech is not cultured, this will remain in the future dancer's memory and will go on stage with him. If the teacher talks to his pupils too softly, too sharply, or even in a crude manner, this will also remain in the dancer's memory and will manifest itself correspondingly in his actions—first in class and eventually on stage.

Everything the pupil hears from his teacher in class—both the good and the bad—will be retained in his memory as a store of impressions and knowledge which he will later use in his work. Of course, the teacher must be strict, demanding and, at times, very pressing. But the cultural level of his spoken word must always be high. Some feel that the most important aspect in the development of memory is in the demonstration of a step. It seems to me that the spoken word is sometimes stronger than any demonstration if it is logical and addressed to the art of dance, its essence and contents, to music and its imagery, emotions, and intonations, and goes to the heart of the pupil and his creative imagination.

MUSICAL MEMORY

If speaking of the education of the pupil's musical memory, the development of his overall musical culture must be kept in mind. If the teacher and accompanist do not create the habit in the pupil of listening with interest to good music played well, his memory will amass impressions and experiences that are not in harmony with the true culture of a performing artist. A sense of variety and inspired feelings for dance are affirmed in the memory by means of good, not mediocre music.

What is important is not how many melodies and musical rhythms the pupil can remember, but *what kind* of music he has heard and how his mind as a performing artist has been trained by it.

If the music, no matter how fine, does not correspond to the character of the exercise being performed, or if it is too complex for the pupil's capabilities, then he will remember the music formally and superficially. In the first case he will experience an inner psychological protest. In the second case, he will simply hear the music poorly and will not be sufficiently attentive. The pupil will remember the music actively and firmly only if it fully corresponds to the movement. Otherwise, the music and dance will not flow into a single whole or arouse emotional and creative strivings.

THE VISUAL MEMORY

Visual memory is developed and strengthened by means of demonstration. The accumulation of precise impressions and experiences in the pupil's memory depends on the attitude the teacher brings to the lesson, as well as how he behaves during the session and demonstrates combinations. Therefore, all the teachers' actions must be distinguished by a strict discretion, restraint, simplicity, taste, and unaffected interest and love for his pupils.

One of the means of explaining the rules of movement is by demonstration, which may be divided into two categories: the demonstration of new steps, and the demonstration of combinations.

In the lower classes, all new movements must be shown in detail, slowly and repeatedly until they are fully comprehended; they must also, of course, be confirmed by a suitable spoken explanation. Demonstration of combinations in the lower classes is also necessary, but it should be done in an ordinary tempo without too many repetitions, and it must be remembered from the first demonstration of the combination. This is obligatory; it is very difficult but it develops the visual or, more accurately, the choreographic memory of the pupil. There may be exceptions, but two or three demonstrations rob the pupil of the chance to memorize independently and actively.

The *creative individuality* of the student begins to grow from the first steps of study. It grows with the development of dance technique, in inseparable union with it. Daily lessons familiarize the pupil with the artistic nature of dance. His consciousness assimilates the first laws of movements, and is penetrated by the laws of rhythm, dynamics, plasticity, gesture and musicality. Hence, it is natural for the pupil to bring to his technique (even the most elementary) his own sense of plasticity of the movement, pose, and the music. This is already a creative process. This process and the strict preservation of all the rules of technique should be the beginning of training of the pupil's creative individuality and its free manifestation in classwork.

A simple inclination of the head, the gaze, a change in hand position, the bending or straightening of the torso must be executed by the student with the utmost precision and lightness in regard to technique but with a variety in regard to a sense of sculpture and musicality. Otherwise, the development of individuality will become a secondary element in the pupil's classwork and, later, in his stage life. The main element will become a mannered, forced, and "alien" manner of movement based on a precise but formal rather than creative method of study. The feeling of dance movement and pose, corresponding to the age and psychological level of the student, must be technically precise and musical but free from blind imitation which leads to the establishment of stencil-like movement and posturing, robbing the dancer of true artistic freedom. While the pupil should follow the example of his teacher and obey his bidding, he should, while assimilating the demonstration, remain true to himself.

Some teachers believe that the pupil must first learn to stand firmly on his own two feet, displaying no performing individuality which, they seem to think, will automatically appear later at the proper time on stage. Of course, the ABC's of dance technique, the elementary ability to manipulate the body without overstressing the muscles, come first. Only then is work on creative activity and musicality introduced. This is all true, but it is also true that the student's individuality is developed not only on stage and in acting class. It is mainly developed in simple physical activities involving the pupil's will, his creative relationship to work, technique, and dance plastique, and his understanding of music and the character of the exercises.

If the student is totally engrossed in the work of his muscles, with exact form and rhythm of movement, then he is far from developing his individuality and far from expressing his creativity. He is then only superficially imitating the performing manner of his teacher, which, admittedly, may be very good.

It is not possible to agree with the opinion that a teacher must prepare, with the help of demonstration, only a good copy of himself and that stage practice will create individuality. The wish to create lives in every pupil. It only needs support, education and development from childhood. Let the pupil's creative "I" or individuality, exist from the beginning even if it is not quite resolute, but free in even the most elementary exercises. This is not to say it should be indulged at the expense of academic exactness. The emergence of individuality does not give a pupil the right to violate the laws of performing classical dance. The expression of individuality should not be interpreted as the right to violate teaching and stage discipline. It is only the training of the pupil's talent. The demonstrations by the teacher must help the pupil grasp the basis of technique, which must be identical for all. But it must not repress his creative individuality. Unnecessary demonstration, and repeating what the pupil already knows, does not strengthen the memory, but wastes time and slows the pace of the lesson. If, however, a combination is not done correctly by the pupil after one clear demonstration, the exercise was either too complicated or the pupil was inattentive.

If the teacher demonstrates the exercise in its entirety ("full out" in the sense of complete details), in the correct tempo from the beginning to the end of the demonstration, he will simply not have time to give a whole class, or to give comments and corrections. Also the pauses between separate combinations will be too long.

For instance, in demonstrating a barre exercise, the teacher should show the basic pattern of the entire combination with no further repetition. It is best to show the adagio in its entirety. Simple jumps should be demonstrated like the barre exercises, while complex jumps should be shown in their entirety. One must economize on time, but not at the expense of the correctness or the musicality of the movement during the demonstration. A demonstration after the performance of the combination may be necessary as well. In such case, mistakes must be corrected by the demonstration to help the pupil understand and correct the movement quickly.

ADJUSTING THE DEMONSTRATION TO THE LEVEL OF THE CLASS

Every demonstration in the lower levels (nine to eleven years of age), must be at the adjusted level of the nine-to-eleven-year-olds, not adult dancers. Otherwise the valuable aspect of the demonstration will be reversed as the pupil, imitating his teacher, will affirm in his memory the very unpleasant and unnatural manner of movement of an adult dancing "dwarf."

In the intermediate classes (twelve to sixteen years of age), demonstration is also necessary but less so, even though the program for these classes is quite extensive and difficult. The age of the pupil, his awareness, and technical preparedness, permit him to remember and assimilate new movements faster. It is worthwhile mentioning again that the teacher should repeat a demonstration only when absolutely necessary. Demonstration must not replace spoken instructions and comments, which the teacher is able to make much more concisely and vividly.

In the senior classes (sixteen to eighteen or nineteen years of age), demonstration is just as valuable but must be used more sparingly in relation to spoken words. Overuse of demonstration at this point reveals the teacher's inability to evoke an inner impulse to action in the pupil. One need not, however, reduce demonstration to a deaf-mute language. Thinking and memory must be developed on the basis of an independent and active understanding of the combination, reinforced visually by demonstration, not the reverse.

In summary: Demonstration is the best method for the development of a memory for performing and stage manner, but only if it is done in union with the expressive force of spoken instructions and music. In addition, the point behind demonstration is to develop well-rounded expression and perfection of the individual and creative possibilities of the student, not to create imitators of the teacher. The performer in the teacher must retire to the background and defer to the pedagogue.

REFLEX OR MOTOR MEMORY

The motor memory of the pupil is worked on, developed and strengthened on the basis of a precise performing technique. The future dancer cannot achieve mastery if choreographic and technical errors are fixed in his mind in every class.

Experience has shown that relearning is more difficult than learning correctly in the beginning.

The development of a motor or reflex memory in the student demands from the teacher the scrupulously fine work of a jeweler, great restraint and, most important, excellent knowledge of the school of classical dance. *Haste, a lack of system and irregularity in class work are absolutely unacceptable.*

The motor memory is strengthened with difficulty through many repetitions of exercises during the entire course of study. But without a well-developed motor memory, the future dancer cannot possess good aplomb, flexibility, lightness, softness, simplicity and freedom of movement. Naturally, none of these qualities are possible in a pupil without well-developed physical strength, endurance, will, restraint, attention, musicality, correct training and professional ability.

A fully developed motor memory allows the dancer to move with the greatest creative freedom, true musicality, and technical perfection.

All the elements of performance from the school of classical dance discussed here must be learned by the future artist of the professional ballet theater on the basis of planned classwork, not arbitrarily.

PLANNING THE TEACHING COURSE

In choreographic schools, all work is conducted in accordance with a document called the syllabus. The content of the syllabus is determined by the aims and goals of training the versatile, highly qualified artist of the Soviet ballet theater.

The syllabus contains a number of academic and dance-related disciplines, states the number of hours required for their study, and contains a system for getting through the material during the course of study.

It is important to point out that there are two syllabuses in the USSR choreographic schools: one for the eight-year course and another for the accelerated six-year course. The decision for which course to use is based upon the age of the pupil and the goals set by the school. No matter what these goals may be, it may be boldly stated that future ballet dancers must begin to assimilate the school of classical dance at the age of nine or ten and finish at the age of eighteen or nineteen. It is specifically during this period that the body of the pupil is at its most pliable and receptive psychological and physical development, which allows him to master the school of classical dance, most naturally, thoroughly, unhurriedly and to acquire the most secure and deep understanding.

At the same time, teenagers, twelve to fourteen years of age, who begin the accelerated six-year course, may be able to understand and remember more of the first two or three years, but as result of the extreme condensation of the course (and it is quite extensive, physically difficult and complex), they do not have the time to penetrate the true musical feeling of dance as organically as the future dancer who began studying at nine or ten. (The study of musical instruments, such as the piano, violin, or cello, should also begin in the childhood

years.) It is in the childhood years that the pupil must become thoroughly accustomed to the technique of classical dance and its elements in order that later
he not have to think on stage about overcoming physical difficulties and can
devote his forces to the creation of an image in dance. Of course, there are rare
exceptions, when an especially talented pupil begins dance training at the age of
fourteen, sixteen or even eighteen years and acquires an excellent knowledge of
classical dance. But this only confirms once again the experience of the oldest
choreographic schools, those of Moscow and Leningrad, that fast *and* good occur
together very rarely and not with everyone. The technical mastery and culture
of dance are developed not because of the acceleration of the course, the condensation of the syllabus, and the greater age of the pupil, but because of the free
distribution and mastery of the material in the syllabus over the entire course of
study and the normal physical and psychological development of the pupil—
approximately from nine or ten to eighteen years of age.

It is not a question of how many years of study are necessary, but a matter of
at what age the student must begin to know the expressive means of dance, which,
of course, the future artist must master with a perfect technique, artistic freedom,
flexibility and musicality. Those lost young years will surely show somehow and
somewhere as a shaded and not fully developed area of growth. After all, childhood
is a time especially receptive to the beauties of dance and music. It is a time of
emotional fullness, impressionableness, dreams and physical action.

Soviet ballet demands from the professional school thoroughly, not hurriedly,
trained actor-dancers. All the more so as the male performer in the past few years
has assumed such an important position in choreographic composition of great
originality, impressive characterizations, and virtuoso technique. This is most
clearly revealed in the production of *Spartacus* by Yuri Grigorovich, winner of
the Lenin Prize, to the music of Aram Khachaturian.

And, if the theater continues to perfect the art of the young dancer, the school
is obliged to produce the professional matured dancer trained on a time-proven
basis, from childhood throughout the teens and on to early adulthood.

In short, experience has shown that in all choreographic schools the most ex-
pedient method of training is through the eight-year course with a separate year,
a preparatory period, before professional work is begun. All this is explained
because the new as well as the experienced teacher must know how to assess the
details of the course, how to make corrections and how to participate in its perfection. The success of the teacher and the pupil depends upon that understanding
as does the school and most of all, the ballet stage itself.

Lowering the number of hours is not desirable. The amount of time devoted
to the study of classical dance in the eight-year course should equal twelve academic
hours a week. This number of hours is essential, as classical dance in the system
of choreographic education occupies a leading position among the other dance
disciplines, which were discussed earlier. Shortening the course results, as a rule,
in a lower level of professional preparedness and a superficial comprehension of
the syllabus.

The six-year course has a positive side: it allows for the acceptance of a talented
youngster, who, for whatever reason, has been unable to enter the eight-year

course in his childhood years. These students must be accepted into the six-year program and trained perhaps individually and under a special syllabus and by the best teachers.

If the school graduates one leading soloist each year, that is considered an excellent record. In the eight-year course, it is possible to produce the strongest group of leading dancers.

The next item in the organization of the teacher's "work" is the subject program, which is based on the syllabus and which establishes the content, system, and the volume of knowledge the pupils must learn.

Each year in the program is inextricably linked to the next. In years one through three, the elementary basis is established, without which it would be impossible to strengthen and develop the skills of the future dancer. In years four through six, the pupils learn more difficult performing movements, relying on the earlier foundation. In the final years, seven and eight, the most complex portion of the program is finished and perfected, based on the accomplishments of the preceding years.

If any portion of the program is skimped by the teacher, either artistically or technically, there will be a weakness in that area that it is not always possible to correct successfully. Therefore, one must not consider one part of the program more responsible or important than another. Each period of study is equally difficult and responsible, for the completion of the entire program depends on the sum of knowledge and skills acquired by the pupils in school; the faculty, which is capable of succeeding in this task; and the artistic directorship of the choreographic school which must methodically and creatively unite the faculty.

While fulfilling the annual program, it is necessary to strengthen and develop all that was properly learned, and to work very carefully on what has not been quite mastered. If for some reason, the previous material was not properly learned, the addition of new material must be delayed, and it may be necessary even to go back and correct previous errors. Only after this can new material be covered.

As previously stated, the program is put together taking into account the age of the pupil and the particular demands of ballet training, and consists of the minimum requirements which must be unwaveringly strived for. But since not all the children who study in school are equally gifted, the results of their study will not be the same for all. Not all of them can master a high degree of technique. When this happens, the teacher is obliged to do everything he can to help the pupil achieve the highest results. If this is impossible, then the program for that pupil must be considered finished.

The results may differ, but all those who graduated from the school must possess an ability to perform within the limits of their professional capacity. The course of study, therefore, must be looked upon not only as the teaching of a technique of movement but as the education of a future dancer who will be able to use his mastery of technique for the creation of artistic dance images.

The successful fulfillment of the program depends upon the correct and well-timed learning of new material. The order in which to thoroughly cover new movements in each class is set forth in the sequence of the program. But the program does not state how to go about teaching any specific movements, or which classroom steps or musical and rhythmic examples to use in learning dance technique or which way to develop the pupil's musicality, artistry and individuality.

Such knowledge can be gained in textbooks, and class materials or from experienced masters of the school. All this enables the new teacher to study the course program more systematically and to understand his profession with more confidence.

However, not every borrowed teaching method turns out to be useful in practice if it is too complex or too simple for the professional capabilities of the students and is not in strict accordance with the age, knowledge, capabilities and length of study of the future dancer.

For this reason, as the teacher gains experience, he must find his own individual creativity based on his own opinions, his own work methods developed in practice in the field and his upbringing as well as his training. To regard the same certain recommended methods as unchangeable in all cases, is to reduce the teacher's art to a standardized, immutable recipe.

The school's best traditions of methods must not only be carefully preserved, they must be developed with creative interest.

In general, the course of classical dance in the choreographic schools provides a ballet dancer with the complete, finished performing education he needs to be a professionally literate person who knows the school and the stage. Otherwise no recommended teaching method even from the most authoritative, qualified pedagogue will help the teacher carry out his work thoroughly and with the necessary quality.

The program also does not state exactly when—at what point in the second year—any given step should be studied. That is, there is no calendar schedule to follow. Correct planning of the program into the teaching schedule will help the pupil's success to a considerable extent. By taking into consideration the number of hours set aside for learning the program, as well as the capacities of the pupils, the teacher can make a calendar schedule of work for the entire year.

SCHEDULING THE MATERIAL FOR THE SCHOOL YEAR*

In the first quarter of the year, on every level (with the exception of the very first year), enough time must be given to repeat movements learned the previous year and to return the pupil's bodies gradually to full professional working form. About two to three weeks is needed for this. The rest of the first quarter may be given to the study of the most simple elements of the program and to previously learned material in more complex combinations.

In the second quarter of the year, the teacher may plan the study of more complex elements of the program along with more complex combinations than given in the first quarter.

* Tarasov takes for granted that lessons will be given six days a week, beginning with forty-five-minute sessions, then extending in a year or two to two hours.

In the third quarter of the year (after winter vacation) it is recommended that the body be conditioned back to full capacity once again and the material of the second quarter be repeated. This should require an estimated two weeks.

In the third quarter of the year, the most difficult movements of the program and the most complex work include the study of coordinating movements learned during the first half of the year. (Actually, I would recommend that all new material for the year be covered on all levels by the third-quarter mark with the exception of the first year of study. The entire first year provides the foundation of classical dance, and the work of coordinating those movements is not too great. Therefore, the last quarter of the first year may include the complex movements scheduled for that level at that time.)

In the fourth quarter (which begins after spring vacation), about one week should be given to return pupils to full capacity, just as after winter vacation. Then the coordination of material and all elements learned that year may begin as a preparation for the examinations.

These are the basic principles of the calendar schedule, which may require some modification depending upon the ability of the students to master the material and depending upon how the teacher copes with his work. Unjustified accelerating or slowing down in reaching goals does not aid the pupil's progress. Some teachers give all the material for the year during the first half of the year, reserving the second half for perfecting its execution. While this method usually interests pupils, it does not give them solid professional knowledge and skills. By the same token, excessive drawing out of the presentation of new elements cannot be considered good planning. Slowness forces the teacher to skimp in work on combinations in the last quarter. Consequently, the completion of the program will not be of high quality. And in addition the normal course of study during preparation for examinations will be disrupted.

Each teacher can establish the form of his own calendar schedule. It is important to designate deadlines for the fulfillment of the entire program. In this way, the calendar plan will regulate and direct the teacher's work for the entire year. This is its methodological significance and strength. But even a well-scheduled plan may not produce the desired quality in the work if the teacher does not prepare himself thoroughly for each lesson.

The degree of success of the pupil's comprehension and fulfillment of the calendar schedule largely depends not only upon the teacher's experience, knowledge and gifts, but on the degree of his preparedness for each lesson. While preparing the lesson, the teacher must first of all determine its content, that is the teaching material upon which the class is constructed. Each lesson will change depending upon the different combinations.

It is most advisable for young teachers to be guided by the following rules: (1) Include new examples in coordination with the problems of each part of the lesson to further consolidate and perfect the knowledge and skills already amassed and practiced by the students; (2) Evaluate the new material for study and determine whether the students are sufficiently prepared to understand it; (3) Introduce this new material into combinations to further strengthen and develop skills; (4) Together with the accompanist, determine the suitable meter and the character of the musical accompaniment for each part of the lesson.

It is recommended that the new teacher plan his lessons in writing, putting down the most complex teaching material. In this way, he will gradually acquire the necessary skill of planning every lesson. Later, the teacher should decide exactly when written preparation will no longer be necessary, although each class must still be very carefully thought out in regard to content and form.

However, the fixed plan should not suppress the creativity of the teacher. In practice, this means that while maintaining the methodological intent of his original idea, he may somewhat change a combination in each section of the lesson or make it more complex. In short, the teacher who is well prepared for his lesson will be able to conduct it freely and surely but with such corrections as may be necessary.

In preparing for the lesson, one must plan why, how and what must be told the pupil, not only about technique, but about the art of dance, creativity in the ballet artist, stagework, music, gesture, and so on.

Good organization is still not enough. One must breathe into the heart and consciousness of the pupil the beginning of creativity which will lead him to understand the poetry of dance. And, finally, the new teacher must know that an excellently constructed program is not all—he must possess a highly professional and artistic method of teaching. Only a constant creative search, labor, conscientious teaching and awareness of educational and artistic problems, may bring the teacher and his students the desired results.

A program for the subject, a calendar schedule and well-planned lessons are only a guide to action. To become a good teacher, one needs more than to know the subject. One must be able to apply knowledge in practice. I repeat that the mastery of teaching evolves slowly through self-perfection, relentless work, strict criticism of one's own work and a demanding attitude toward one's pupils.

We all know that any teacher may convey to his pupils only the knowledge and skills that he himself possesses. But the teacher of classical dance, in addition to having high professional qualifications, must be armed with a knowledge of aesthetics, ethics, pedagogy, music, history and theory of the ballet theater, acting, anatomy, physiology and psychology. In short, classical dance as a subject requires education and culture from the teacher. In teaching, constructing a correct lesson is very important. Every lesson is based upon natural development and is linked with the principles of going from the simple to the complex, from the small to the large, and seems to become gradually more complicated in the chain of study.

CONTENT OF THE LESSON

Every lesson in classical dance consists of four parts. The first part, exercises, involves the study of elementary movements from which complicated forms are later evolved. Exercises must be learned thoroughly or a precise technique cannot be mastered.

It is a great mistake to look upon exercises as secondary in importance or as a means of warming up the legs. Exercises are necessary to the student as well as the professional dancer for a constant strengthening and perfecting the foundations of his technique.

While executing these exercises, the teacher should require that the pupil: (1) Perform all movements at the barre and in the center first working one leg, then the other, in order to gain even strength in both legs; (2) Perform in the center all movements first studied at the barre, in order to perfect an elementary technique; (3) Begin all exercises with a suitable preparation; (4) Execute a proper ending, in addition to a proper preparation and performance of the movement. This develops the student's ability to finish each given task correctly and attentively, which assures the performance of a clear finish, a very important factor in the development of aplomb. The ability to clearly fix the end of an exercise is first introduced into the dancer's training in these exercises and it enters as well, into a more complicated part of the lesson at a later time. This disciplines the student's attention to a place where he is prone to be inexact in his performance—the end of an exercise.

The subject program suggests a sequence for the study of all movements of classical dance. But as these movements are learned the sequence is somewhat altered.

The sequence of exercises at the barre and in the center may be as follows: (1) Grands pliés (2) Various forms of battements tendus (3) Ronds de jambes par terre (4) Battements fondus and battements soutenus (5) Forms of battements frappés (6) Battement relevé lent and battements développés (7) Ronds de jambes en l'air (8) Grands battements jetés (9) Petits battements sur le cou-de-pied.

Included in these exercises are various poses, ports de bras, dance steps, turns, pirouettes which all make the sequence more complex and varied, depending upon the preparedness of the pupil and the personal method of the teacher. For instance, some teachers prefer to give battement développé at the end of the barre and grand battement jeté in the middle of the barre. Or, some prefer to begin the barre exercises with battement tendu instead of grand plié.

Exercises in the center, as a rule, are constructed in a more compact, shorter, and more technical form. From year to year, the content of this portion of the lesson must become gradually more complex and the number of separate exercises smaller. But no matter how the center exercises are structured, they are only the preparation for the next part of the lesson and never a substitute for it.

The second part of the lesson, the adagio, involves work on the overall mastery of poses of classical dance linked together in a great variety of ways. While the exercises through repetition of different kinds of battements and other movements in single exercises provides the elementary technique of dance, it is the adagio portion where the character, manner and technique necessary for performing long and flowing dance phrases, is learned.

The adagio in the different class levels is composed from previously learned poses and movements. But in the first year, there is as yet no adagio as such. Here the pupils only begin to learn different small poses with the working leg not yet off the floor. From the second year, the pupil begins to learn poses at 90 degrees, and to connect them with simple movements; this is the simplest form of adagio which is done after the exercises in the center.

Gradually, about the fourth or fifth year, the adagios acquire a more difficult and demanding character that reflects the increased capacity of the student and the increased complexity of movements: connecting steps, tours lents, and big and small pirouettes. In this manner, the academic form of the grand adagio is established.

Finally, in the fifth and sixth year, when the pupil's requirements are heavier and after the adagio has been introduced into this portion of the class, a so-called second adagio is added which consists of a sequence of gradually more and more complex turns on the floor. In a technical sense, this second adagio must be more complicated and mobile, but lighter in forcefulness and shorter in length than the grand adagio.

The second adagio may start with small pirouettes finishing in various big poses, and later go on to pirouettes beginning with a big pose. Later both methods may be combined and joined with a transitional demi-plié. Other uninterrupted turns, such as tours chaînés may be included. In the senior classes it may be helpful to use certain jumps such as pas failli or sissonne tombée as a preparation for pirouettes in big or small poses. These jumps may be introduced along with a pas échappé to second position as a preparation for small pirouettes, or the small pirouettes may begin from the open position of the leg after a jeté passé or grand jeté. These jumps may be done en tournant but usually only in the second adagio for the senior classes and especially the graduating class.

In planning the first and second adagios, it is necessary that movements join progressively and logically, forming a finished exercise, and not a haphazard collection of movements. Each adagio should have a definite aim—work on a specific step, not merely the development of strength, aplomb, and plasticity.

The third part of the lesson, allegro, involves the mastery of the various jumps of classical dance. While the students learn technique in the exercises, elementary technique and work on poses and dance phrases in a slow tempo in the adagio, the allegro is the portion of the class where all is summarized and executed in the tempos of jumps—small or large, simple or complex, soft or bounding in character, impetuous or restrained.

Jumps, like all other movements, are in the sequence set forth by the program. At a later time, this sequence will be somewhat changed. Except in the first year, the pupils first do combinations consisting of small jumps—for example, temps sauté, pas échappé, pas glissade, petit pas assemblé, petit pas jeté, sissonne simple and sissonne tombée as well as beats, petite cabriole, various turns, and small pirouettes. Each jump must be repeated in the same combination and in the order of difficulty of performance.

The pupils are then recommended to do big jumps without approaches (preparatory steps), in the order of difficulty: grande sissonne ouverte, grande sissonne fermée, pas ballotté, temps levé in big poses, jeté passé, and big jumps from two legs to two legs as in tour en l'air, etc.

Then, energetic approaches may proceed the big jumps such as pas chassé, pas glissade, pas failli, pas coupé, pas de bourrée, etc. These big jumps may be grand assemblé, grand jeté, grand jeté entrelacé (jeté dessus en tournant), grand fouetté, grand cabriole, saut de basque, various turns, batterie, complex tours en l'air, etc. These jumps are characterized by high elevation and travel a considerable distance in straight, diagonal or curving lines. These jumps are combined gradually in more and more complex forms.

Finally, for the second time, small jumps are executed again, but in more complex combinations than earlier in the lesson. Now virtuoso batterie with turns, for example, in brisé, pas jeté, etc., are performed. These jumps are followed by simple steps such as changement de pied, combined with entrechats quatre, to bring the body and breathing of the pupil into a quieter state.

It must be noted that as the number of learned jumps increases, especially in the higher levels, the jumps seem to acquire greater "mobility" in the sense of variety of combined steps and intensity of performance.

In the fourth part of the lesson, the purpose is to permit the body of the pupil, after strenuous work, to come to a state of quiet by performing forms of port de bras.

Organizing the lesson in this manner permits progressive complexity without sharp increases and decreases in difficulty. In addition, each part of the lesson should have its own curve, reflecting a gradual increase and a certain decrease in intensity, allowing the pupils to regain their strength for the next part of the lesson.

This construction of a lesson, organized to complement the body's physical capacity, guards against injury to joints and stress on the heart. At the same time it must be noted that the structure of various movements and the rules of performing these movements, will produce in the student different degrees of physical and psychological stress. For that reason, it is necessary in each portion of the lesson not to complicate the structure of each combination or to place an undue strain on the memory or attention of the pupil, when the physical difficulty increases. Then, when the combination requires maximum attention, it should allow for less physical demand. Complex, forceful exercises must be alternated with easier exercises, so that the pupil may regain his strength and more easily and freely overcome the difficulties of the lesson.

These are the points that I consider necessary for the teacher just beginning his profession. It is impossible to establish an absolute order for the work on movements. Even if it *were* possible, the lesson would acquire a standardized form which would not allow for the development of the pupil's comprehension of technique, nor would it allow for the pupil's individuality, not to mention the teacher's creativity. Remember that, on the whole, the construction of the lesson indicates the progression in the study of the movements, in each separate part of the lesson.

ALLOTMENT OF TIME FOR PORTIONS OF THE LESSON

The next consideration in constructing a proper lesson in classical dance is to determine the duration of time to be given each portion of the class. The overall time for the daily lesson is generally two hours. Within the limits of this time, from the beginning to the end of the course of study, the amount of time given to the first portion of the class will gradually shorten as the exercises increase in complexity and difficulty. The second, and especially the third portion of the class, must gradually increase in time as they increase in complexity and difficulty. The fourth portion takes the shortest amount of time and its complexity is not greatly increased.

At the end of the first year, the first portion of the lesson (the barre and center floor exercises) will take half of the allotted time to complete. In the higher levels and the last year of study, the time should be gradually lessened to one quarter of the class time. The second portion of the lesson, the adagio, should increase in allotted time to double the original amount, while the third portion, the allegro, should increase to three times its original amount or more.

This apportioning of time in the lesson is approximate, and deviations from this norm can, and must, be based upon the conditions of the work. If, for instance, the students are fatigued from theatrical or school stage practice, the time for the second and third portions of the lesson should be shortened. Especially after summer vacations, the length of the entire lesson in the second and third portion must be gradually increased, and then shortened at the end of the year after the examinations. The teacher must pay special attention to a pupil who has missed lessons because of illness and increase his lesson time very gradually.

PACE OF THE CLASS

The next condition to consider in planning the class is the correct pace. One may establish a sensible progression of the study of different movements, construct the combinations in a useful and good professional manner, hold to the correct time allotment for each portion of the class *and still not achieve systematic development*.

Students periodically fall out of normal working condition during class or become excessively fatigued, that is, the body does not remain warmed-up. This occurs if the class is not conducted at the proper pace.

Gradually increasing the physical effort of the student to his maximum calls upon effort from the nervous system as well. The greater the effort, the greater the fatigue of the body. To avoid this condition, the teacher must alternate periods of effort with periods of rest. That will enable the students to regain their strength and become prepared for the performance of more complicated elements of the lesson. Therefore, these alternating periods must be very strictly observed, since they determine the correct pace of the lesson.

If the period of rest for renewal of energy is insufficient, and the exercises bring too much fatigue, then the lesson was led at too fast a pace. In such a case, perfectly healthy children will appear to be exhausted, weak, be inattentive and unable to coordinate the movements correctly and be unable to react to the remarks of the teacher. If, however, the students cool off, then the lesson's pace is slow and the time is not allotted properly. This kind of slowness during the lesson does not promote the development of strength and endurance in the pupils. The time between the exercises, for instance, should be short because the physical load in this part of the lesson is not great.

In the adagio portion, the students should be divided into two groups, as the physical burden is noticeably greater. While one group works, the other rests.

In the allegro portion, small jumps may be performed by all the students at the same time. But as the allegro section progresses, the group should be divided into two or three sections to give the students ample time to rest while others are working, since this portion requires the utmost effort.

In addition to the general pace of the lesson, there is great teaching value in the correct pace of separate exercises and combinations. The movements of classical dance differ in the pace of performance depending upon the complexity of the construction of the combinations, upon the conditions of the performance and upon the degree to which the student is prepared for the given task.

For the best understanding of a movement, the teacher must establish the most useful and practical tempo for the purpose. Any recommendation of pace here is useless since determining a pace depends, to a great measure, upon the preparedness and ability of the pupils. But it should be remembered that a slower tempo is more conducive to the development of technique, since it permits time for thorough work on all details within the movements and on the structure of those movements as a whole.

To strengthen the muscles, a moment is necessary to direct the body's muscular tension. The slower tempo exercises the attention span, memory, the exactness of the rhythm, precision, pliability, stability and cantilena quality of the movements. The higher level the class, the faster the pace of performance of the given tasks, but the teaching approach must never be changed.

Therefore, for the most part, the working through of any movement must be done at the slowest possible tempo, so that at a later time, in a combination, it will be correctly executed. In adagio, for instance, a pose must be held for some time in order to check and confirm the correct position of the arms, head, torso, the entire structure of the pose, its pliability, its sculptural look, etc. Even the study of various forms of turns should not be taken at a quick tempo. The student must first learn the correct form during the turn, and only then be asked to perform it in the proper tempo.

For a better grasp of jumps at the beginning of the study, the movements should be stopped after each jump and the combinations performed with sufficient demi-pliés.

This does not mean that the student should be kept for a long time in a slow performance of the work. On the contrary, when a step or exercise has been learned well in each class, it must then be performed at its normal tempo, being careful that the student does not get carried away by a faster tempo, which is not the way to learn exact and stable jumps.

While keeping a normal and useful tempo during the lesson, the performing demands must not be lowered. The student must not only be well "warmed up," but the teacher must demand that the student use what he already knows, and must give him what he must know in order to possess a high level of technique and culture. Not to do so would be to commit a gross teaching error.

CREATING COMBINATIONS FOR THE LESSON

No less important in the structure of the lesson is the method used in creating combinations. These combinations may be small or large, elementary or complex, but they must all be part of the development within a definite performing technique for mastery of classical dance.

The structure of the combinations in general cannot be fixed within the framework of a method. While the separate movements are based upon an established progression and a division of parts, combinations, in essence, depend upon the ability of the teacher to bring the teaching material into definite relationships.

The creative individuality and the mastery and experience of the teacher play the most important role in creating the combinations. While teachers may be united in the direction of their teaching goal, there are inevitable individual differences in the methods and manner of building combinations.

The creation of a textbook for combinations is a task for the future for a group of teachers. But some short and general suggestions may be recommended to new teachers. For instance, in building a combination the teacher should consider if the course is to be six or eight years; the aims of the teaching program; the age and level of preparation of the students. In each part of the lesson, the movements that will form the *basis* of the proposed combinations should be executed first. This means those movements entering into the contents of *any part* of the lesson. In this manner, the progressive performance of these combinations will gradually increase in complexity with no superfluous or haphazard steps.

The position of the body at the end of each movement must become the starting position for the performance of the next movement. In this way, each movement not only has an independent meaning but serves as a link to other movements. If this rule is not observed, the combinations will be sloppy and vague, not flowing or compact in structure.

These recommendations do not exclude combining small movements with large movements as linking steps. On the contrary, this kind of combining imparts contrast in the combinations and variety, but it is a method which should be used so that the movement which is serving as a basis for the combination can be clearly seen and does not become obscured.

The teacher must not be carried away with extremely complicated and confusing combinations which may be effective from the viewpoint of choreographic inventiveness, but are inadmissible for the teaching aim. Often an inexperienced teacher will create excessively complicated and confused combinations, the result being that movements which were well learned and familiar to the student are then performed somewhat incorrectly and unmusically. On the other hand, combinations that are too simple are not advisable since each task must contain a sufficient degree of difficulty.

The most correctly devised combinations are those that the pupil is able to master on the basis of material already learned, since this material is not above the ability of the pupil or the level of his professional preparedness.

Additionally, movements used within a combination must be repeated. This will permit the pupil to concentrate his attention more closely on the movement under study, and acquire firmer skills and a deeper knowledge of its performance. It also permits the teacher to correct errors in the combination. Should the teacher notice that certain movements within a combination are not being correctly performed by the pupils, the teacher must repeat these movements separately for several lessons, then include them once again into the same or new combinations.

Movements that have gone through various forms must be included in enough combinations to ensure their retention in the memory and understanding and become better in quality of performance. Recently learned movements must be performed often enough in combinations to become a sort of basic rest when combined with previously learned movements in a variety of couplings.

It is absolutely necessary that all the combinations of the lesson follow one common line of development. One must not scatter or fragment the learning of the movements being studied, and the method of the dance program. Of course, all the learned material cannot be put into one lesson, especially into the classes of the middle and later levels, but one should not give combinations in the first part of the lesson that have nothing to do with the adagio and allegro portions of the class. Everything must be interdependent for the integrity of the method and the choreographic unfolding of its development. *It must not be a scattered lesson of uncoordinated parts.*

REPEATED COMBINATIONS

Work on combinations requires their repetition for a definite period of time— about three lessons. The first lesson is given to learning new combinations. The second lesson is given to repeating the combination with added complications and the third lesson is a final affirmation of the material learned with shortened periods of rest between the repetitions.

This procedure permits the pupils to become accustomed to the work under study in a more sensible way in better progression. In this way, too, time is not spent in giving attention at every lesson to the learning of new material or combinations which are only of one day's duration. These may be useful in construction, but have no chance to undergo repetition or to increase gradually in complexity which is very important for acquiring strong dance habits. This is the way to master the performance of dance in a thorough, progressive and planned manner.

After the three above mentioned repetitions, a completely new lesson must be constructed on a concrete, repeating theme to keep developing the performing art of the students while taking into consideration whatever lack has been revealed in the preceding lesson.

At the end of each month about three lessons of completely new combinations will help the teacher sum up the value of the previous periods and expose the weaknesses of the students. This summing up will help the teacher create better combinations based on the exposure of the weaknesses, and aid the students to affirm their knowledge and good habits.

The repetition of an entire lesson is useful to the accomplished artist as well. It prepares the artist perfectly for his next stage appearance, restores his nervous and physical strength, as well as his precision and plasticity, especially for principal dancers. Artists must continue to learn in a class of artists, and not just repeat daily various combinations and exercises. The old masters of classical ballet used to say: "Today we learned well and productively because we repeated yesterday's lesson."

Teaching is sometimes called training. This is wrong. Dance is an art and remains an art even in an ordinary lesson. How can one say that a singer trains to sing or a musician is training on the piano or violin? One must say that he must work and study every day in addition to performing and rehearsing, but not train, since that is not actually true and sounds dilettantish.

It must be remembered that when students go on to the next class, with a new teacher, they do not become immediately comfortable with combinations constructed in an unfamiliar way. Consequently, they do not always perform well. But this unfamiliarity soon passes with the least expenditure of time if the teacher at first gives simple combinations, allowing the students to understand his method faster and more thoroughly.

Preparing the lessons for the yearly examination in the intermediate and senior classes should begin a few days before the examination time. These combinations must show the entire course of study for the year and give the students a chance, without too much worry, to show how well they know the material. It is useful to get the opinion of other teachers to determine if the material can be "sight read," so to speak, by the students. While it is true that there are no unrehearsed appearances on stage, all graduates of the choreographic school must know all the elements of technique and must possess excellent attention. They must especially have the command of their instrument, the body.

INDIVIDUALITY OF THE TEACHER IN THE COMBINATIONS

The new teacher usually cannot create combinations that meet the demands for the construction of a lesson as just described. This uncertainty is natural and arises from a lack of experience and knowledge. It is wise at first, to use those combinations that the teacher himself performed during his school years, perhaps not exactly the same ones, but along the same plan. It is also useful to observe and take notes on the classes of experienced teachers and to use this material as a source, not as a script for directing a lesson.

No lesson, observed and notated, can substitute for live creations by a teacher who has the ability to build a lesson correctly, lead it ably and directly and, at the same time, demand the utmost from himself as well as his pupils.

Notes on combinations by other teachers may not answer the needs of the new teacher's class and may not answer the demands of their stage of study. Each combination constructed for a previous lesson which does not take into consideration the abilities of the students, nor has a sensible appraisal of the aims of the task, is in danger of being used in a mechanical and formal way. It does not contribute to the development of the teacher's knowledge, his creative thought, and the feeling of responsibility for his own work.

Textbooks intentionally do not give examples of combinations, since the gift and experience of the teacher who is artistically able to develop the performing mastery of the future dancer would be missing. The performing capacity and musicality of the student is developed not only by useful combinations but by the necessary creative independence in the work of every teacher. To use the examples of another teacher means a refusal of one's own direction and individuality in the approach to each new group of students. Rather let the first combinations be modest and imperfect, but one's own, with one's own creative thought on the subject.

One's own "signature" in combinations has a great meaning in the development of technique and the professional education of the future artist. The new and the experienced teacher must constantly strive to perfect his "signature" and aim for the greatest brevity, artistic simplicity, strictness and variety, avoiding all confused and tricky accumulations. The "signature" of combinations by men differs in style and character from that of women, just as the work in classes for girls emphasizes grace and elegance in movements of the head, neck, shoulders, back, waist, elbows, wrists and hands. This is evident in the feeling of the movements as well, just as the movements for the legs prepare the girls to dance on pointe.

Male teachers who have studied for a long time or even occasionally in classes for girls, are sometimes apt to use female "signatures." This, of course, is a drawback in the education of males and especially in virtuoso steps such as big jumps and complex batterie.

Inexperienced teachers usually become overly interested in the special characteristics of their creative "signature," which actually has not yet taken shape. This interest is a drawback to good teaching. At the same time, each teacher strengthens his pupils' mastery of dance through these combinations, constructed artistically, not from a choreographer's imagination, but from his own. The consequence of this is the free and comprehending use of the body, since the greater the technical mastery, the more possibilities for expressive dancing.

In summation, the correct structure and direction of the lesson depends upon the following conditions: 1. Placing movements of progressive difficulty in each part of the lesson. 2. Allowing proper duration for each part of the lesson. 3. Choosing the correct pacing of the lesson. 4. Constructing combinations correctly. All these conditions are brought together organically and require strict coordination.

Let us suppose that the duration of a portion of the lesson is incorrect while the placement of the movement is correct. The time for the lesson is therefore being used incorrectly. If the duration of a portion is correct but the movements are haphazardly placed, there will not be a gradual increase in the complexity of the lesson. If the first two conditions are correct, but the pace of the class is incorrect, it will lower the working level and the progress of the pupils. If all three conditions are correct but the combinations are scattered and not in a teaching plan, the pupils will not acquire reliable skills. It is therefore very important to have a well-planned lesson, with suitable time given to each portion and led at the proper pace. A lesson makes definite demands on the pupils without asking what is beyond their physical ability to perform.

COMBINING CLASSWORK WITH REHEARSALS

In the choreographic schools, there is a special section of the program called Stage Practice. The aim of this section is to help the pupil understand, develop and perfect his performing mastery by rehearsals and performances on stage. This section is consequently an integral and finishing sector of the teaching process.

This book is concerned with the problems of uniting the lessons in classical dance with stage rehearsals. As a rule, students begin rehearsals from the second year of study. This demands of the student a certain amount of professional knowledge and ability, although that demand is, as yet, very elementary. Yet that demand requires the ability to be exact and well rehearsed. By knowing the structure of the stage work, it is a good idea to relate the combinations given in the lessons to these appearances. At first, the most complicated elements, consisting of perhaps two or three movements, can be included in the combinations in a manner close to the stage requirement in rhythm, form and character. While these elements should not exclude the teaching problems given to each portion of the lesson, they will aid in preparing the student for a freer, more exact and technically perfect comprehension of performing choreography.

It is also useful in these combinations, to direct the attention of the pupil to the various dancing methods used in choreography to deepen and widen the connection of the teaching program with performances. And finally, after the lesson, if it is necessary and if time permits, the teacher may work separately with the pupils on solo variations that are technically highly complex or that present problems in breathing or endurance. In this way, the teaching process supports, as an elementary preparation, the rehearsals and performances. Hopefully, all this work is assumed *by the same teacher*, since that would best help the student prepare for performance.

MAKING CORRECTIONS DURING CLASS

There are a number of conditions necessary for directing the class properly. For instance, in order to better observe the pupils, the teacher should change the place of the students who work on the barre along the sides of the classroom with the students who work on the barres in the middle of the classroom. This can reveal faults that may have gone unnoticed when the pupil was always in the same place.

For the center work, pupils must be placed in chessboard formation so all of them may be seen. After one or two lessons, the lines must change so that each one has a chance to be in front of the mirror. The placement of the pupils in the lines must be constant and the selection of the placement made by the teacher independent of the pupil's ability. This permits each to feel himself equal and creates a feeling of camaraderie.

For the combinations, the pupils should be divided into groups that permit them to move along the floor without interfering with each other. Those not working at the moment should be standing to the right or left of the classroom, near the barres, so that the back of the room is free. These rules of positioning are basic to the conduct of a class.

It is very important that pupils on stage keep a correct distance from one another. This ability to keep the correct distance is necessary for stage work. Although the lesson is ideally conducted in front of a mirror to permit the pupil to observe and correct himself, it is useful from time to time to stop working before the mirror. These periods improve self-control in the pupil and bring him closer to stage conditions, where there are no mirrors.

The content, character and form of remarks during the lesson have an especially important meaning for successful work as a teacher. Remarks may be made to the entire class or to a single pupil. In both cases, it is useful to first make some remarks of a preventive character. Knowing the weaknesses of the class or the pupil, the teacher first must point out what needs special attention, what must be strengthened and what should be avoided. These remarks are made when the performance of a movement is repeated on the other leg or other side, when executed in reverse, or repeated. Remarks may be made during the exercise and adagio portions of the class during the performance of these sections. Take advantage of the duration and repetition of movements in this portion of the class to make remarks. The fast tempo of the allegro sections give no opportunity for remarks, which must be made at a later time. When the performance does not call for a remark, the teacher should compliment the class or pupil without encouraging complacence.

In the beginning levels, along with the remarks, it is useful to physically, carefully, yet firmly, round the hand, lead the leg into a turned-out position, or position the trunk, head, arms, etc. to give the pupil quicker understanding of the use of the body. However, the teacher must not go to extremes, since the pupil must strive himself to achieve the position for the best performance. Correcting one pupil too often makes the teacher lose sight of the others. While it is very difficult to watch all the pupils, the teacher should be aware of gross errors from the beginning.

This does not mean that the teacher may overlook mistakes of lesser importance. On the contrary, the pupil must know and feel that he is under constant supervision and the smallest of his mistakes does not go unnoticed by the teacher. It is best for the teacher to be in the center of the classroom, near the mirror, where all the pupils can be observed. The new teacher must develop these abilities from the very first lesson. Remarks and corrections must be made in the lower classes in a simple, short, clear, confirming and progressive manner. One remark must not contain every correction. The teacher must clearly separate the comments, which must be in a suitable form. For instance, the teacher should make a comment on the mistakes in the use of the legs, then the use of the trunk, arms and head. Or he should first remark on the choreography, then the music, the attention and memory of the pupil, the need for stability, softness, etc.

It is not recommended that the remarks be long and wordy. This leads to a loss of class time, and the students cool off for too long a time. The subject itself demands that remarks be to the point, imaginative, clear and concise. They must touch upon the essence of the problem and be presented for quick and easy understanding of what is demanded of the pupil.

The pupil's progress is dependent, to a considerable measure, upon the content and timeliness of the remarks. If, however, the remark was to the point and timely as well as short, and an improvable mistake appears again in the work, it means that the teacher succeeded in pointing out the error but not in helping the pupil correct it. In this case the new teacher may find fault with the pupil, but it does not release the teacher from fault. He must remember that the most important part of his work is to have his remarks acted upon even if they are harsh demands. Otherwise his remarks will not reach their goal, and the pupils, accustomed to lesser demands, will perform carelessly. Once that happens, timely and valuable remarks will be of no use whatsoever. At the same time, strict demands must not be made a system. The relationship between the pupil and the teacher must always contain the utmost clarity and mutual respect. If the pupils, or even one pupil, are lazy, show a lack of energy, and an imbalance in the level of the work, etc., it is the teacher's fault, for he is responsible for everything that happens during the lesson as well as teaching and maintaining discipline. A teacher must show strictness and be demanding, but not roughly or crudely in order not to hurt the pupil's psyche.

Naturally, requiring exactness does not mean that the teacher must at all times force knowledge on his pupil. One must strive for a condition where the pupil and the teacher help each other to achieve the best results. Of course, talented and obedient students are pleasanter to teach, but it is the difficult students who shape the growth of the mastery of teaching. In short, the new teacher must observe the activity of the psyche, learn psychology and, in general, aid the pupil to develop his personality.

EVALUATING A CLASS

The young teacher usually finds it difficult to analyze the work of his colleagues. In taking part in discussions he should be open to new suggestions and exact in his explanations. First, he should determine how a co-worker constructs his lesson, asking himself: "Was it sufficiently complicated? Strict teaching? Without ornamentation or superficial effects? Or was it too simple, elementary and dominated by choreographic detail which hides technical and other lacks or mistakes in the pupils?"

The young teacher should observe how the body was aligned—arms, legs, head, torso—and what mistakes in performing or misunderstandings of the principles were made. Which of them were well or badly understood? Then, the young teacher should evaluate the education of the musicality, the individuality and the artistry of the pupils. Was diligence and conscientiousness developed in the pupils? Rate the value of the teacher's and the accompanist's contribution to the pupils in an objective fashion.

This outline will aid the young teacher to express his opinion of the observed class clearly and accurately, and will allow him to rate his own work critically.

Good or excellent work must, of course, be praised and given great respect and thanks. But excessive rapture is out of place since it serves no practical use, wastes time and, at times, interferes with the pedagogic growth of the teacher and, consequently, with the progress of his pupils.

When showing his own work, the young teacher must be able to explain clearly to the members of the examining committee how he worked with the pupils, what problems he put before himself, what his creative contact was with the accompanist, what his difficulties are at the present time and to what extent he has fulfilled the teaching program.

The young teacher must understand the benefits of frank criticism of his work especially from older, more experienced teachers. He must listen to the criticism, whatever it may be, with restraint and thankfulness. Self-satisfaction and complacency have never resulted in growth.

DIFFERENCES IN TEACHING BOYS AND TEACHING GIRLS

Classical dance is studied in the schools by girls and boys in separate classes because they differ in their performing styles, methods and program material.

In the first two years, from ages nine to eleven, this difference is not yet very noticeable, but later it becomes quite marked. While girls, especially teenagers from twelve to sixteen, already show a desire to be graceful and elegant, the boys of the same age still show a certain boyishness and awkwardness. Girls, as a rule, move more sensibly, aptly and surely than boys and develop psychologically and physically earlier.

At the age of seventeen to nineteen, the young boy begins to acquire a certain masculinity and coordination while the girls at that age are already much more independent, assured and active.

With all due respect for the grace of the girls, the male pupil must move in a way natural for his age, while not hindering his technical development. During the lesson, the teacher must direct each one of them, the uncouth as well as the elegant, to avoid that gracefulness so welcome in girls, and so unwelcome in males.

Boys and girls in all classes must be reared in good taste, musicality, nobility of movement, artistry, etc., but in accordance with their age group.

The teaching profession knows that experienced female teachers conducting classes of boys from the first through the third levels, develop exactness of movement and other performing skills in the pupils. That is, of course, very important and valuable. We should be grateful for their contribution. However, the boy's psychological outlook may be somewhat damaged. Since the basis for the male performing style is laid in those early years, the appearance of effeminate mannerisms may be the result of wrong teaching at this early stage.

By the same token, one cannot entrust the earlier classes of girls to even the most highly qualified male teachers, because these classes require a specific teaching system with its own style, character and performing finesse that the male teacher cannot know and will overlook in the teaching.

To conduct a few classes of boys or girls on the lower levels is not very complicated. But directing for a protracted period of time, devoting oneself to the education and discovery of individuality, musicality, taste and artistry in the future dancer, is a very difficult, refined and demanding task requiring feeling for the true nature of male and female dance.

Remember that a too refined performing style that copies the grace of women, contradicts the nature of male dance and only gives rise to effeteness and falseness, which is contrary to the realistic school of Soviet classical ballet.

The difference between male and female performing styles may be described as follows: In doing any battement, port de bras, pose or jump, etc., the form and tempo of movement is basically the same for both, but the character is changed. With boys, the movement has more resolve, physical force, simplicity, terseness and vigor in performance. If a boy and a girl execute an identical turn of the head, the boy will do it with more definite resoluteness than will the girl. And so throughout the education of the male, the performing style based upon his own psychological direction and the strict teaching of good taste, will result in a virtuoso manner of movement free of prettiness. For this reason, the professional school must be very discerning, scrupulous in selecting and preparing new personnel for male classes, especially the lower levels, and not leave this work to even the most highly qualified female teachers. Perhaps the teaching program of classical dance ought to be compiled separately for boys and girls, including the necessary explanations and corrections. This would best help to clarify the essence and character of teaching and educating future dancers and to widen the methods of the subject as a whole.

CHOOSING THE TEACHER'S TEACHING LEVEL

The teaching future of every teacher is formed differently. Some, because of their leanings and abilities, specialize in teaching the middle classes; others, in teaching the lower or higher levels. Experience has shown that a teacher who can conduct all levels of an entire course equally well is rare. To determine his best level as an excellent specialist, the teacher should begin by teaching the lower levels, which, unfortunately, is not always possible. Nonetheless, it would give the new teacher a chance to understand and grasp ABC's of schoolwork so that in higher levels he would be able to develop his art of teaching with more assurance and better planning, under the guidance of an experienced teacher. Finally, after amassing sufficient experience in various classes for a length of time, he may finally discover his teaching level.

Some new teachers find themselves rather quickly, others find themselves slowly and with difficulty. There are a number of causes for this. One of them is based upon haphazard placements and transfers by the school that occur too frequently. This is harmful to the new teacher and his pupils, and to the school as a whole.

Altogether, the education of a new teacher is a complicated job demanding from its artistic leaders and from co-workers much care, attention, restraint and knowledge. To entrust a class to a new teacher means helping him systematically, steadily and in a professional way. Otherwise, excellent performers cannot become excellent teachers, masters of a new specialty.

And still, some choreographers assert that one cannot master pedagogy, one must be born with it. Of course, talent is needed for each specialty, but along with talent must be professional knowledge, true love of work, and culture. Knowledge, ability, labor, as well as talent, are needed for every specialty of the choreographer. Talent alone is only a precious possibility which is formed and developed with preparation and education. And let us have as many excellent and different teachers as possible. Let the creative individuality of each one of them be formed and developed independently, differing in inimitable talent, style and method in conducting the teaching of the subject. Let them all be unified in the excellent training they give their pupils and also by the high artistic principles of the Soviet school and the Soviet ballet.

Some of the methods and peculiarities of the work of the teacher of classical dance in the male classes have been given here as a starting point, a direction in helping to educate the performing style of the future artist of Soviet ballet.

EVALUATING PROGRESS THROUGH
A GRADING SYSTEM

Periodically, and at established times, the teacher must evaluate the progress of the pupils and give marks or grades in a school grade book or in his own papers.

Grades are not just a formal indication of the quality of progress; they are an active symbol of education which spurs the attitude of the student to more active and conscientious work. The teacher is personally responsible for the quality of the progress as well as for the evaluation of it.

Permit me to give short but essential information and advice on the subject:

There are intermediate and concluding grades for the year. The first grade checks the current progress of the students, the second is the sum total of a definite period of time: a quarter, half or entire year. In addition, there are examination grades and general grades which form the yearly and exam ratings.

The intermediate grade is a very important link in the system of grading, for on this basis the teacher makes his conclusion as to the rate of progress being made.

Each student will show greater diligence in his work if he knows that grades indicating his progress are calculated in toto and not from case to case. Even the laziest pupil usually pulls himself together toward the end, hoping to catch up for lost time and to get a higher mark.

This intermediate grade allows the teacher to note carelessness in a pupil in time to take suitable measures in school or at home, and to help a pupil who is progressing poorly as a result of sickness, and to give him additional lessons. Evaluation of the class should be made every two weeks and posted in the class grade book. In this way, each quarter is divided into four parts controlled by the teacher. The teacher cannot rely entirely on the current evaluations since they represent only short periods of study (in general, twelve lessons of two hours each). The concluding rating should be included in the overall evaluation, since it indicates the pupil's progress during the quarter, half or entire year. It indicates if the pupil has worked diligently and sufficiently during the entire period.

In determining the concluding rating of progress, the teacher must pay attention to the intermediate mark received for the finished quarter. At the same time, the fourth rating must not be just an arithmetic addition of intermediate ratings. It must be compiled on the basis of the student's actual knowledge. Therefore, the greatest importance is given to the last intermediate mark.

The same principle applies to yearly ratings. Whatever the grade, it should not be excessively soft or exceedingly hard. Objectivity and exactness are principles for evaluation. In the final analysis, the results of progress are indications of the teacher's work. The ratings, for this reason, must not be over or under the exact mark. On the contrary, the students must be shown that only a fair evaluation brings them the most good and that they can achieve best results if they themselves learn to have an objective and correct attitude to their grades.

This attitude does not come by itself! It must be systematically engendered by the teacher's fair yet demanding attitude to the level of progress made by all his pupils.

In rating the yearly progress, the teacher must consider not only the performing ability of the pupil but his knowledge, which is determined by oral examination. These questions concern artistic taste, music, elements of technique, etc.

Classical dance is very much a practical discipline, not a theoretical one. There exists a viewpoint that if the teacher shows and explains the teaching problem well and the pupils perform well, there is no use for an oral test. They suggest that it is a waste of precious time, since every pupil, in performing the learned elements, is actually accounting for his knowledge and ability. This seems to me to be not quite true, since the teacher can gain more comprehension and objectivity in his grade if he knows the real truth and depth of understanding in his pupil, in addition to his performance and attitude to the daily work. Without oral testing, it is very difficult and sometimes impossible to establish whether the student performed his given tasks consciously or intuitively.

Oral questions must be posed to each pupil, but only those which have direct meaning to the performance of a current task. In listening to the answers, the teacher must require that the pupil reply in clear, imaginative and brief explanations. He must correct the pronunciation of the dance and music terms.

There is still another method of checking and strengthening the knowledge, but, unfortunately, it is rarely used. It is written homework. I have used this method in my own work and I recommend its use in this way: In all classes, once a week or once every two weeks, give a written assignment. This grade is given to the pupil for his own evaluation, but is considered in the teacher's intermediate rating.

(In the first year, the written assignment may be given only from the second half of the year, after enough teaching material has been given the student to become acquainted with the specifics of the subject.)

Themes for a written assignment might be: In the lower levels—writing the terms used in the class, describing the rules for their performance and the time signature and character of the music used. In the intermediate levels—the above assignment adding a description of the combinations and the student's own combinations with the musical material for them. In the senior levels—the above assignment for the middle level, adding the description of the lesson last given, the construction of separate parts of the lesson, and finally, the construction of an entire lesson. This last assignment may be entrusted to a pupil once a quarter, and only in the last two levels.

Unfortunately, methods of homework are as yet not sufficiently worked out, and in practice, they are insufficiently tested. There is no doubt as to the value of homework, since it develops in the student self-control and a more attentive attitude to dance and music materials and fosters a creative understanding of the teaching problems.

This kind of written homework is useful for future dancers and future teachers, choreographers or répétiteurs, because each one of them must know the school of classical dance very well. It is therefore necessary to set aside some time in the choreographic school for a critical analysis of the written work. At these sessions the teacher must analyze the work of every pupil, observe how it is presented and, by considering its good and bad qualities, determine a rating. This is a time when the teacher can share with his pupils those of his teaching and stage experiences that are directly tied to the learning and comprehension of the art of classical dance. This kind of work cannot be done during regular lessons.

Our grades are made on a 5-mark system, which means that a grade of 5 indicates excellent progress; 4—good progress; 3—satisfactory progress; 2—poor progress; and 1—very bad progress. The basic considerations for the marks are: (1) the degree to which the pupil assimilated the program; (2) the degree to which he *comprehended* it; (3) how he was able to perform the material he learned.

At the same time, the number and character of his mistakes in performing the material add to the determination of the student's progress. Mistakes in performance may be divided into *gross errors:* when the basic rules of elementary technique are often broken and the rhythm and character of the music poorly comprehended.

Or *secondary mistakes:* when the pupil occasionally misses technical details or is unrhythmic or unmusical.

Or *mistakes of little importance:* accidental and rare errors in technique, unimportant musical and rhythmic errors.

The number of mistakes and the character of the mistakes may be different. Not all of them should be counted in the evaluation of progress, only those which, in spite of constant demands, do not improve and continue to be repeated in following lessons. Mistakes that a pupil cannot improve because of insufficiently strong physical attributes despite extraordinary musical and acting ability must be judged very strictly. His other qualities must not be underestimated, however, since, objectively speaking, classical dance prepares pupils for other forms of dance disciplines, for acting and stage careers in general.

Progress owes much to diligence, but it must not be judged in the same way as talent. Talent, without a proper attitude toward work, is unused potential. There are instances when a very gifted pupil, with excellent qualities, does not want to labor. A serious attitude toward daily obligations depends, in great measure, on the teacher. His personal example, his experience, his demands and his pedagogic art shape the attitude of his students to the work and in the end reflect in their progress. While considering the diligence of the pupil, the teacher must be especially objective and critical of himself. If diligence is insufficient and inconsistant, the teacher must first find the reason for it and then sum up the situation and correct *his* own personal shortcomings, or persuade or even penalize the pupil, to force him to change his mistaken attitude toward work. This attitude is sometimes due to outside causes.

If the pupil stubbornly refuses to change his attitude toward work, the teacher must lower his rating.

No less important to his attitude is his appearance. He must at all times be dressed neatly in a well-fitting dance costume and slippers, etc. In short, one must watch over the appearances of the student, his personal hygiene and his manner in associating with his fellow students and adults. All this is necessary to the future artist, not only in his private life, but also on stage.

Pupils must progress in their general educational studies as well. This may be checked directly with the class director.

If necessary the pupil must be reminded that an artist of the Soviet ballet theater must be well educated and well mannered and the insufficiencies in his knowledge, carelessness in his behavior and outward appearance, will tell in the most negative way in his performance.

EVALUATING PERFORMANCES

The professional qualities of the student must be evaluated since they are reflected in his progress in class and in the quality of his work on stage. The professional qualities include physical gifts and body build, proportions and height, psycho-physical qualities, attention, memory, will, energy, adroitness (that is, free and precise coordination of movements); muscular strength, musicality and emotional range, and creative imagination.

All these qualities are conventional, but they determine the factors which form the complex professional qualities of the pupil.

Stage practice shows that some dancers with very modest outer physical gifts at times achieve highly artistic results. And on the contrary, some pupils who possess good physical gifts and an excellent technique cannot as yet create a live or moving stage image. Therefore, an artistic gift must be highly rated by the teacher. Not to note this gift, not to consider it, is to miss what is important in the pupil. In evaluating professional qualities, some teachers make a mistake in expecting the pupil to be a future performer of leading roles, forgetting that the inclination and qualifications of the ballet artist may be different. The performing gifts of each pupil must be valued by the teacher, as this is the purpose of the choreographic education. The teacher must know how his pupil is progressing in all subjects. This will help him define more truly and deeply the direction of his future stage activity, revealed while still in school, and the special aspects of his professional gift.

The teacher may consider that a pupil's future might be in folk dance, and to lower his mark would not be right, since it might do the pupil harm and create a traumatic situation. Similarly, a pupil may have an excellent gift for acting but a mediocre physical gift. For the same reasons, he also must not be given a lower mark.

Guided by these suggestions, the pupil must be given the mark of 5 if he knows in depth the volume of material presented, if he has learned all the rules of performance for those movements; is able with no difficulty exactly, energetically, with stability, plasticity and softness, to perform those elements of technique in all their variations, making only unimportant mistakes in combinations; is faultless in his attitude to his daily work; takes all his teacher's remarks attentively; asks questions on occasion with the teacher's permission; has a harmonious build, a strong body, endurance, suppleness and ease in motion. This pupil has excellent attention, excellent musical comprehension and memory for choreography, an inborn sense of rhythm, emotional comprehension of music, a live, clear and creative imagination, a character that aims at a goal and a vivid performing individuality!

The mark of 3 may be given to the pupil if he knows the volume of material presented very well and the rules of their performance; acquits himself well in performing simple and repeated combinations; but does not always correctly or economically use his forces. He commits some mistakes—sometimes of the gross variety; has a good attitude to his daily work; does not break the rules of discipline in class; takes the remarks of the teacher for the most part for his use; has a proportioned body; general ease in motion but is not sufficiently strong or enduring; is attentive; has a good memory and a satisfactory sense of rhythm; is sufficiently musical; creatively active; but does not possess performing individuality or a remarkable outward appearance.

These ratings of 5 and 3 give a sufficient idea of the demands made on pupils in the evaluation of their progress. These examples must not be considered standard, but only examples containing the sum of indications in the formation of the grades of progress. The ratings may be further refined in more detail on the methods and separate movements, or just the opposite, based upon just a few points and fewer words.

Finally, the rating must not be determined dryly, arithmetically, but should have a creative approach and should of course be constructive. It must not be an evaluation separate from future stage activity, but as an evaluation of a young, not yet strong, future performer who is steadily growing. The younger the pupil, the more carefully, and lovingly he must be rated.

The teacher must explain to each pupil why he received his mark and how he can improve it. Only then will the grades become truly strong as an educational means that will stimulate each pupil to reach the best results.

The choreographic profession is divided into four specialties: the ballet master (choreographer), the performer, the répétiteur, and the teacher. They are a tightly knit group and yet they differ from one another. The ballet master creates choreographic works. The dancer with his art embodies the idea of the ballet master. The répétiteur prepares the dancer for the stage appearances. The teacher in the theater preserves and heightens the abilities of the dancer. The teacher in the school prepares the performers of the future.

So the question of what is most important in the work of the teacher in the school is, in short, Everything! However, one must separate the specific peculiarities of each professional in order to understand the whole.

It is necessary to know classical ballet excellently, to know trends and methods of its work and to be able to plan and summarize the work, to love the pupils but be exacting to the utmost degree. All these things, plus true professional responsibility, diligence, will, restraint, and talent will help the new teacher in time to become an experienced master of his craft. Performing talent and experience are extremely important to the work of the new teacher, as the nature of dance and its technique is understood through performance. But to understand and therefore to master the art of teaching is truly impossible without knowledge and ability for teaching.

Methodical self-analysis is obligatory in the work of the teacher. Copying others is directly alien both to the Soviet pedagogic thought and to the school of classical dance. The deeper the new teacher penetrates into the essence of this specialty, the more creative and productive his work will become.

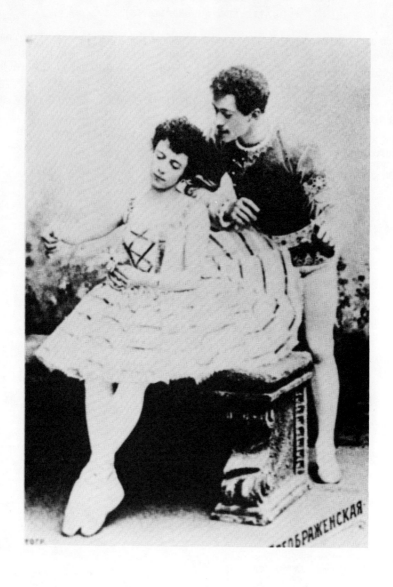

Nikolai Legat, Tarasov's teacher, with Olga Preobrajenska, a pupil of Cecchetti's, about the turn of the century. Tarasov was graduated from Legat's class at the Moscow Choreographic School in 1920.

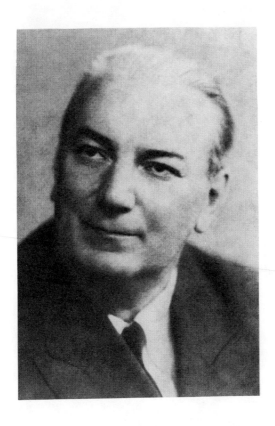

Nikolai Ivanovich Tarasov performed in the Bolshoi Ballet from 1920 to 1935 in classical roles. He taught at the Moscow Choreographic School (the official school of the Bolshoi Ballet) from 1923 to 1960. He was its general director and its artistic director from 1942 to 1945 and again its artistic director in 1953.

In addition to teaching the "Classe de Perfection" at the Bolshoi Theater and the Moscow Artistic Ballet, 1929–30, Tarasov served as the artistic director of the Technicam (Lunacharsky) from 1933 to 1937. From 1946 he was a teacher and artistic director of the Department for Pedagogues and Choreographers at GITIS (State Institute of Theatrical Arts), and was given the rank of professor in 1962.

Tarasov was a co-author of the Methodology of Classical Training, 1940, and in 1971 wrote Classical Dance: School of Male Technique (Ballet Technique for the Male Dancer) for which he won the State Prize of the USSR. Tarasov, born December 6, 1902, died February 8, 1975, the same year he won the State Prize.

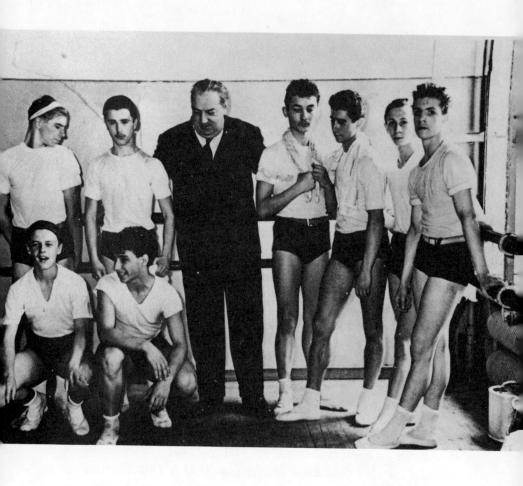

Nikolai Tarasov (center) in 1958, with his graduating class of 1961. Left to right, Valery Antonov, Ivachenko, Mikhail Lavrovsky, Dinor, Alexander Prokofiev, Vlasov. Kneeling are Meknelo and Nikolai Tagunov.

Tarasov's most famous pupils were performers: Mikhail Lavrovsky, Yuri Zhdanov, Alexander Lapauri, Maris Liepa and Yaroslav Sekh.

Current choreographers and teachers from Tarasov classes are: A. Chichinadze, P. A. Pestov, A. Prokofiev, A. A. Khercul and Evegoni Valukhin.

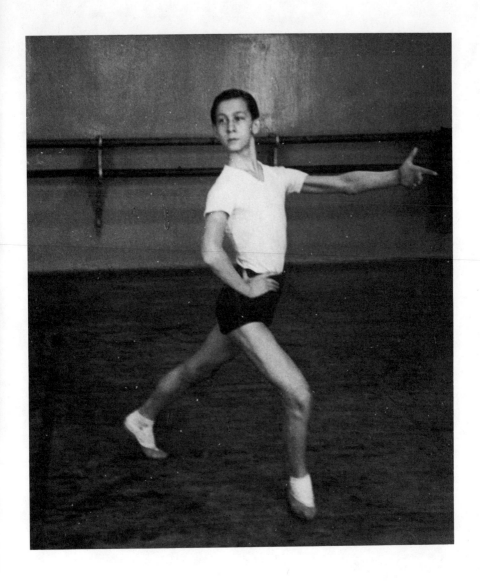

Alexander Prokofiev in 1956, as a young student of Tarasov in the Bolshoi Ballet school. Prokofiev has produced his own famous pupils: young Andris Liepa (son of Maris Liepa), Irek Mukhammedov and Anatoly Kucheruk, all medal winners in the competitions and members of the Bolshoi Ballet.

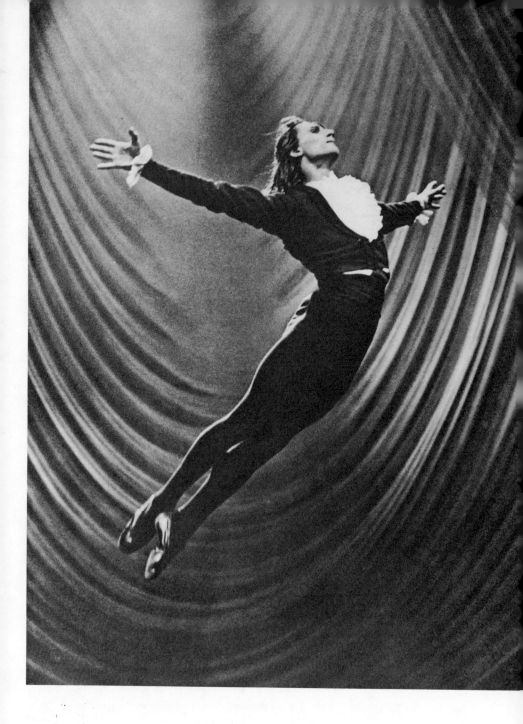

Yaroslav Sekh in the title role of Paganini, *created for the Bolshoi Ballet in 1961 by Leonid Lavrovsky. Sekh (b. 1930) is known for his strong portrayals of dramatic characters. At right, Sekh as the matador in* Don Quixote. *At far right, Sekh as Mercutio in* Romeo and Juliet.

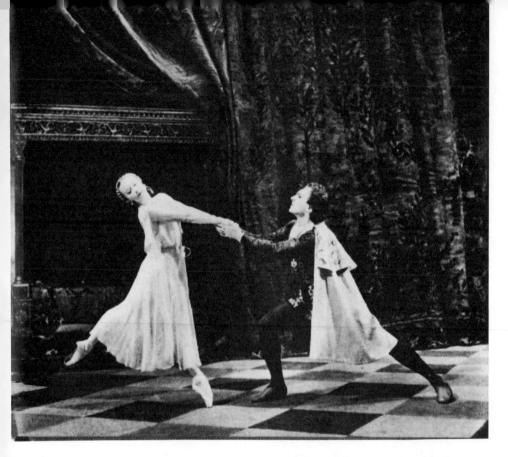

Yuri Zhdanov is Romeo to the incomparable Galina Ulanova's Juliet in the Leonid Lavrovsky version of Shakespeare's Romeo and Juliet. *Zhdanov, born in Moscow in 1925, graduated from the Bolshoi Ballet school in 1944 and immediately joined the Bolshoi Ballet.*

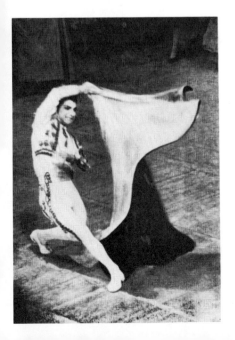

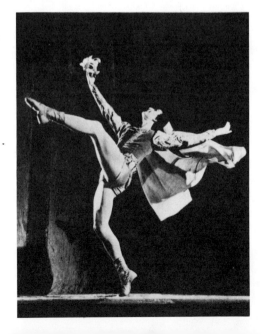

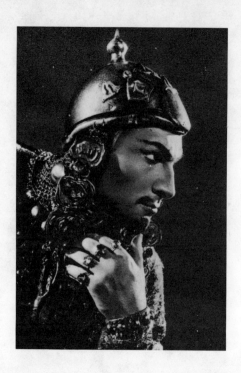

Alexander Lapauri as Girei in The Fountain of Bakhchisarai. *This most famous version marked the choreographic debut of Rostislav Zakharov in 1934, and is still performed.*

The Pushkin poem of the same name was considered as a libretto for choreography by Filippo Taglioni in 1838, but it never reached the stage. Foma (Thomas) Nijinsky, father of the great dancer, produced in Kiev a grand ballet, A Victim of Jealousy, *based upon the poem.*

At right, Cinderella, *with Alexander Lapauri (b. 1926) and Raissa Struchkova (b. 1925), Lapauri's wife and classmate in the Bolshoi Ballet school, in the title role.*

While still at the height of his performing career, Lapauri studied choreography at GITIS and produced his first ballet, Tale of the Woods, *in 1961. In 1963, Lapauri scored a success with his* Lieutenant Kiji, *set to the Prokofiev score, for a film, then for a ballet. Struchkova displayed her sense of humor in the principal role of the ballet, the Lady-in-Waiting.*

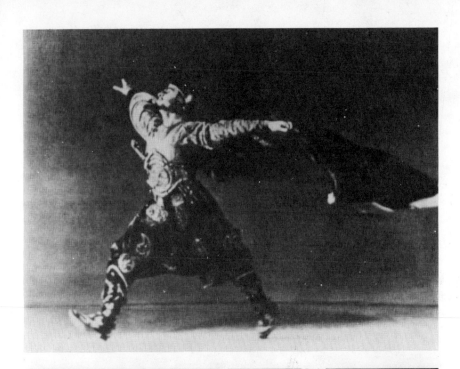

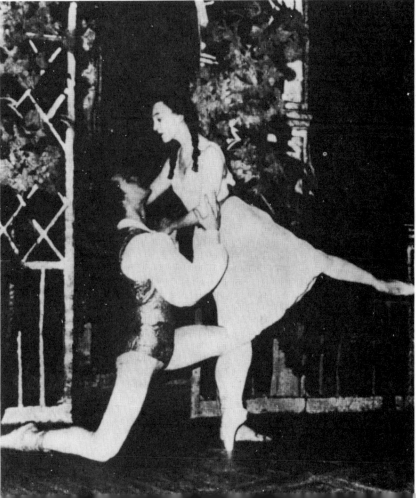

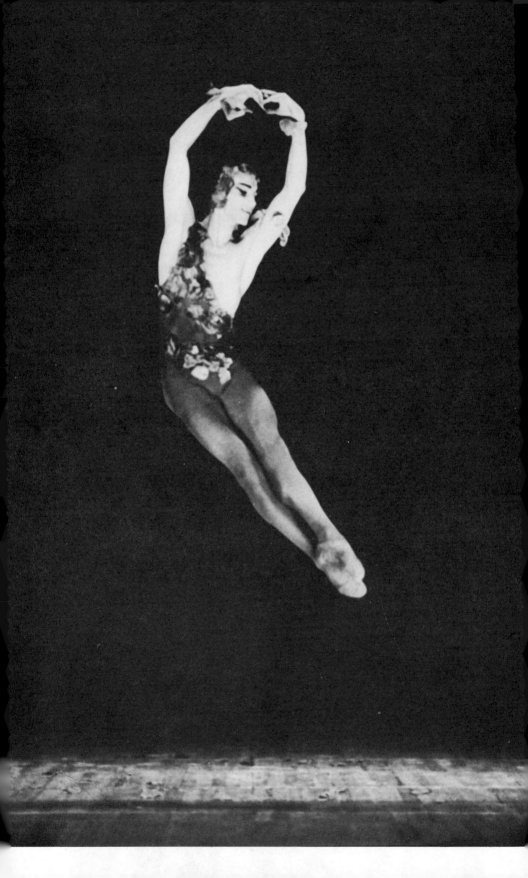

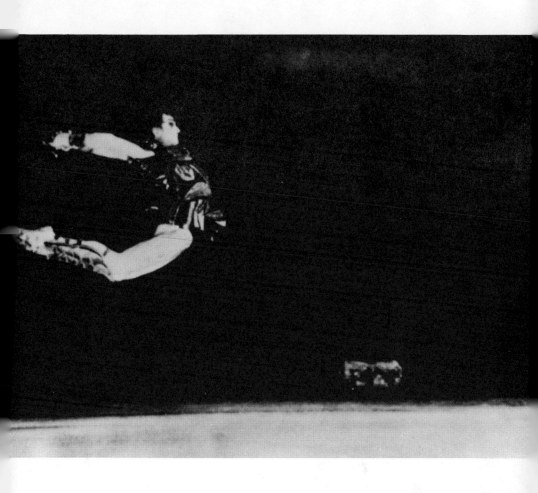

Maris Liepa, Latvian-born (1936) leading dancer in the role of Crassus in Spartacus. *Liepa graduated from Tarasov's class in 1955, joined the Riga Opera House, was invited to the Nemirovich-Danchenko Lyric Theatre, and in 1960 joined the Bolshoi Ballet.*

At left, Maris Liepa in a more classical role, Le Spectre de la Rose, *displays Tarasov's training in his aplomb and easy, contained upper body.*

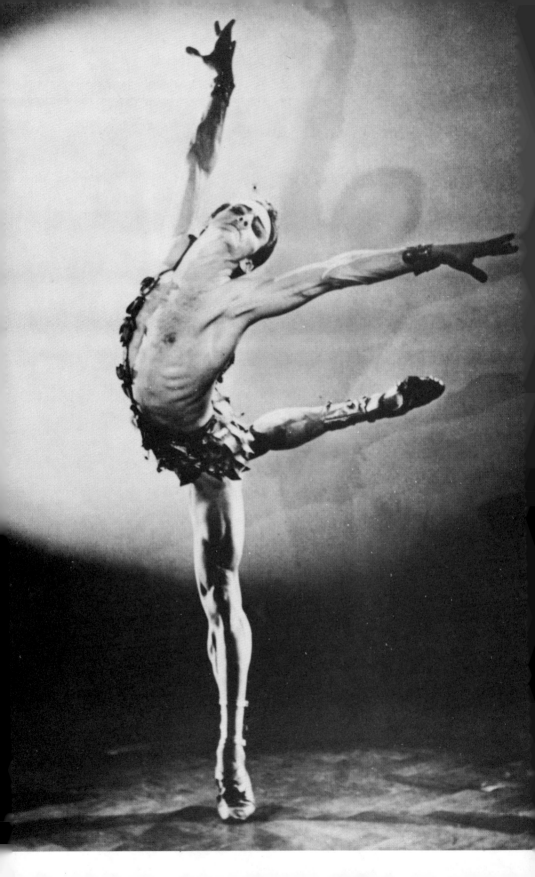

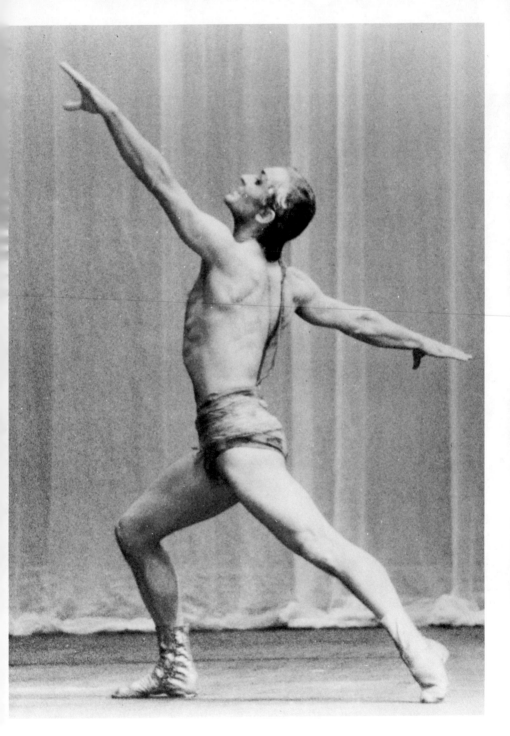

Mikhail Lavrovsky, son of choreographer Leonid Lavrovsky, in the Diana and Acteon pas de deux from the ballet Esmeralda, *choreographed by A. Vaganova.*

At left, Maris Liepa in Walpurgis Night.

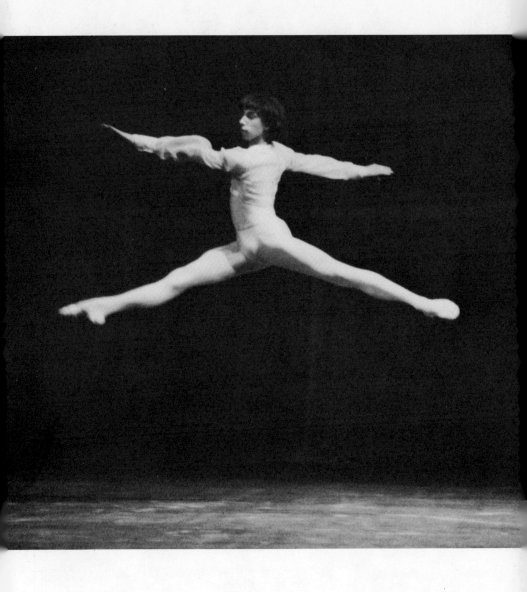

Alexander Vetrov, a student of A. A. Pestov (a Tarasov pupil) was taken into the Bolshoi Ballet in 1980. The twenty-year-old medal winner excels in the Bluebird pas de deux in The Sleeping Beauty, *and as Tybalt in* Romeo and Juliet.

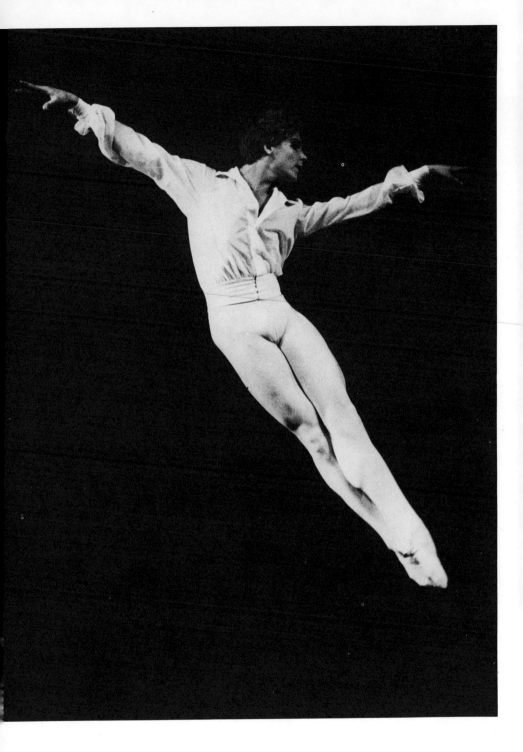

*Andris Liepa, twenty-one-year-old son of the celebrated Maris Liepa,
in* Homage to Ulanova, *choreographed by Vladimir Vasiliev.*

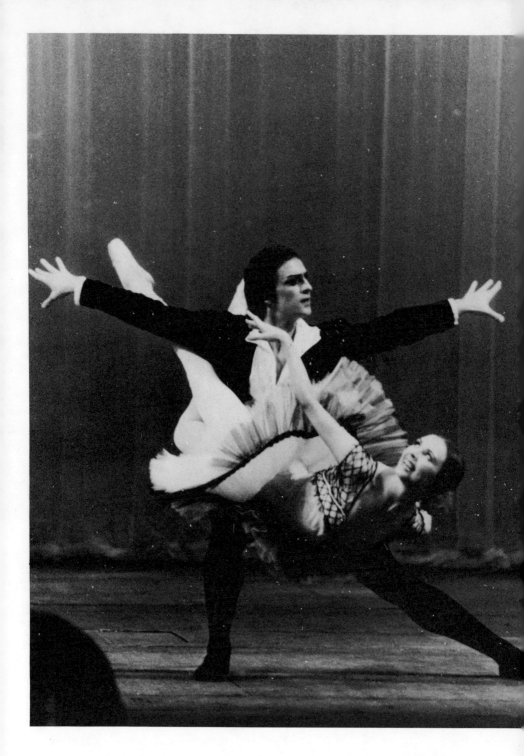

Irek Mukhammedov, with Ludmilla Semenyaka in Don Quixote. *A principal of the Bolshoi Ballet, the twenty-one-year-old dancer who performed in the Young Classical Company before entering the Bolshoi, is already performing leading roles, such as Crassus in* Spartacus.

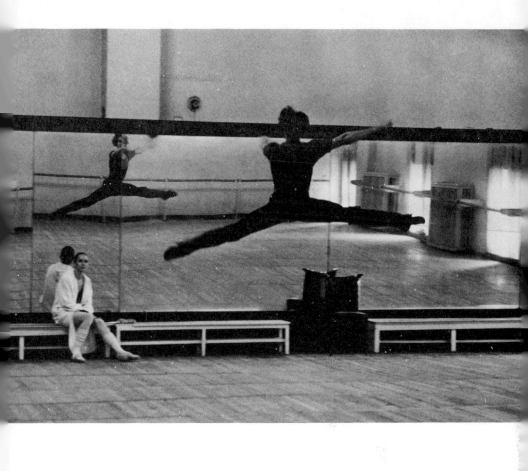

Irek Mukhammedov executes a grand jeté in the classroom while Bolshoi ballerina Natalia Bessmertnova watches.

PART TWO

ELEMENTARY MOVEMENTS OF CLASSICAL DANCE

In this section, the movements of classical dance used in teaching the system are described. First, the movements of the legs, then of the arms, torso and head are described to reveal greater detail, as in a musical score, and to facilitate a fuller understanding of the whole.

Similarly, the rules for the execution of the movements and the method of study for those movements are described. At the end of the description, any existing variation of the movement is given.

The drawings only outline the correct poses and movements, and only those that lend themselves to pictorialization. Pirouettes, lifts, tours en l'air, etc., are not illustrated: they would take too much room and serve no appreciable purpose. In any case, the most complicated movements are based on movements illustrated in preceding pages, which do not need to be repeated.

This textbook is not meant for self-teaching. The drawings are included as an aid to the new teacher.

ELEMENTARY MOVEMENTS
OF CLASSICAL DANCE

All elementary movements are grouped together and discussed in one of two sections:
1. the diverse forms of plié, relevé, battement and rond de jambe;
2. the various forms of port de bras.
First the basic positions of the legs are given, then the positions of the arms.

POSITIONS OF THE LEGS

There are five basic positions of the legs in classical dance. (See illustration #2.)
In the First Position, the feet are joined at the heels and form a straight line.
In the Second Position, the feet are still in a straight line, but there is a distance of one foot—about 12 inches—between them.
In the Third Position, the turned-out feet are close together, with one heel adjoining the other at the halfway point of the length of the foot. (At a later time, the Third Position will be used as a transitory position in demi-plié, grand plié, as an approach to a lift, and with battement tendu for batterie. In some instances, there is no need for this auxiliary position because the technique of performing a Fifth Position, in all its complexity, will have been fully learned.)
In the Fourth Position, the turned-out feet are parallel to each other with the distance of one foot—about 12 inches—between them.
In the Fifth Position, the turned-out feet are joined together, covering each other, the heel of one touching the toe of the other.

In all five positions, the legs are turned out and the feet are placed *firmly and evenly* on the floor without overstressing the big toe. (The weight is evenly distributed on the large toe, the small toe and the heel.) The center of gravity of the body comes exactly between the legs. The knees are gently pulled up, and in the Second and Fourth positions they form a straight line without any looseness or locking of the knee joint.

At first, the student must learn the First and Second positions facing the barre, holding each position for eight measures of music. The arms are free and the hands rest lightly on the barre at the same width as the shoulders, with the elbows hanging loosely along the sides of the body. The trunk is kept straight, with the diaphragm and ilium region pulled up. The shoulders are free, open, and lowered and kept in a straight line. The head is kept facing the barre with the eyes looking straight ahead and the neck and face muscles free of tension. It is not permissible to lean or "hang" onto the barre, or to look down or sideways.

The First and Second positions may be strengthened with the addition of demi-plié. The student is then introduced to the Third and Fourth positions using the same method: holding the position through eight measures and adding a demi-plié to each position.

The positions of the legs are also learned as preparations and as finishing positions.

---

2   Positions of the feet

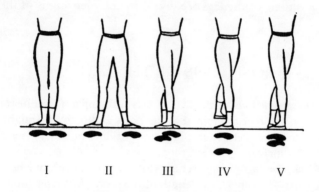

          I   II   III   IV   V

The last to be studied is the Fifth Position, since it is the most difficult. All the rules must be observed without exception while learning the positions as well as throughout the course of study. The least inaccuracy in performing these positions will lead to the loss of the turnout and the entire figure as well.

Positions, in classical dance, teach correct posture on both legs. At the same time, many of the exercises are executed on one leg. The free leg moves in fixed positions along very strict rules. If, for instance, while standing in Fifth Position, the front leg is lifted to 25 degrees, 45 degrees or 90 degrees in one of the three possible directions (front, back or side), the working leg is in Second Position, (if it is to the side) or in Fourth Position (if it is front or back). The leg, bent at the knee, may be placed on the standing leg only at the ankle (sur le cou-de-pied), at the calf, or at the knee, while the standing leg may remain straight or execute a demi-plié or relevé to demi-pointe. All this forms the elementary basis for leg movements as accepted by the school of classical dance and is learned through special exercises.

PLIÉ

The plié is an element of almost all the movements of classical dance. It develops elasticity, flexibility, the turnout of the legs, facilitates the smooth and soft joining of stability and elevation, and gives a pliable character to exercises and to choreography. It is one of the most technically forceful and expressive elements in the art of classical dance.

Pliés are divided into demi-pliés and grand pliés.

DEMI-PLIÉ

The student, while standing on both legs in one of the positions (First through Fifth), bends the knees and ankles smoothly, with equal pressure on both feet. (The depth of the demi-plié is about half the way to a full bending of the knees, or a grand plié.) The knees and ankles are thus bent to the utmost without the heels being lifted from the floor. (See illustration #3.)

The demi-plié is done turned out, with no pressure on either the big or the little toe and with the heels pressed firmly to the floor. The bent knees should be in a straight line and directly over the toes, the buttocks pulled up but not pressed together, and the entire movement executed with ease and elasticity. The knees and ankles are then straightened, following the same rules in reverse, to complete the demi-plié.

The hands, if the student is facing the barre, are placed lightly on the barre at shoulder width, and the elbows are lowered and held freely, along the sides of the body.

If the demi-plié is executed with one hand on the barre, the other arm is in Second Position (directly side). (The hand on the barre is held with the shoulder and elbow lowered and the hand placed lightly on the barre about six inches in front of the student or a distance that does not unduly bend or extend the elbow.)

The torso is kept straight, the buttocks pulled up; the shoulders are kept freely open and lowered and the weight of the body is equally distributed on both legs during the descent and the return.

The demi-plié begins by executing the movement four times in each position—First, Second, Third and Fifth. Later, the Fourth Position is used. The time signature for the music is 2/4, with one measure for a smooth bending of the knees and ankles, and one measure for the return.

Next, the demi-plié is executed twice in each position (except Third Position) with a battement tendu making the change to the next position. The change through battement tendu is done together with the ending of every second demi-plié, and in the fourth measure of the music. The straightening of the knees and the battement tendu take one measure, and in the next measure the leg is moved to the next position and the whole foot is lowered to the floor. The entire exercise is performed as eight demi-pliés and four changes of position with the right leg in battement tendu.

After a slight pause, the entire exercise is repeated with the changes made to another position by the left leg.

Later, the student executes the exercise holding the barre with one hand and using the right leg (outer leg with the left hand on the barre) and then executes the exercise using the left leg for the changes. (The student turns *toward* the barre in order to reverse the exercise, then places the right hand on the barre to begin the demi-pliés on the other side, using the left leg for battement tendu changes.)

Before the start of the exercises, the free arm and the head perform the accepted preparation. (The free arm moves from Preparatory Position at the side of the thigh, to First Position of the arms, then to Second Position of the arms, where it remains at this level of the student's comprehension.)

---

3   Demi-plié in five positions

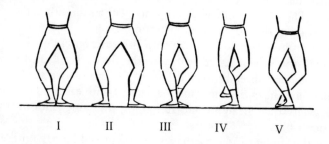

I   II   III   IV   V

Somewhat later an arm movement may be added during every second demi-plié. The arm moves from Second Position through the Preparatory Position into First then Second positions. At the same time as the deepest bend of the demi-plié, the hand should be above and slightly in front of the knee. As the legs begin to straighten, the arm is moved into Preparatory Position and moves continously to First then Second Position of the arms. The arm movement must begin strictly with the bending of the knees and end in the Second Position at the same time as the straightening of the knees. As the arm lowers into Preparatory Position, the head follows the arm by leaning slightly forward. When the arm moves into First Position, the head turns slightly to the barre, inclined lightly and barely to the shoulder. As the arm moves to Second Position, the head returns to its former position at the start of the exercise. (Turned toward the open arm.) The eyes follow the hand.

When the demi-plié has been well learned at the barre, it is executed in the center of the floor, keeping the same rules of performance. This exercise should begin in the center of the floor with a preparation.

For some time, all demi-plié exercises should be done en face in the center, then in Fifth and Fourth positions, in épaulement. (Shoulders turned, along with the hips, to face corners #2 or #8.) The arms and head are also held in the épaulement position.

Demi-pliés in the épaulement position in Fourth Position are executed with a different movement of the arms. When the right leg is in front, the left arm moves from Second Position into First Position and remains there. When the knees are straightened, the left arm moves from First to Second Position, and the eyes follow the left hand.

Later, the demi-plié is not done as an exercise but becomes an additional element in various movements.

GRAND PLIÉ

The grand plié is a development of the demi-plié. The grand plié is executed like the demi-plié on both legs in the same position, except for the full bending of the knees and ankles. The grand plié must be done smoothly and evenly (using the same number of counts to descend as to return). In all positions, *except the Second Position,* the student must raise the heels as if in a low demi-pointe position. (See illustration #4.) The student must not "sit" on the heels, which are slightly raised from the floor. In the Second Position, during the bending of the knees, the heels must not leave the floor and the hips (pelvic region) must be kept in a horizontal line, not tilted forward or back. (See illustration #5.)

The straightening of the knees begins smoothly and evenly and *at once* after the full bend is reached, with no stop made at the deepest point of the bend. Except for the grand plié in Second Position, the heels are returned firmly to the floor.

As in the demi-plié, the weight of the body is placed evenly onto both legs with no leaning on the large or small toe and with the turnout maintained throughout the movement. The knees, during the bending, are opened to form a line from the shoulders, and the buttocks are pulled up, not left in a flabby state.

The arms, torso and head are moved as for the demi-plié.

At the barre and in the center floor, this movement is executed twice in each position as for demi-plié. The change of arms becomes part of each grand plié. In the middle and higher levels, the students may be introduced to various changes of arms. For instance, while bending the knees and in Fifth Position, the arms

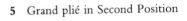

4 Grand plié in First Position   **5** Grand plié in Second Position

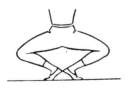   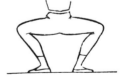

may move lightly and smoothly to the Preparatory Position, and while the knees are straightened, move smoothly to return to the Second Position. The head keeps the épaulement position.

Another example: When executing a grand plié from the Fifth Position, the arms may perform the Second Port de Bras. (See port de bras section.)

On the first level, it is recommended to grand plié in a slow 4/4 time signature using one measure to bend, one measure to return. Later the tempo may be changed to a 3/4 or 6/8 time signature.

RELEVÉ TO DEMI-POINTE

This movement consists of rising smoothly to a high demi-pointe position while standing on both legs in any of the foot positions, and then lowering to the whole foot. (Some schools call the smooth rise to the demi-pointe, élevé—a rising—while the Italian School calls the spring to the demi-pointe from demi-plié a relevé. The lowering is called abaisser.) (See illustration #6.) The relevé is an excellent exercise for the development of elasticity of the foot, flexibility of the toes and resilience in the ankle. These qualities support difficult technical maneuvers from elementary exercises to complex turns. The relevé to demi-pointe, like the demi-plié, is an integral element of many movements of classical dance. Correctly performed, the relevé gives the entire body a look of lift and lightness. The relevé,

6   Relevé to demi-pointe in First Position de face

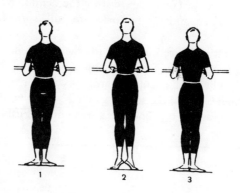

in some exercises, may be combined with demi-plié. The exercise is done in First, Second and Fifth positions. Beginning in First Position, with the tempo 4/4 and facing the barre, the student executes three relevés in First Position, then changes to the Second Position by doing a battement tendu with the right leg to the side. After the foot is lowered to the floor from the battement tendu, three relevés are executed in Second Position, and a change with the right foot in battement tendu to Fifth Position ends with the right foot front in Fifth Position. Three relevés in Fifth Position are followed by battement tendu to the right closing right foot back in Fifth Position, followed by three more relevés. The right foot then changes with a battement tendu, back to First Position. The exercise is repeated with the left foot making the changes of position in battement tendu.

The arms are kept on the barre and the torso and head held directly front or en face. In performing this movement, the student must raise his heels evenly and smoothly *both at the same time,* lifting high onto the demi-pointe position with the ankles free and not rigid, with no pressure on the big toes, maintaining the turnout and pulling up from both legs. Lowering back to the floor, the return must be smooth, elastic, with both heels arriving on the floor at the same time, especially when the relevé is done in Fifth Position.

The arms must be kept free from tension, hands resting lightly on the barre, the torso pulled up at all times, especially when rising onto demi-pointe. The shoulders are free, lowered and open. The weight of the body is evenly divided on both legs. The head is kept free and the eyes forward. The relevé must be done lightly and without unneeded exertion.

Each relevé is executed in two measures of 4/4 tempo: rising to demi-pointe in 2/4, staying in demi-pointe for 4/4, and lowering for 2/4. Each battement tendu is executed in two measures. When the exercise has been mastered at the barre and on the floor, it may be done in one measure of 4/4. A change of arm position is recommended. For instance, while executing relevés in First and Second positions, the arms may be opened through First and Second arm positions. When the relevé is done in Fifth Position, in épaulement croisé, the arms may be lifted through First Position into Third Position. (The Third Arm Position in this school is directly overhead. It is known as the Fifth Position in the Italian School.)

Later, the relevé is not used as an independent exercise but, like the demi-plié, enters into various movements.

BATTEMENTS

BATTEMENT TENDU

Battement tendu consists of a slide by a turned-out leg, along the floor with the toes never leaving the floor, from the First or Fifth positions, into one of the three possible directions: forward, side or back. The same sliding movement is made with the turned-out leg in bringing the leg back to the starting position.

This movement must be done strictly in a straight line from the heel of the standing leg to the toes of the moving leg and back. No deviations from this direct line are admissible.

The battement tendu is the primary element in achieving the proper stretch of the leg from the knee to the tips of the toes. This movement is most important since it is found in literally all movements of classical dance, especially in transitional movements. (See illustration #7.)

While the leg is being extended, the student must strive for an especially clear line connecting the instep and toes and well-stretched knee. The slide begins with the heel, and as it extends, the toes skim along the floor until the leg and toes are fully extended. *At the final point, there is no pressure on the toes.* The leg returns along the floor and the heels gradually lower onto the floor as the leg nears the starting position. No overcrossing of the foot, unextended toes or turned heels are to be permitted. In order to better maintain the turnout during the movement, it is necessary to begin the movement with the heel and begin the return with the toes. When executing a battement tendu back, the student begins with a movement of the toes. The closing movement is begun with the heel. If the movement is done from the Fifth Position, to the front or to the back, it is necessary that the returning foot, when it has returned to the starting point, be pressed lightly to the floor, with the entire foot reaching the Fifth Position at the same time. When the movement is done to the side, the foot must slide evenly along the standing foot along a straight line and return along that same straight line to the front or back Fifth Position as designated. The standing leg must at all times have a stretched knee and be kept in a turned-out position, with the entire foot on the floor without undue pressure on the big toe.

---

7   Battement tendu, front, back, side

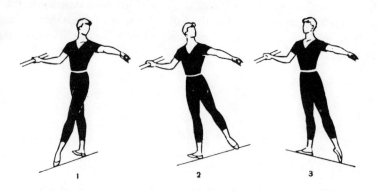

Arms, as a rule, during the performance of the battement in all directions, are kept in the Second Position and placed before the start of the movement. The center of gravity is at all times on the standing leg. The head, when the right leg moves toward a battement tendu front or back, is turned toward the same shoulder and is slightly bent away from the open leg. When the battement tendu is done to the side, the head is kept en face. The eyes always follow the direction of the head. No glancing sideways or pronounced bending or turning of the head is permissible. All movements of the head and eyes must be strictly observed, kept simple and in harmony with the pupil's age.

Movements of the head connected with the change of direction of the moving leg must be done smoothly. The teacher must not introduce any turning or bending of the head before all the details of the leg movements have been mastered. The battement tendu is learned facing the barre and executed from First Position to the side. This gives a better understanding and attainment of a turnout during the movement of the leg.

The musical tempo is 4/4 and the starting position the First Position. The hands rest on the barre with the elbows lightly lowered, the trunk and head kept straight. The leg smoothly, without pushing, slides to the side, using an entire measure of music. The fully extended position to the side is held for one measure, and another measure is used to return the leg to the First Position, where it stays for another measure. All exercises for battement tendu are repeated four times on the right leg and then on the left leg. In the same manner, battement tendu forward, then back, is executed. Throughout the movement, the turnout must be maintained and the hips kept in a straight line. The standing leg is pulled up over the hip. The standing leg is in a straight line that runs from the foot to the shoulder. This alignment must be strictly kept, *especially when executing the movement to the back.* (Any tilting of the pelvis when executing the movement to the back must be avoided.)

After the battement tendu has been properly learned facing the barre, it may be done with one hand on the barre. This exercise is executed with the student standing with his left side at the barre, his hand placed lightly on it, and his standing leg in the proper position. Then he puts his free leg into First Position and his arm in Preparatory Position (lightly touching the side of the thigh) at the same time.

This entire preparation must be done quietly, and without looking at legs or arms. Later, the preparation for the beginning of the exercise is done in two measures. During the first measure the pupil raises *both* arms into First Position, and during the second measure he opens the arms into Second Position. His left arm opens during the Second Position to the barre, and he places his hand lightly on the barre, elbows lowered.

On the first measure, the head turns from its en face position and leans lightly toward the left shoulder, eyes following the hands. During the second measure the head turns to the right, eyes following the hands, and as soon as the working leg begins the movement, the head returns smoothly to the en face position. At the end of the exercise, the free arm lowers into Preparatory Position and, at the same time, the head turns to the right. After quietly freeing the body from its closing position, the student turns toward the barre and begins the exercise on the other leg. It is necessary to free the body after working, particularly in later, more complicated movements.

Later, the battement tendu is performed separately in each direction in two measures instead of four. One measure is used for the slide, the second measure for the close into First or Fifth Position. This way the number of battements in each direction increases to eight. Following the mastery of this tempo, the battement is then performed in one measure, 1/4 note for the slide, 1/4 note for the closing position.

Finally the battement is performed on each quarter with the slide occurring *before the measure* (on the "and" count, which makes the first beat of the music the closing position). In the higher levels, the battement tendu is performed in combinations at times in 1/8 of a measure.

The study of battement tendu from the Fifth Position should begin facing the barre and be executed in the same sequence and tempos only after the First Position movements have been mastered.

Later, the battement tendu may be done en croix (in the shape of a cross opening front, side, back and side), varying the number of movements in each direction. First, only one en croix direction may be given: four battements tendus to the front, two to the side, four to the back. Battement tendu en croix in First Position may be done somewhat differently: 1. to the side, forward, side again and back. 2. to the side, forward, back and then side again. 3. forward, back, to the side and again to the side.

In the Fifth Position, the movement is possible en croix in all possible variations, changing direction a number of times and returning the leg from the side position to the front or the back of the standing leg. The use of the en croix in all variations at the barre or center floor may be part of the following movements: battement relevé lent, grand battement jeté, battement frappé, battement fondu, battement soutenu and battement développé.

Battement tendu may be done through First Position without stopping in that position. In this case, the leg moving from the First or Fifth Position slides forward to the Fourth Position and then in a straight line moves in an uninterrupted and gliding movement past the heel of the standing foot (heels meet in passing) through First Position and continues back into Fourth Position and returns to the starting First Position. This movement may be done in reverse (opening backward first) or after repeating the movement two or three times, closing into the starting position.

Battement tendu is a useful movement to perform alternating legs from Fifth Position. The movement may begin with three battements tendus with the right leg to the front, followed by three with the left leg toward the back, three with the right leg to the side (closing behind the left leg) ending with three to the front with the left leg.

The arms are kept in the Second Position, and the center of gravity (weight shift) is transferred to the standing leg before the working leg moves. The trunk is maintained level or square, and the head movements are done according to the previously given rules.

This method is studied with the battement performed in 1/8 note tempo. Or the tempo may be varied, as well as the number of movements and directions. This same method of study, beginning at the barre and then in center, may be used for the study of grand battement lent, grand battement jeté and battement développé.

The use of this method must not be overdone to the detriment of other forms of battement tendu and each must be done in accordance with the preparedness of the pupil for the exercise.

BATTEMENT TENDU DOUBLÉ

There is another form of battement tendu, with pressure—a lowering of the heel to the floor then stretching the foot once more before returning it to the starting position. At this point in the teaching, it is executed only in the Second Position and returned to the First or Fifth positions. This movement must be clear and elastic, with the toes never leaving the floor. (This movement is sometimes called battement tendu doublé or battement tendu relevé.) The arms are kept in Second Position, the hips straight, and the center of gravity over the standing leg. The head, after the preparatory movement, turns en face.

At first, this battement with "pressure" is learned facing the barre from First Position and executed four times with each leg to the side. Each battement is done in two measures of 2/4 tempo: 1/4 note each is used to lead the leg, lower the heel, stretch the instep, and close the leg into the starting position. Then the movement is executed the same way to the side with one hand on the barre.

Then this battement form may be done from the Fifth Position in one measure with the leg sliding *before the first beat:* 1/8 for the lowering of the heel, 1/8 for the stretch of the instep, 1/8 for the return to the position. In this way the battement tendu doublé is performed eight times on each leg. All the rules of performance of the battement tendu in its simple form are strictly kept for this form of battement tendu as well. (See illustration #8.)

Finally, the battement tendu must be studied as a small pose (croisée, effacée and écartée). First as a small pose in a given position, it is taught at the barre, then for perfection, in the center. The poses are decided by the teacher and incorporated with the battements tendus. At first, the combinations should be simple with repetitions in one direction then increased to four repetitions of battement tendu. It must be remembered that the enthusiasm of the pupil in striving to perfect the work begins with the simplest exercises, including the battement tendu.

8 Battement tendu doublé

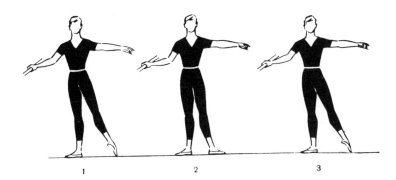

1   2   3

The battement tendu may be performed in combination with demi-plié. In this exercise, both elements combine into one whole, which is reached *at the moment* of the return of the open leg to the starting First or Fifth Position. The demi-plié starts a little later and is deepened when both feet have joined at the starting position. The slide of the leg is executed according to the same principles, but the unbending of the knees from demi-plié starts a bit earlier and is completely straightened by the time the leading leg reaches the fully stretched tendu position in its given direction. This is the basic form of execution of this exercise and is used in a multitude of movements in classical dance.

To master the correct combination of tendu and demi-plié, the exercise must be learned slowly and separately. At first the exercise is performed from First Position facing the barre, four times to the right and then to the left. The tempo is a slow 2/4; 1/4 for the leg to slide to the side, 1/4 to close back into First Position, 1/4 for demi-plié and 1/4 to straighten the knees. The leg in this exercise leads and closes with stretched knees, but the flow into demi-plié is without stops or haste.

Then the exercise may be studied facing the barre with the tendu forward and back, four times in each direction in the same tempo.

Then the exercise is performed with one hand on the barre and from First Position separately in each direction, then en croix, twice in each direction. The arms are kept in Second Position, the torso remains erect and the head en face.

At the next stage, the battement tendu with demi-plié is studied en croix from Fifth Position with the hand on the barre in a 2/4 tempo. The leg slides before the measure, 1/4 note to close in demi-plié, 1/4 to straighten the knee *and open the leg to the given direction.* (The beat is in the demi-plié position and the tendu starts before the count.) In this exercise the head follows the rules of battement tendu, but it becomes more complicated at a later time. When the leg leads forward or backward, the head keeps its turn and bend, but in demi-plié the bending is done away from the direction of the closed leg in Fifth Position. (See illustrations #9 and #10.) All these turns and bends of the head must not be done roughly or deliberately, but in a simple and clear manner.

In battement tendu from Fifth Position, it is useful to lower the arm into Preparatory Position or open it through First into Second Position. In that case, the head turns and leans toward the movement of the hand with the accent on the deepest point of the demi-plié. (See illustration #11.)

Finally, the battement tendu with demi-plié must be practiced at a faster tempo, performing every movement of the leg two or three times in the same direction. The arm remains in Second Position and the head at this tempo does not lean away during the demi-plié itself.

One must strive in this exercise for total togetherness of the movements, with the bending or stretching of the knees occurring somewhat earlier when the leg closes into Fifth Position. This faster tempo leads to a still greater togetherness of both elements and prepares a flexible and clear finish for jumps such as sissonne fermée, jeté fermé, cabriole fermée, etc.

This exercise may be done en croix and with a change of standing leg or done

9 Battement tendu devant closing in demi-plié Fifth Position

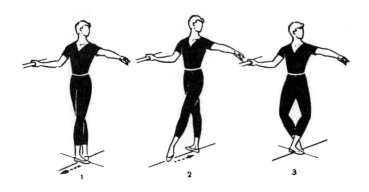

10 Battement tendu to the side closing in demi-plié Fifth Position

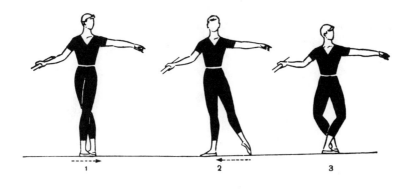

11 Head movement for battement tendu with arm in Preparatory Position and in Second Position

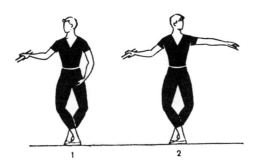

on both legs in Second and Fourth positions. The working leg opens to the position, the toes and heels lower into a demi-plié in Second or Fourth Position, and the knees unbend and the change of weight to the standing leg is made at the same time that the working leg is stretched, toes touching the floor. Finally, the working leg returns from the Second or Fourth Position to the starting Fifth Position. The arm, when the working leg is sliding into its stretch position, is in Second, and during the demi-plié in Second or Fourth Position it is changed along a horizontal line to Second Position. (See illustrations #12a and #12b.)

The torso is kept erect at all times and the buttocks pulled up. The weight of the body in demi-plié is evenly divided on both legs; the head, during the change of the arms from Second into First Position, turns toward the barre and leans lightly toward it. At the opening of the arm from First Position into Second, the head turns after the hand and leans back a little.

The exercise must be done with flexibility and with an effort to coordinate all the elements.

12a Battement tendu with demi-plié in Second Position

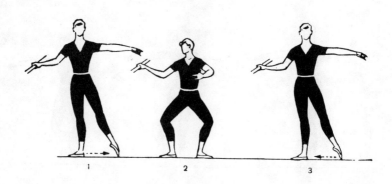

12b Battement tendu with demi-plié in Fourth Position devant

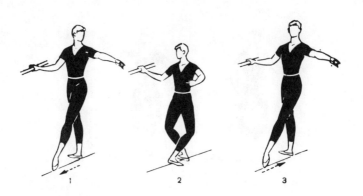

This movement is studied at first in Second Position, with one hand on the barre. The tempo is 2/4 and the starting position Fifth. At the first two measures, the arms open from the Preparatory Position through First and into Second Position. On the first 1/4 note, the leg slides to the side and does a plié on the next 1/4 note, the plié is released on the next 1/4 note and the leg slides behind the standing leg into Fifth Position on the last 1/4 note. This movement is repeated four times, and at the two final chords the arm is lowered into Preparatory Position. Then, this battement is studied en croix, with the tendu done twice in each direction, in the same tempo. Finally, the movement is studied with the leg sliding out before the count. (This places the accent on the demi-plié and the tendu on the "and" count.)

These exercises may be done with a change of weight during the straightening of the knees from demi-plié, into a Second or Fourth Position or, with an additional demi-plié, a return to the starting Fifth Position.

It is good to join both of these movements and the methods only after all the previous forms have been mastered, especially in maintaining the turnout and coordinating the movement.

BATTEMENT TENDU SOUTENU

The battement tendu may become still more complicated by doing a demi-plié on the standing leg at the same time the working leg slides into Second or Fourth Position. As the working leg returns to the starting position in First or Fifth Position, the standing leg straightens from the demi-plié. The working leg is straight at all times. This exercise is called battement tendu soutenu (battement soutenu in the French and Italian schools). It is widely used in many movements.

The arms, in this form of battement, are kept in Second Position. The torso, when the working leg is to the side, is kept straight, but when the leg is moved forward or back, the top of the back leans a little in the opposite direction of the working leg. In the Second Position the head is en face. When the working leg moves forward or back, the head turns toward the open arm, leaning slightly in the same direction as the trunk. (See illustration #13.) The demi-plié in this exercise must be started in First or Fifth Position and be fully stretched when the extended leg is in its given direction with the knee, toes and instep stretched. Battement tendu soutenu must be done flexibly, lightly, sliding the entire foot along the floor until it reaches its fullest extended instep, heel off the floor, toes on the floor. At the same time, the standing leg softly deepens the demi-plié at the finish of the movement of the working leg, while preserving the turnout and the correct pressure on the entire foot.

The return of the working leg to the starting position must be done lightly and smoothly, with the foot gliding along the floor at the same time the standing leg straightens. This battement form is studied like the previous battements, first facing the barre, in the following manner: In a 2/4 tempo, beginning from First Position, the leg is moved to the side on the first 1/4 note; on the second 1/4 note the demi-plié begins on the standing leg as the working leg continues to slide along the floor with the toes; the next 1/4 is used to straighten up from the demi-plié; and the last 1/4 is used to close the leg in First Position. (Care must be taken to keep the weight directly over the standing leg in the demi-plié position.)

This exercise is repeated four times on the right leg, then four times on the left leg, then forward and backward. Then the exercise must be studied holding the barre with one hand in the same 2/4 tempo and beginning in First Position. Each leg movement is done twice in each direction en croix.

The arms move during the two measures of the introduction of the music, from the Preparatory Position through First Position and open to the Second Position where they stay during the exercise. At the end of the exercise, on the last two musical chords, the arm is lowered into Preparatory Position. The torso and head are kept erect and the buttocks pulled up and the center of gravity kept strictly on the standing leg.

Then, the battement tendu soutenu must be studied *with the demi-plié as the starting position,* in First Position and then performed en croix: demi-plié in 1/4 count, slide the leg on the next 1/4 count, straighten the knee from demi-plié; on the next 1/4 count return the leg to the starting First Position and rest 1/4 count.

---

13 Battement tendu soutenu side, front, back

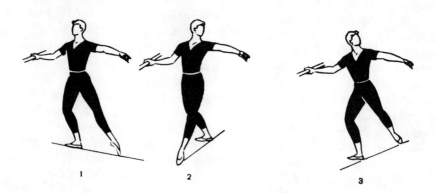

In the final stage, this exercise is performed en croix from Fifth Position. The demi-plié and slide of the leg are performed together to 1/4 count; the return and straightening of the knee of the standing leg, on the next 1/4 count.

The arms remain in Second Position, the trunk is kept erect with the head en face in the slide to the side, leaning forward or backward and turned toward the open arm as it leans slightly away from the open leg.

Later, when this movement is mastered, very insignificant leanings of the torso may be introduced into the movement. In addition, the arms may be moved at the same time as the leg. Remember that this exercise must be coordinated smoothly and with no extra exertions.

There is still another battement tendu movement which is performed from Fourth to Fourth Position passing through First Position in demi-plié. This form, already described, requires that the demi-plié fully coincide with the change of the free leg from Fourth into Fourth and that the deepest portion of the plié fall in the First Position. The movement of the standing leg follows the same tempo in the passing. On the whole, the movement is done together, elastically with light gliding of the foot through First Position.

The arms, head and torso follow the battement tendu rules and the exercise, with the hand on the barre, is executed as follows: Two battements tendus are done to the side from the Fifth Position; then battement tendu back and forward passing through First Position in demi-plié. After that, the leg extended to the front, closes into Fifth Position and the entire movement is done in reverse (opening to the front, then back-passing through the demi-plié in First Position). The tempo is 2/4. The extending and closing of the leg is done to 1/4 counts and after being mastered at that tempo is performed to 1/8 of the measure.

This kind of battement tendu in combination with demi-plié as an element is incorporated in the rond de jambe par terre, small pas de basque, pas failli, etc.

The battement tendu with demi-plié is useful in combination with relevé on demi-pointe starting in First or Fifth Position. It should be done after two or three battements, but no more often in order not to get distracted from teaching useful exercises while introducing variety.

The arms, head and torso follow battement tendu rules, and the exercise is done in 2/4 tempo. Beginning in the Fifth Position, three battements tendus front are done with demi-plié with the accent on the first 1/4 of the measure in demi-plié. Then the three battements are followed by a relevé on demi-pointe lowering into a demi-plié. The exercise is performed en croix. All this must be done evenly, together and with flexibility according to all the rules that are indicated for each separate movement.

Battements tendus with demi-plié in Second and Fourth positions are useful when joined to relevé on demi-pointe. For instance, after a demi-plié in Second Position, there may follow a relevé on demi-pointe followed by another demi-plié in Second Position, tendu to the side from the demi-plié in Second, and a close to Fifth Position with demi-plié. The same pattern may be followed in Fourth Position front or back or en croix.

The tempo is 2/4 and the tendu opens *before* the count (on the "and" count), demi-plié and relevé on demi-pointe are on the first 1/4 beat; demi-plié is on the second 1/4 beat; tendu in Second to Fifth Position is before the beat; Fifth Position demi-plié is on the second 1/4 beat.

The arm opens to Second Position in the relevé, the torso is kept straight, the head turned toward the open arm, eyes on the hand. All else is performed according to the rules described previously.

The combining of the demi-plié and the relevé must be done elastically without a jumping movement onto the toes or with a flabby lowering from the demi-pointe.

Battement tendu soutenu, like the two previous movements, may be joined

14   Battement tendu soutenu ending in demi-pointe

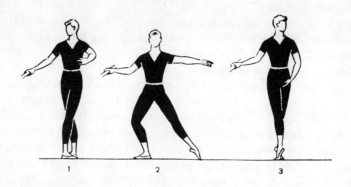

15   Battement tendu front and back with demi-plié in First Position

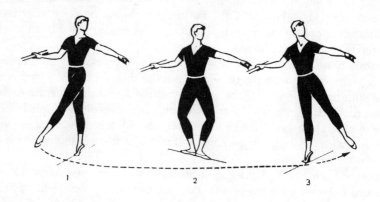

16   Battement tendu jeté to the side

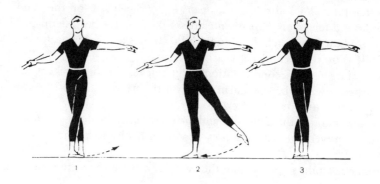

with relevé on demi-pointe when the working leg returns to the beginning position. (See illustration #14.)

The arms, head and torso follow the rules of battement tendu soutenu and the relevé is added to the exercise only when the other movements are mastered.

Finally, battement tendu from Fourth into Fourth Position passing through First Position in demi-plié, may have an added relevé on demi-pointe as the working leg reaches the front or back in the Fourth Position. The toes lift from the floor as high as the heel of the standing leg. (See illustration #15.) Remember that the entire movement must be done on a high demi-pointe, turned out and with no pressing onto the big toe.

BATTEMENT TENDU JETÉ

This battement is different from the previously described battement tendu because it is clearly thrown (jeté) to the height of 25 degrees. It is performed in the same tempo, returns to the starting position, and is thrown with a quick, sliding movement keeping to the exact height of 25 degrees. (See illustration #16.)

The return to the starting position is made without stopping, as the stretched toes energetically touch the floor and the foot returns to starting position with a sliding movement.

The throw and return of the leg must be done smoothly and *energetically* while the supporting leg is pulled up off the hip and the knee is kept stretched. Both legs remain turned out throughout the movement.

The arms are usually held in Second Position, the torso is erect and pulled up and the center of gravity is over the supporting leg.

The head is turned toward the open arm if the movement is performed backward and forward, but if the movement is done to the side, the head is kept en face. This position may be held as a small pose at the barre and in the center floor work.

The movement is studied at first facing the barre in 2/4 tempo. Beginning in First Position, the leg is thrown to the side on the first 1/4 count; held to fix the position on the next 1/4 count; returned to the First Position on 1/4 count; and rests for 1/4 count. It is performed four times on the right leg, then on the left. The battement tendu jeté is then studied with one hand on the barre, executed to the side, then forward and backward. It may be done from a starting position in Fifth, or en croix with the throw executed before the count and without a stop at 25 degrees. When the leg is in the 25-degree position, there is a pause for 1/4 of the count. Later this pause is no longer held and the entire battement tendu jeté is executed in 1/4 of the measure.

In the middle and higher levels, this battement is performed with speed, which provides excellent mobility of the hip and ankle joints and provides force and lightness to the whole leg.

The battement tendu jeté may be joined in demi-plié or relevé to demi-pointe in the starting First or Fifth Position after the third throw.

Three jetés, including the demi-plié, are done to 1/4 counts. The fourth 1/4 count is used to unbend from demi-plié as the leg is simultaneously thrown to the next direction.

Both of these exercises may be performed en croix and exchanging the standing leg to perform some of the jetés.

Further, battement tendu jeté may be done with the relevé to demi-pointe at the same moment the leg is thrown to 25 degrees, and returned to Second or Fourth Position. Beginning in First Position, three battements tendus jetés are performed to the side, with the third jeté in relevé on demi-pointe. The relevé ends in demi-plié in the First Position and the knees straighten on the fourth count. This exercise may then be executed to the front or back. The tempo is 2/4 and each jeté is done on a 1/4 note with the accent in First Position. The relevé is on the 1/4 note of the second measure, and the demi-plié and pause returning to straightened knees is on the last 1/4 count or note. Or two measures may be given to demi-plié: one to plié and one to straighten the knees.

17 Battement tendu jeté piqué

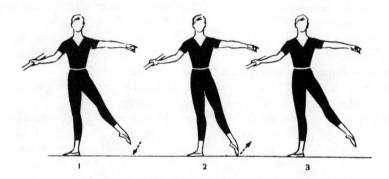

Battement tendu jeté should be executed in Fifth Position as well, on a high demi-pointe, making sure that the throw of the leg is with fully stretched toes each time, and that the foot returns to the floor lightly.

This exercise may be done en croix, with four jetés in each direction from Fifth Position.

The arm is kept in Second Position; the torso and head movements are as usual.

Finally, this movement may be complicated by the addition of a small piqué, or striking motion by the toes, onto the floor before the leg is closed into the starting Fifth Position. The movement is called battement tendu piqué. This movement may be done two or three times in succession before the leg returns to Fifth Position. (See illustration #17.) Battement tendu piqué may be further complicated by moving the leg along a low height from Fourth Position into Second Position, or from the side to the back, or en croix. This moving of the leg, or transfer to another direction, is executed between the second and third piqué movements, followed by a close to the starting position or a continuation in another transfer to a different direction. The piqué is executed at first on 1/4 notes, then on 1/8 of the beat. Each piqué must be done clearly, with a strongly stretched leg, without stop. The standing leg is kept straight, the arms and trunk held according to the rules of battement tendu.

BATTEMENT TENDU POUR BATTERIE

This exercise is a preparatory exercise for batterie (beats). It must be done energetically and clearly in a quick tempo. Starting in Fifth Position with the right leg forward, the working leg is thrown to the side to 25 degrees with the knee, instep and toes stretched. Then it makes a forceful return to the standing leg into Third Position behind the standing leg (foot flexed), transfers in front of the leg in Third Position, then energetically returns to the side at 25 degrees. (See illus-

18   Battement tendu pour batterie

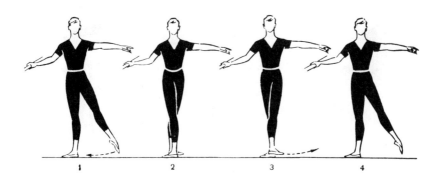

tration #18.) When the leg closes the transfer is executed with a "lift," the foot never touching the floor, knees stretched. The foot in Third Position back is parallel to the floor, knees stretched. The foot in Third Position front is parallel to the floor and very slightly lifted or separated from it. Both transfers into Third Position are followed by a short rebound from striking the calf. *Absolutely no movement of the body must accompany this performance.* It is studied facing the barre in a 2/4 tempo. The leg is thrown to 25 degrees to the side before the measure, and each strike of the calf or close to Third Position is done on 1/8 count, with the opening to the side as the starting position, on 1/4 of the beat. When the exercise is mastered, and performed with a jump, it is no longer necessary to use this preparatory exercise.

(Teaching this exercise on the first level to boys is an important factor in their training. Meticulous execution in making the transfer to the side and with a completely quiet body is an immeasurable technical contribution at this early stage.)

BATTEMENT RELEVÉ LENT

This exercise evolves from battement tendu and is a lift to 90 degrees, thereby enlarging the step and requiring an exact position different from the previous battements. It is executed as a smooth lift with a stretched leg to 90 degrees forward, to the side, or backward. The position is fixed and the leg returns just as smoothly into the starting First or Fifth Position. (See illustration #19.)

The working leg has a stretched knee, stretched toes and instep and moves turned out without stopping to 90 degrees. It returns in the same position, smoothing and without bending or stopping and still turned out to the battement tendu.

19　Battement relevé lent

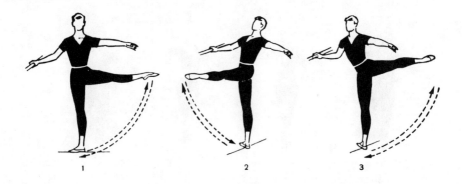

Special attention must be given to the correct placement of the hips as the leg moves forward or backward. The hips must not turn in the same direction, or lean to the side of the moving leg when the leg moves to the Second Position. The center of gravity must be kept over the standing leg throughout. The torso during the movement of the leg to the front and to the side is kept erect, lifted. When the leg moves backward the torso leans *slightly* forward. When the leg returns to the starting position, the torso resumes its erect position. The shoulders are always kept free, even, unlifted, not turned in the direction of the moving leg.

The arms first open from the Preparatory Position, through First and into Second Position, or open together with the working leg. The head moves at the same time with the arm into First Position, then leans slightly forward; the head moves with the arm movement turning to the right and leans a little backward. When the right leg moves backward, the head turns toward the right but leans a bit forward. When the movement is performed to the side, the head stays en face.

This exercise may be done in combination with demi-plié and relevé on demi-pointe. For instance: at the moment the leg is lifted, the standing leg may rise to demi-pointe, or after a demi-plié, there may be a relevé to demi-pointe. After the leg is lifted, the standing leg may rise to demi-pointe and into demi-plié, or the reverse.

The closing of the leg may join the demi-plié as the leg lowers, or at the moment the leg closes from demi-pointe into the starting position. This exercise may be reversed: the closing of the leg may end in demi-pointe, or may end in demi-pointe in the starting position.

These variations may be given in sequence, but not overdone in number or complication at the expense of a smooth movement, a clearly fixed position in 90 degrees, incorrect arm, head, or torso positions.

Battement tendu lent (lent means slowly) is also performed in large poses at the barre and at the floor. (Large poses are held positions at the end of an exercise or combination, and they become part of adagio movements at a later level.)

Studied first, back to the barre, the exercise is done to a 4/4 tempo in two measures. On the first 1/4 beat the leg slides to the tendu position front; lifted to 45 degrees on the second 1/4 beat; continued to 90 degrees on the third 1/4 beat; *stays in that position* for 1/4 beat; lowers to 45 degrees on the first 1/4 of the second measure; lowers to the toes in the tendu position on the second 1/4 beat of the second measure; closes into the starting position on the third 1/4; and rests or pauses on the last 1/4 beat.

For a while, each part of the movements must be fixed, then performed smoothly, keeping the lifting and lowering uninterrupted.

Then, the movement may be executed with one hand on the barre, moving the leg forward without breaking the lift into separate parts.

The arms move from the Preparatory Position through First into Second Position. The head turns toward the open arm.

Then the exercise may be learned with the leg lifting backward facing the barre, then learned to the side facing the barre. This is followed with the performance of the exercise with one hand on the barre, and then in the center of the floor.

Battement tendu lent may be done in one measure of 4/4: 2/4 to lift to 90 degrees, 1/4 to fix the position, 1/4 to return to the starting position.

Battement tendu lent may be useful when teaching battement développé. The flowing and smooth character of these movements permits a diverse method of performing large poses in adagio movements at the barre and on the center of the floor.

GRAND BATTEMENT JETÉ

This movement is similar to battement relevé lent but is executed as a quick, smooth throw of the leg to 90 degrees. (See illustration #19.) This movement develops force and strength in the leg, and a high and flexible extension, which is useful in later movements like grand fouetté and big complicated jumps.

The grand battement jeté begins with a light, gliding movement along the floor, rising to and increasing in force until it reaches a height of 90 degrees. The movement should be light and free. The return is more restrained, and slightly slower, and the toes touch the floor lightly in the descent, closing in the manner of the battement tendu, into the starting position. The thrust of the leg must be done with energy and smoothly, turned out, with straight knees, pointed toes, and exactly along a direct line forward, side, or back. The standing leg must be kept turned out and the knee kept straight. Pressure on the big toe is inadmissible and moving the foot from its position, especially in executing the battement backward, is not permitted.

The position of the hips and the center of gravity apply as for the battement relevé lent. The arms are usually held in Second Position. The torso must be kept erect when the leg is thrust forward and to the side, but tilts a bit forward in thrust to the back. At the moment the leg returns, the trunk once again assumes its erect position. The shoulders are kept even and free and the head at the time of the thrust forward and backward is turned toward the open arm in Second Position. At the thrust to the side, the head is kept en face.

The study of grand battement jeté begins first facing the barre, with the movement to the side. Then it is studied with the thrust of the leg forward, while holding the barre with one hand. Next, the movement is studied with the thrust to the back, facing the barre. The time signature should be two measures in 2/4 and the character of the music energetic. The first 1/4 note is used for the thrust, the second 1/4 note for the lowering of the leg and toes to the floor, 1/4 for the close to the starting position, and 1/4 rest.

It is then executed flowingly, without a stop in the tendu position on the floor, but without stop to the starting position, now the Fifth Position. The movement is performed in one measure: 1/4 to thrust the leg upward, 1/4 to close in the starting position.

Later, this movement is performed en croix with the exchanging of the standing leg, as in the manner of battement tendu described earlier. This faster form requires the same exactness and change of weight to the standing leg in the manner as battement tendu jeté.

The arm, during the grand battement jeté en croix and with an exchange of weight and standing legs, remains in Second Position.

When the exactness of the movement and the timing are mastered, the movements may be added to big poses at the barre, then to the work in the center of the floor.

Grand battement jeté, like the other battements, may be done combined with demi-plié and with relevé on demi-pointe. Demi-plié may be introduced into the movement before the movement from the starting position. The relevé to demi-pointe is combined with the thrust on demi-pointe or with the return to the starting position on demi-pointe. And, relevé to demi-pointe may be combined with a demi-plié before or after the thrust in a starting Fifth Position.

These elements may be used in a sequence, but not to the detriment of the exactness, lightness or tempo of the jeté itself.

GRAND BATTEMENT JETÉ POINTÉ

There are, as well, more complicated forms of this battement:

1. The leg is thrust into Second or Fourth Position at 90 degrees and lowered to the tendu position, raised again in battement to 90 degrees, and then closed to the starting position. This exercise should be executed in a flowing, light passing movement of the toes along the floor. The tempo, force and other elements remain the same as in the above description. Special attention must be given to maintaining the tautness and lightness of the movement of the leg. This exercise as described is called battement jeté pointé. (The position on the floor is known as piqué à terre in the French School and is the same as pointe tendu. The movement is called grand battement fini piqué.) (See illustration #20.) It is done first to each 1/4 note in a 2/4 tempo and later to 1/8 of a beat. The introduction of relevé and demi-plié is not obligatory here as they will hamper the tempo of the thrust, the lightness and forcefulness of the movement which should be almost trampoline-like in the departure of the toes from the floor. This version of battement may be combined with grand battement jeté in this manner: A grand battement jeté forward from Fifth Position may be followed by grand battement jeté pointé done twice in the same direction or the entire exercise may be done en croix.

---

20 Grand battement jeté pointé

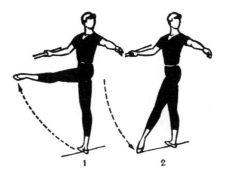

GRAND BATTEMENT JETÉ POINTÉ IN AN ARC

Additionally, this battement may be done in an arc-like swing at the moment of the thrust, when the leg transfers from a throw from Fourth Position into Second Position in the pointe position; or a throw into Second Position ending in a pointe position in Fourth Position front or back in the pointe position. This movement keeps to all the rules of the grand battement jeté pointé.

This movement may be further complicated by a transfer of the leg from Fourth Position in the front to Fourth Position backward through the Second Position. This bow-line movement, because of its complexity, may be executed only in the higher levels if the exact arc is preserved and it is executed with lightness, force and in the correct tempo.

The arm is kept in Second Position, the trunk is kept straight, the head turned away from the standing leg.

2. Another complication to this exercise may be added in starting and finishing the movement for grand battement jeté in Fourth Position with a leg stretched backward, toes on the floor. In this movement, the working leg glides through First Position, is thrust forward to 90 degrees and returns through First Position to the starting position. The movement may be reversed starting with the position to the front, the thrust to the back and the return to the front starting position. This exercise is called grand battement jeté from Fourth into Fourth. In this movement the working leg must be turned out and glide lightly along the floor through First Position, making a somewhat restrained return to the starting position. The arms, head and torso conform to the grand battement jeté requirements. In the study of this movement, a rest or a pause must be kept in the Fourth Position after the thrust, which is executed before the movement. Later, the movement may be executed without a stop but with the accent on the leg at the moment it returns to the starting position.

This battement may be combined with demi-plié at the moment the leg returns through First Position into Fourth Position. Next, the thrust may be executed with the demi-plié, and the moment the leg glides through First Position the knees are straightened as the leg passes into Fourth Position. This movement increases the force of the leg into Fourth Position and the entire body lowers swiftly in its execution. The name, "the roll," describes this movement.

In the higher levels, it is useful to add to "the roll" a movement of the arms into Third Position (overhead, or Fourth Position en haut in the Cecchetti method, with the inside hand on the barre). After passing through Preparatory Position into First and Second positions, the arm rises to Third Position at the time of the 90-degree thrust and opens from Third Position into Second Position. When the thrust is backward, the arm rises to Third Position from Second Position and, at the moment of the return, opens from Third to Second Position.

In all of these movements, the head is turned toward the hand. The torso is kept firm and bends slightly away from the open leg, but the turnout is maintained. The movement should be done energetically, accurately, lightly and without dragging the tempo in demi-plié. The thrust is before the measure of 2/4 (on the "and" count before the beat).

GRAND BATTEMENT JETÉ BALANÇOIRE

3. Another form of grand battement jeté is the balançoire (this movement is similar to grand battement en cloche—like a swinging bell—during which, unlike balançoire, the body is kept erect).

The movement begins with the toes of the working leg stretched on the floor in Fourth Position back. From this position, the leg is thrown through the First Position forward to 90 degrees without stop, thrown backward through First Position to 90 degrees, and, for the third time, thrown again through First Position to 90 degrees front, and passed through First Position to the starting Fourth Position in tendu back. The number of grands battements balançoires may be increased to eight times. It may be reversed as well and begin in Fourth Position tendu forward, with the first throw to the back.

The arm is usually kept in Second Position. The head is turned toward the open hand. The trunk, during the throw to 90 degrees, leans evenly and energetically in the *opposite* direction to 45 degrees. The simultaneous lean of the body as the leg is thrown to 90 degrees in the opposite direction to 45 degrees gave the step its name, balançoire (seesaw). (See illustration #21.) This movement may be executed alternately front, back and side. When the leg moves to the side the starting position is First or Fifth Position and the movement is performed without stop. The arms are still held in a horizontal position and the torso moves

21 Grand battement jeté balançoire in Fourth Position

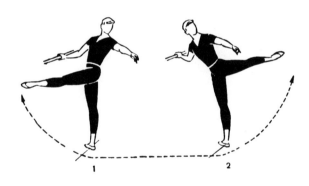

22 Grand battement jeté balançoire in Second Position

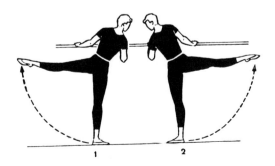

to the side opposite the leg to 45 degrees. The head turns toward the side opposite the leg at each throw. (See illustration #22.) The balançoire to the side is only performed by the middle and higher levels.

All the described forms of grand battement jeté (with the exception of the pointé movement with the leg transfer to another position) may be done with a pause of the leg at 90 degrees. It must remain turned out and stretched to the limit and must not go higher if it loses freedom and aplomb. The pause is not in the lowering of the leg, but at its height at 90 degrees and may be held for 1/4 count or longer.

To this exercise may be added a light and fast additional swing of the leg in the air. The leg is thrown to 90 degrees; pauses there; lowers to 70 degrees; pauses there; and is once more returned to 90 degrees. The swing is done with the accent on 90 degrees and with firm resolution. This exercise must be *seldom used* and only as a small addition, despite the fact that it creates force and accuracy for the working leg fixed at 90 degrees.

The balançoire may be inserted in battement relevé lent movements or in battement développé at the barre.

---

23   Battement frappé

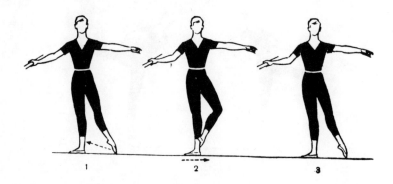

1   2   3

BATTEMENT FRAPPÉ

The battement frappé exercises a fast, exact and energetic bending of the working leg into the sur le cou-de-pied position and its opening front, side or back to the floor or to 45 degrees. (See illustration #23.) This movement starts with a preparation from Fifth Position. The arm moves from the Preparatory Position to First Position and into Second Position. At the moment the arm moves to the side, the leg moves to the battement tendu position to the side.

The head follows the arm from First Position, turns toward the hand and leans slightly to the barre. The torso is kept erect.

From the tendu forward, the frappé is executed by bending the knee of the working leg into the cou-de-pied position with a light strike to the standing leg. When the tendu is begun backward, the frappé executes the same motion clearly, but with more restraint. When the knee is straightened from the sur le cou-de-pied position, it does so with a pushing movement and a small gliding of the toes along the floor to the final point of the tendu. If the frappé is executed at 45 degrees, this glide along the floor is omitted and the leg opens at the last moment with tautness and stretched insteps and toes. When the battement frappé is performed to the side, with the toes to the floor in tendu position or opened to 45 degrees, *the thigh and knee remain turned out and immovable in this position.* If the exercise includes front and back battements frappés, the thigh and knee are moved in the same direction and must be immovable when the knee is straightened and when it returns to the starting point. The standing leg, as well, must maintain the turned-out position with a pulled-up knee (lifted kneecap). The arm is kept freely in Second Position and the torso erect and shapely. The head follows the rules of previous battements.

Before the study of battement frappé, the position of sur le cou-de-pied must be learned separately, standing facing the barre. The movement is done in a slow

24 The sur le cou-de-pied position in front	**25** The sur le cou-de-pied position in back

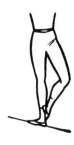 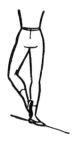

tempo without accents in two measures of 2/4. Beginning in Fifth Position, the working leg moves smoothly to the side, according to the rules of battement tendu to the two measures of music which precede the beginning of the exercise (the introduction). This is the preparation for a battement frappé exercise. On the first count of 1/4, the knee bends to the cou-de-pied position forward; is held for 1/4 count; straightened to the tendu position to the side on the next 1/4; and is held in that position on the last 1/4 count. The same exercise is repeated to the sur le cou-de-pied position behind the ankle. The exercise is then repeated to the front and to the back for a given number of times. The two final chords of music accompany the return of the foot into Fifth Position. The exercise is then repeated on the other leg.

The bending and straightening of the knee in this exercise must be done in an even movement holding strictly to the Second Position. The sur le cou-de-pied position must be fixed tightly to the supporting leg especially in the forward position and without pressure on the big toe of the supporting foot. The hips are pulled up (care must be taken not to "sit" on the hips). The hand rests easily on the barre and the torso is kept erect and immovable. The shoulders are kept open and lowered. The center of gravity is over the standing leg. The head and eyes are kept forward.

The battement frappé is then studied with the tendu forward between the cou-de-pied positions, then with the tendu backward. This is done in the same slow tempo and with pauses in the tendu position as well as in the sur le cou-de-pied position.

Later, this exercise may be studied with two frappés in each direction, en croix. The preparation and the finishing movements are obligatory.

At the next stage, the battement frappé is performed in one 2/4 measure. Then the sur le cou-de-pied position is taken *before* the measure with a soft strike to the standing leg. The straightening speed is somewhat increased to 1/8 of a count; the pause in the tendu position is 2/8. (The beat is now in the tendu position with the cou-de-pied on the "and" count.) Finally, the pause is eliminated while the accent remains in the tendu position and the exercise is executed with full force.

The final tempo of this movement alternates with a 1/4 and a 1/8 count: after two battements frappés are done to 1/4 count they may be followed by three of the same movement to 1/8. The last movement of the battement frappé is kept in the open position in tendu.

When the battement frappé has been mastered with the toes to the floor on the 1/4 counts, it is studied at 45 degrees according to the same rules but with a stronger accent in the straightened position. In this exercise the strike to the ankle of the standing leg is done with more resilience. When the movement is executed at 45 degrees and on demi-pointe, the preparation is also done with relevé on demi-pointe. The relevé to demi-pointe occurs when the leg moves to sur le cou-de-pied and lowers when the leg straightens. This method may be used when the leg lowers to tendu on the floor and when it rises to 45 degrees.

Before studying battement frappé on demi-pointe, it is necessary to practice relevé on demi-pointe on both legs, then alternating on one leg, facing the barre in a 2/4 tempo. Starting in Fifth Position, the relevé is done in one measure as the front foot is transferred to the sur le cou-de-pied position; the next measure is used for the standing leg to lower smoothly while the front foot remains in its position. This is followed by two more relevés to demi-pointe with the last one ending with a lowering of the free foot back into Fifth Position forward.

Finally, at the end of the exercise, the last two chords are used for battement tendu to the side with the close into Fifth Position behind the standing leg. The exercise is then repeated on the other leg and with the foot back in the sur le cou-de-pied position.

All these exercises must be done smoothly, turned out, lightly, and with knees held immovable and a flexible foot. The torso and head are kept erect and straight and the center of gravity over the standing leg. The hands lie freely on the barre and the body is pulled up off the legs especially upon rising to demi-pointe.

BATTEMENT FRAPPÉ DOUBLE

A more complicated form of battement frappé is *battement frappé double* or double frappé. It is different from the single battement frappé because of an added transfer of the foot to a sur le cou-de-pied position by the use of petit battement.

The first exercise in the study of battement frappé double begins holding the barre with one hand. The tempo is 4/4 and the exercise is done in one measure. The leg is bent to the sur le cou-de-pied position in 1/4 count; the foot transfers on the next 1/4, straightens on the next 1/4 and pauses on the last 1/4. It is then done twice as fast, or 1/8 count for each part of the movement. Later, the exercise may be begun before the count of one, or before the measure with the sur le cou-de-pied and the transfer beginning the movement; the straightening on 1/8; pause 1/8. The pause is then eliminated in order to execute the following exercise: Do battement frappé double to the side, then forward and back, or en croix in various combinations. (Care should be taken that the area from knee to hip remains immovable and the action of the transfer to the side be made without disturbing the turned-out position.)

At first this exercise is studied with the toes to the floor in a tendu position; then at 45 degrees; then standing on demi-pointe; and in combination with relevé to demi-pointe. All the rules that apply to the execution of the battement frappé and petit battement sur le cou-de-pied apply to the execution of the battement frappé double.

Finally, this frappé, with the toes on the floor, must be combined with demi-plié at the moment the leg opens, which may be done *with or without lowering the heel to the floor.*

This form is learned at first, en croix, with the same port de bras, torso posture and head position. Then small poses are added at the end of the frappé. For instance, two double frappés may be done to the side, one forward ending in the pose of tendu effacé. (This position in the French School is called quatrieme devant ouverte.) Each frappé is done to 1/4 beat with a pause on 1/4 beat.

Or two frappés may be done to the side, one double frappé à terre ending effacé à terre devant (toes on the floor in tendu position in effacé) and one double frappé ending effacé derrière (quatrième derrière ouverte, in the French School). Each frappé is done to a 1/4 beat.

Another example of this exercise is to perform one double frappé to the side, one devant in effacé, one ending in écarté devant; one to the side. Each frappé is done to 1/4 count. All three of these examples may be done in reverse.

The arm movement in the effacé devant pose is a rounded line in First Position with a bending of the torso forward to 45 degrees. The head is turned toward the hand. The change in the pose is done with the head turning toward the standing leg at the same time the foot makes its double beat (petits battements). Each frappé ending backward (derrière) is done with the arms in the position of a second arabesque with a bend backward of the torso. The transfer into this pose is done with a turn of the head toward the standing leg at the same time the foot makes its double beat. This method of study will develop fast and exact coordination of all the elements from which it is formed. The performance of the frappé movements must be light, exact, with no unnecessary accents and performed strictly in the character of the frappé.

PETIT BATTEMENT SUR LE COU-DE-PIED

This movement consists of fast and clear exchanges of the sur le cou-de-pied position front to sur le cou-de-pied back. (See illustration #26.) The exchange must be executed at the same height in front as well as in back. The working foot *moves only to the side* in the smallest possible distance around the standing leg and with the utmost accuracy in placing the foot in the correct sur le cou-de-pied position each time, front and back, with a strongly held foot. The thigh and knee are kept totally turned out and immovable. The ankle performs its movement freely with a resilient accent on the cou-de-pied front. Although there is an accent on striking the foot in the back sur le cou-de-pied position, the heavier accent is on the accent in front as the foot grasps the ankle. The standing leg is turned out, well pulled up, and holds each grasp of its ankle. The arm is fixed into a quiet Second Position and should show no sign of strain during the fast movements of the working foot.

The torso is held erect, pulled up and held easily. The center of gravity is over the standing leg. The head clearly moves toward the open arm, which is in Second Position. The neck and face should also be independent of the foot movements and the eyes kept toward the open arm. (See illustration #27.) The preparation for this movement consists of two parts: the usual preparation to the tendu side; then the transfer of the leg from the side to the sur le cou-de-pied position front. This preparation is done in two introductory measures in 2/4 tempo with the arm rising to First Position, then Second Position in the introductory measures. Each portion of the preparation for petit battement uses one measure.

At the beginning of the study, the leg must bend from Second Position freely into hanging position (see illustration #27) and then, just as freely, continues to bend into the sur le cou-de-pied forward position and so on with two movements, back and front, considered one transfer. All this is done in a quiet tempo without accents. The tempo is 2/4, with each leg movement to a 1/4 note of the measure and a pause of a 1/4 note.

The exercise is studied at first, facing the barre and from Fifth Position. During two introductory measures, the leg in the front position of the Fifth Position makes the preparation as described above. Then eight transfers are executed and the exercise finishes with the leg to the side on the floor, followed by a close to Fifth Position back into Fifth Position on the last two chords of music. The exercise is repeated on the other leg. The exercise is then done with one hand on the barre and in the same slow tempo. Later, it is practiced without the pauses with a

26 Petit battement sur le cou-de-pied

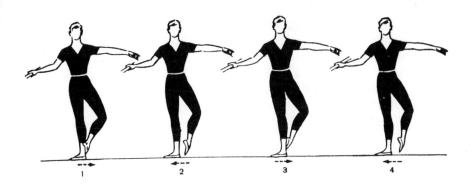

1   2   3   4

27 Petit battement sur le cou-de-pied in transition

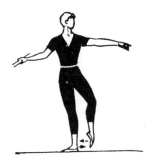

transfer of the foot on each 1/4 note, but with an accent in cou-de-pied front. When that form is mastered, the exercise is performed with a pause only in the cou-de-pied front, while the transfer to the leg back is executed before the beat. In this form, both transfers are done on 1/8 of the first 1/4 note and the pause is 3/8 of the second 1/4 note. (The first transfer, or beat, is before the first count on the "and" like an upbeat, and the pause in front is on the count.) Finally, this pause is eliminated, and while the movement is still done to 1/8 of a count, the tempo becomes gradually faster.

The whole movement takes on a virtuosic character, like a tremolo on a stringed instrument, when performed very quickly. (It is sometimes known as petit battement suivi—one following another.) This exercise develops excellent mobility in the ankle *while maintaining total immobility of the working thigh*.

This movement, too, is extended to include its execution in the demi-pointe position and should be practiced with relevés as well. Here, the transfer of the leg occurs on the rise to demi-pointe, and the return of the foot to the front position occurs at the same time the heel is lowered to the floor. The procedure may be reversed with the rise when the transfer goes to the back. The form may be combined: four petits battements on demi-pointe; four with relevé, etc.

Finally, the relevé is combined with a short and flexible demi-plié at the moment of the lowering from demi-pointe. The exercise is executed to 1/4 count for each portion: Two petits battements on demi-pointe are performed to 1/8 of the measure ending in demi-plié to 1/4 of the measure. The exercise may be performed four times front and four times back.

In each demi-plié the working foot is fully stretched at the instep in battement fondu position (coupé). The fondu position must be clear and done accurately in tempo. When the knee unbends from the demi-plié, the foot resumes the sur le cou-de-pied position. This series of exercises becomes a component of the faster movements in classical dance, such as jumps.

The head is turned toward the free arm, and bends slightly toward the working foot in sur le cou-de-pied position front and back. Finally, when the movement is mastered, it may be combined with the forms of battement frappé described previously.

---

28 Battement battu in the front position, on demi-pointe

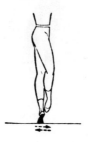

BATTEMENT BATTU

This movement is practiced in the higher levels by girls, but is useful for boys because it develops speed and clarity of movement in the working leg. The speed reaches 1/16 of a measure in 2/4 tempo.

The movement consists of uninterrupted and very short beats by the toes of the working foot on the heel of the standing leg, which is on a high demi-pointe. (See illustration #28.) (In the French School, the term for this movement is battement serré—tight. It is also called petit battement sur le talon—heel.)

The free arm is fixed in the Preparatory, Second or Third Position (over the head. When one arm is overhead and the other to the side, not on the barre, the

French School calls it the Third Position. The Cecchetti School calls it the Fourth Position en haut.).

The torso is erect and the body pulled up off the standing leg regardless of the speed of the movement of the working foot. The center of gravity is over the standing leg and the head is turned toward the shoulder of the free arm.

The working knee, regardless of the speed of the movement, must move freely, lightly, strictly turned out and remain immobile in the hip joint. Movement from the hip forward or backward by the leg is not acceptable. Only the slightest bending and unbending of the knee is admissible for the correct execution of this exercise. The standing leg must be turned out, with a stretched knee, and remain immobile at the ankle.

When learning the battement battu, it is recommended to restrain the tempo at first to 1/8 count for each beat, gradually increasing the speed to 1/16 count for each beat. The battement battu may be done with beats in back. In this movement, the heel of the free leg beats the ankle of the standing leg, with less force, but just as lightly and clearly. (The foot is kept in the coupé or fondu position and the inside of the heel nearest the standing leg beats the ankle of the supporting leg.) Battement battu is usually performed effacé front and effacé back.

---

29   Battement fondu

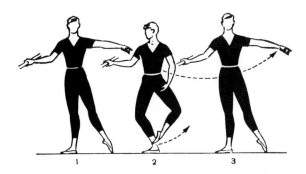

1   2   3

BATTEMENT FONDU

This movement belongs to the group of complex and smooth movements that develop strength, turnout and flexibility of the legs. It begins from a preparation in Second Position with the toes on the floor (tendu). The movement is begun with a demi-plié of the supporting leg as the working leg *simultaneously* goes to the sur le cou-de-pied position (toes downward) front or back. Then, as the knee straightens from plié, the working leg simultaneously opens to a tendu position, toes on the floor, or to 45 or 90 degrees. When the leg is open, it remains fixed, but the rest of the movement is performed flowingly. (See illustration #29.)

When this battement fondu is done with toes on the floor or to 45 degrees, the working and standing legs begin and finish the movement at the same time. This means that the beginning of the demi-plié and the joining of the leg in the cou-de-pied position occur together, just as the stretching of the knee of the standing leg and the opening of the working leg happen at the same time. When the battement fondu is done at 90 degrees, the working leg begins its descent to 45 degrees before the standing leg bends into demi-plié. The rest of the movement is executed in the same manner.

The opening to 90 degrees may also be done somewhat differently: The straightening of the standing leg and the raising of the working leg *to the knee* of the supporting leg begin at the same time. The standing leg then straightens completely and the working leg opens to 90 degrees like a développé. This entire movement must be done smoothly, flexibly, with the turnout maintained throughout, *with even hips* (the hip of the working leg must not be raised) and according to all the rules of the demi-plié.

The arms may stay in Second Position or lower into the Preparatory Position when the fondu bending begins, then, together with the opening of the leg, the arm rises through First Position into Second Position. The torso is kept straight, and the body pulled up off the legs. The shoulders are kept even and the center of gravity is over the standing leg. The head turns toward the open arm of the working leg; stays en face when the movement is done à la second (to the side) and during the demi-plié portion of the movement the head turns slightly toward the barre independent of the arm staying in Second Position or moving through the positions just described. When the standing leg straightens and the développé begins with the working leg, the head turns to its starting position, en face, if the movements are executed to the side.

A variation on the use of the head follows the rules of battement tendu in the demi-plié movements. As the leg bends, the head gently bends forward or backward according to the final position of the tendu. (The head inclines forward when the tendu is to the back.) The arm, in this variation, is in the Second Position. As the foot reaches the sur le cou-de-pied position forward, the head leans gently forward and leans back as the foot opens to the front. The reverse applies to tendu front. Battement fondu is done in small poses with the toes on the floor, at 45 degrees, and in large poses opening the leg to 90 degrees. Battement fondu at 45 degrees and 90 degrees may be done with relevé to demi-pointe according to the rules of both elements. The rise to the demi-pointe occurs the moment the knee of the standing leg has straightened from the demi-plié. The following demi-plié, which is the beginning of the next battement fondu, begins only after the heel has been lowered to the floor from the high demi-pointe. Both of these movements must be joined in one single tempo.

Battement fondu is studied at first, facing the barre with the working leg opening to the side and with a separation of the sur le cou-de-pied movement and the demi-plié. The sur le cou-de-pied in this movement is somewhat changed and, in teaching practice, it is termed "conditional." It is done as follows: The working foot, with the instep and toes well stretched, lightly touches the standing leg with its small toe at the inner ankle bone of the turned-out standing leg. (See illustration #30.) When the movement is done to the back, the position of the instep and toes of the working foot touch the outer ankle bone with the metatarsal bone of the large toe.* (See illustration #31.)

This conditional form may be practiced with exactness with the aid of the following exercise: In a slow 2/4 tempo, and from a starting Fifth Position, the forward foot extends to the Second Position in battement tendu during the two introductory measures. During one measure, the working leg moves to the cou-de-pied front; on the next measure, the standing leg does a demi-plié. On the next measure the knee straightens, and on the last measure the foot opens to the side with the toes on the floor. Each leg movement uses 1/4 note of a measure. Then the same movement is done with the cou-de-pied to the back and repeated once more, from the beginning with the foot in front in sur le cou-de-pied, etc.

30-31   Conditional form of sur le cou-de-pied front and back (coupé position)

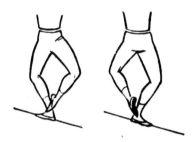

Then the movement is learned facing the barre with the working leg opening forward, and also with the leg opening backward.

Later, the battement fondu is executed with the bending and straightening done with both knees bending and straightening at the same time. The tempo is then changed to using two measures of music in 2/4 tempo: one measure for an uninterrupted demi-plié, and one measure for the straightening of the knee of the supporting leg.

Subsequently, battement fondu is studied with one hand holding the barre executing the movement in each direction separately; then en croix with two movements in each direction.

Later the complexity may vary, including an opening to 45 degrees, then to 45 degrees on demi-pointe, and eventually to 90 degrees. It is useful to exchange standing legs when executing the movement on demi-pointe.

At the barre and in the center floor, the battement fondu, combined with other movements, brings rhythmic and choreographic variety to the teaching problems. One may combine it with rond de jambe en l'air, pas tombé, battement frappé, partial turns, and pirouettes. Combined with small jumps, it can be combined in the sur le cou-de-pied position as temps levé, pas coupé, etc.

* It must be observed that the basic form of this movement is assumed in battement frappé and petit battement sur le cou-de-pied. In the following movement, the form is always "conditional" with or without a demi-plié.

32 Battement fondu doublé

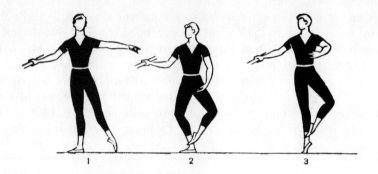

BATTEMENT FONDU DOUBLÉ

There is another form called the double battement fondu. It begins with the previously described demi-plié movement. The standing leg rises to demi-pointe, while the working leg does not open to a given direction but remains in sur le cou-de-pied position, and the second plié is done when the working leg opens to the extended position. This is a peculiarity of the double fondu. It may be executed in all directions and en croix. The arms, torso and head follow the rules of battement. The double form is studied when the regular form has been well mastered on demi-pointe. Coordination, elasticity and all the rules of technique are the same for the correct execution of this movement. It is necessary for the accuracy of the movement that the second plié of the standing leg coincides with the straightening of the working leg and that they both end the movement in a straightened position—the standing leg on demi-pointe and the working leg at 45 degrees. The tempo is a quiet 2/4. The first demi-plié is on the first 1/4 note; the relevé on the 1/4; the second plié on the next 1/4; and the fondu opening on the next 1/4 count. The double battement fondu may be combined with the regular form of fondu. Both forms may begin from the Fifth Position. In such a case, the leg transfers to cou-de-pied at the same time as the beginning of the demi-plié and may be done not only at the start of the movement, but also in its combinations. (See illustration #32.)

The double battement fondu is performed at 90 degrees with the principles of the battement développé: 1. During the first relevé the working leg rises from the sur le cou-de-pied position to the front of the knee of the standing leg; 2. During the second plié the working leg opens to 90 degrees; 3. During the second relevé the working leg remains fixed at 90 degrees; 4. The open leg descends in the manner of the battement fondu at 90 degrees, first to 45 degrees with the standing leg on demi-pointe, then with a demi-plié on the standing leg.

This exercise to 90 degrees is done at a slower tempo, 4/4: The first demi-plié

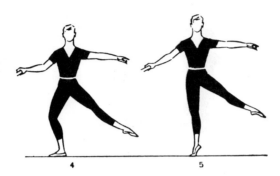

4   5

is on the 1/4 note; the first relevé on the next 1/4; the second demi-plié on 1/4; and the straightening and final opening of the working leg on the next 1/4.

The double battement fondu is learned after battement développé, in combination with demi-plié and relevé to demi-pointe, has been well learned.

BATTEMENT SOUTENU

Battement soutenu, like the battement fondu, is a melting and flowing movement which develops the turnout and flexibility in the legs. (See illustration #33.) It is performed at 45 degrees and at 90 degrees. Beginning in Fifth Position, both feet rise to relevé on demi-pointe smoothly and uninterruptedly and the front foot transfers to the sur le cou-de-pied (conditional form) at the same time. As the standing leg lowers into demi-plié, the working leg opens at the same time to 45 degrees forward (or side, or, if the sur le cou-de-pied began derrière, it may open side or back. The French School would term this portion of the movement as dégagé à demi-hauteur). The working leg lowers, toes to the floor, as the standing leg remains in demi-plié. The working leg then slides along the floor with the stretched toes up to the Fifth Position on demi-pointe *at the same time* the supporting leg rises to meet the working foot in demi-pointe in the Fifth Position. (The movement begins and ends in demi-pointe in the Fifth Position.) The free arm at the time of the transfer to sur le cou-de-pied moves from the Preparatory Position to the First Position and opens to the Second Position when the working leg is opened. It remains in Second Position as the toes lower to the floor and at the moment the working leg is pulled up to the Fifth Position on demi-pointe the arm returns to the Preparatory Position.

The center of gravity is over the supporting leg. The shoulders are open, free and lowered. The head faces the hand in sur le cou-de-pied, which is in First Position, follows the hand to Second and ends leaning slightly backward as the leg opens forward, and slightly forward if the leg opens backward. The head

33   Battement soutenu at 45 degrees

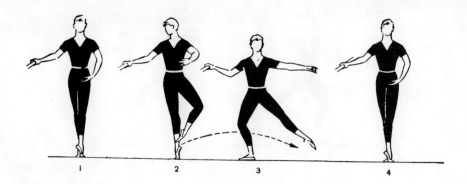

straightens and remains en face if the leg opens to the side. The teacher should remember that all the elements of the movement must be combined smoothly and flexibly. The turnout must be maintained and all the rules of demi-plié and relevé to demi-pointe observed. The lowering from demi-pointe must be to a firm heel on the supporting foot before the demi-plié is begun, as described in battement fondu to 45 degrees. The count is a slow 4/4. The transfer to sur le cou-de-pied is on one count of 1/4; the opening to 45 degrees on the next 1/4 count; the toes lower to the floor on 1/4 and gather to the starting position on the last 1/4 note.

At first the battement soutenu is studied facing the barre extending the foot to the side, then with one hand on the barre en croix. The exercise consists of two battements soutenus in each direction en croix with an exchange of the supporting leg. Finally, the battement soutenu is used in small poses in the center floor exercises.

The battement soutenu at 90 degrees can be added to combinations after the battement développé has been well incorporated in combination with demi-plié and battement fondu with relevé to demi-pointe. The battement soutenu at 90 degrees is studied en croix, then with an exchange of the supporting leg and later in big poses in the center floor.

BATTEMENT DÉVELOPPÉ

The battement développé is a difficult movement which exercises the movements at 90 degrees and is therefore an especially important element to master. It must be executed lightly, freely, energetically but clearly. The battement développé is divided into four components: the transfer of the working leg from the starting Fifth Position through sur le cou-de-pied up the supporting leg to the knee; the opening to 90 degrees front, side or back; fixing the open position of the leg at 90 degrees front or more; lowering the leg to the starting position. (See illustration #34.)

34 Battement développé

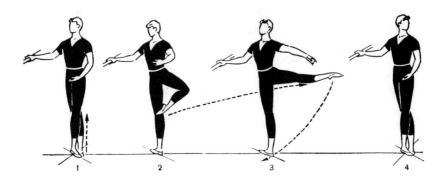

The leg closes to the starting position flowingly and lightly with toes stretched along the floor. When the développé is performed forward or to the side, the torso is kept straight. If it is done to the back, the torso leans slightly forward.

The arm moves from the Preparatory Position as the working leg transfers up the supporting leg to the knee into the First Position, then to Second Position. It lowers to Preparatory Position when the leg lowers to the starting position. The head follows the arm from First Position and follows the arm to Second Position, and when the leg does the développé front, it turns to the right and leans a bit back. When the battement développé is done backward, the head follows through the same as described above, but leans a bit forward when the leg is fully stretched. If the battement développé is to the side, the head stays en face.

The movements may be further complicated with additions at the time the working leg is moving along the supporting leg and when it is straightening. A relevé to demi-pointe may be added to either of those movements. At the opening of the working leg, a demi-plié may be followed with a relevé. When a relevé or a demi-plié is added *with the leg already in the open position,* the open leg must rise a little to give the movement greater lightness and accuracy. The finish may be Fifth Position with a relevé on demi-pointe or in demi-plié.

BATTEMENT DÉVELOPPÉ PASSÉ

Battement développé may be executed with a passé movement. The position of the passé is working-foot toes at the back of the knee of the supporting leg, at the side of the hollow. The position is not in front of, or in back of, the knee but directly to the side but not touching with the toes. (See illustration #35.) From this position, the leg opens into a given direction following the rules described above. The passé position may be done on demi-pointe of the supporting leg. At the next stage, the passé is used in big poses at the barre and in the center floor work.

Battement développé passé is studied facing the barre performing the passé, at first, in front and in back of the supporting knee, ending in a return to the starting position. Then it is learned thoroughly to the side of the knee, no higher than 70 degrees from the vertical axis of the body.

Then, with one hand on the barre, the movement is executed forward. The free arm makes a movement from Preparatory Position through First and into Second Position before the working leg begins. The head turns toward the open arm. Then, the battement développé passé is performed to the back facing the barre. Finally, it is done to the side. When this is properly learned, the leg movements may be at 90 degrees, with a very slight raising of the hip of the working leg. In the study of battement développé, the teacher must take particular care that the students keep an exact direction in the opening of the leg, especially backward into Fourth Position. In this position, the working leg must be kept turned out, hips must be fixed in a straight right angle to the body, and the knee of the working leg kept perfectly straight. No less important is the warning that the student must not "hang" on the barre, but must stand on a turned-out and stretched leg. The torso and upper back are always lifted, the shoulders free, open and lowered. The arms must not tense and the head must move exactly and smoothly together with the arm.

---

35   Passé position

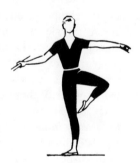

The study of the passé movement is in a slow tempo: 4/4. The sur le cou-de-pied position is assumed on the first 1/4 count; the next 1/4 count is a rest; the next 1/4 finds the foot in the passé position; the last 1/4 count is a pause. The leg lowers to the starting position and resumes the exercise at the given counts.

The battement développé is also performed at a slow 4/4 tempo: 1/4 is used for the sur le cou-de-pied position; 1/4 for the passé position or at the knee; 2/4 are used to unfold the leg in a given direction; 1/4 is used to lower the leg to the stretched toes on the floor; and 1/4 to close to the starting position.

Later, the tempo may be changed to: 1/4 to reach the knee position; 1/4 to open the leg; 1/4 pause in the fixed position; 1/4 to lower to the starting position; or: *starting* at the knee position before the measure or count of "one" *and opening* to the given direction, the position is fixed for 3/4 of the measure and lowered on the remaining 1/4 count.

In general, the rhythmic pattern of performance of this movement is most varied depending upon the nature of the problem confronting the student. In spite of the fact that all the various components of the movement must come together, they must be smoothly executed with the fixed position only in the développé not in the passé position.

It is useful to include a balancé movement into the study of battement développé. It strengthens the ability to lightly and exactly keep the leg at 90 degrees. It is added at a later date. The leg opens to 90 degrees; lowers quickly, lightly and slightly in the open position; and is then returned sharply to 90 degrees.

BATTEMENT DÉVELOPPÉ TOMBÉ

No less important is the battement développé combined with tombé. (See illustration #36.) It begins with a développé to the side, for instance, with the whole foot of the supporting leg on the floor. The supporting foot then does a relevé to demi-pointe. The working leg, then, making a small arc, catches the "fallen"

---

36   Battement développé tombé

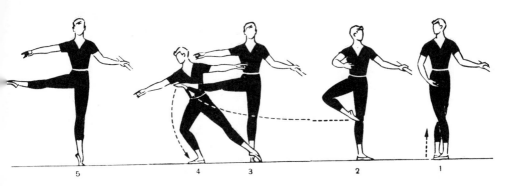

weight in a soft and deepened demi-plié. The supporting leg at the moment of the fall is stretched at the knee, the instep and the toes, with the toes lightly touching the floor. Finally, a strong and energetic push is made to return the weight to the supporting foot which returns to the whole foot position, as the "fallen" leg, stretching and sliding the toes along the floor, is brought up to the supporting leg. It continues through Fifth Position, is extended to 90 degrees when the relevé to demi-pointe begins again on the supporting leg, etc. At the end of this exercise, the leg lowers into Fifth Position and is repeated to the Fourth Position front or back.

The trunk during the tombé leans forward toward the working leg, and the upper back is held in a lifted position. The arms remain in the Second Position.

The rules governing the head and arms of the développé are applied to this movement.

The tombé movement is done at the barre and on the floor in the croisé, effacé and écarté directions. All the movements take two measures of 4/4: 1/4 for the développé; 1/4 for the relevé on demi-pointe; 1/4 for the tombé; 1/4 for the return; 1/4 for the second développé; 2/4 for the fixed open position; 1/4 for the closing into the starting position.

(Note that the hand leaves the barre in the tombé position to the side and is replaced on the return. When the tombé is done to the Fourth Position front, the hand slides along the barre and returns and slides back along the barre when the tombé is to the back. The hand and arm must not be used to push back during the return to the erect position.)

---

37   Rond de jambe par terre en dehors

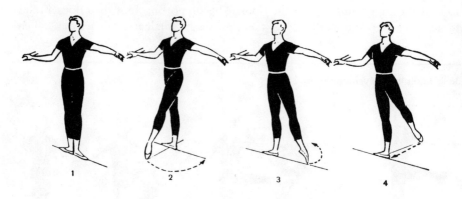

ROND DE JAMBE

ROND DE JAMBE PAR TERRE

Although the word "rond" means circle, it really describes half a circle when applied to the rond de jambe. From the starting point in First Position, the leg, by means of the battement tendu, moves into Fourth Position front; continues uninterruptedly with the toes along the floor, to Second Position; continues to the Fourth Position back; and returns to the starting First Position, thereby completing a half circle motion or arc. The outward direction is called en dehors. When the motion is reversed and the circle moves toward the body, the direction is called en dedans.

As a rule, the arms remain in Second Position. The torso and head are kept straight. (See illustration #37.) When the leg is fixed into Fourth Position forward or backward, the head turns toward the open arm as it does for battement tendu.

The working leg keeps turned out and lightly and evenly glides the toes along the floor, passing accurately through Fourth and Second positions.

With this exercise, the pupil first learns the use of the circular movement of the hip joint which contributes to its development and strength. It must be given special attention.

The supporting leg keeps turned out and its knee and hip are pulled up. The center of gravity stays unchanged over the supporting leg. The arms, torso and head are kept in their exact position with ease.

At first, the rond de jambe par terre is learned facing the barre, moving only one quarter of the half circle and with pauses at fixed points. The working leg moves freely and smoothly from First Position forward (in battement tendu), then just as smoothly transfers en dehors to the side in an arc, and from that point returns to First Position. The exercise is learned in the reverse position, en dedans. The count is 4/4 (flowingly). To the first two 1/4 counts, rests. It is followed by the exercise in reverse, en dedans, in the same rhythm.

The rond de jambe is then learned as a full arc or half circle, but with a pause in each position: Fourth, Second, Fourth back, and First. Each separate movement and each stop receives two 1/4 counts.

The rond de jambe is then learned with one hand on the barre and practiced with the pauses, together in one measure of 4/4, 2/4, 1/4 and 1/8. Regardless of the speed of the movement, the form must not be changed in the Fourth and Second positions. (The tendency with increased speed is to overcross the front tendu almost into a croisé position, and to miss an exact Fourth Position to the back.)

Before the rond de jambe par terre en dehors begins, a preparation is executed which consists of two sections: 1. A demi-plié in First or Fifth Position. The working leg glides forward into Fourth Position while the supporting leg remains in demi-plié; 2. The working leg moves with the toes along the floor, into Second Position, as the supporting leg straightens.

The arm moves from Preparatory Position to the First Position as the supporting leg does the demi-plié, and moves to Second Position as the working leg moves to Second Position and the supporting leg straightens. The torso is kept straight and exactly over the supporting leg.

The head during the first portion of the preparation bends slightly toward the supporting leg, and during the second portion straightens and bends slightly toward the open arm, which is in Second Position. (See illustration #38.)

For the rond de jambe par terre en dedans, the preparation is made in reverse. (The arm, head and body movements are the same.)

The movement is studied in the center as it was at the barre to a measure of 4/4.

ROND DE JAMBE SOUTENU

The rond de jambe par terre done with a demi-plié is called rond de jambe soutenu. It begins in First Position with a demi-plié as the working leg moves forward,

38   Preparation for rond de jambe par terre

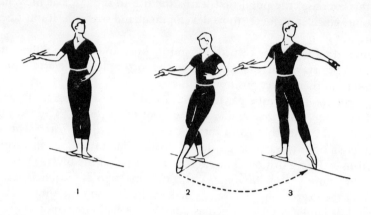

39   Rond de jambe soutenu

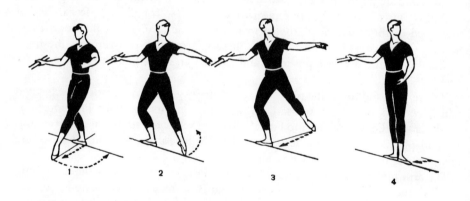

40   Rond de jambe en l'air en dehors and en dedans

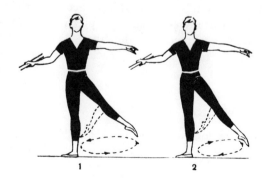

and the demi-plié is maintained as the leg moves side and back. The supporting leg straightens when the leg returns from the Fourth Position to the First Position. The arm, as for rond de jambe without the demi-plié, rises from Preparatory Position as the leg glides forward, and together with the transfer of the leg to Second Position, the arm opens to Second Position as well. The torso is kept straight and exactly over the supporting leg. The head leans a bit to the barre as the arm rises into First Position and, during the change to Second Position, straightens and turns toward the open arm. When the arm lowers into the Preparatory Position, the head stays in this position. (See illustration #39.)

The working leg must move evenly, lightly, and the supporting leg should not be straightened too soon. All the rules of the turnout and demi-plié must be observed with coordination and lightness.

The rond de jambe, as a rule, is alternated in a given combination of four ronds de jambes in its usual form without the demi-plié (soutenu) on the third and fourth rond de jambe. It must be practiced smoothly in each of its forms with the rhythm two measures of 4/4. This combination should be given only when the battement tendu soutenu has been well learned. The demi-plié begins before the measure; 2/4's are used for the forward movement; 2/4's for the movement side; 2/4's for the movement backward; 1/4 to straighten the supporting leg and 1/4 to close to the First Position and demi-plié again if the movement is to be repeated. The combination may consist of four ronds de jambes soutenus, two en dehors and two en dedans. Later, the movement may be done in one measure of 4/4, smoothly and with pauses, then to 2/4, and finally to 1/4 of a measure.

When both forms have been mastered, they may be done to a 3/4 rhythm (waltz) with one measure for each movement (half circle). Both forms are useful combined with rond de jambe jeté, which will be described later.

ROND DE JAMBE EN L'AIR

The word "rond" here, as in the rond de jambe par terre, refers less to a circular outline than to an elongated half circle, or oval. (See illustration #40.) The movement begins in an open Second Position at 45 degrees, which is the preparatory movement for the rond de jambe en l'air. The raised working leg bends at the knee, making a slight arc to the calf of the standing leg and, without stopping, continues the outline by straightening the leg in an arc en dehors until the foot reaches the original raised position at 45 degrees. The arm remains in Second Position and the torso and head are en face.

The knee must maintain its turnout and immobility throughout, neither moving from the line of the shoulders, nor raising or lowering. The foot is brought to the level of the calf of the standing leg but does not touch it. The leg must be stretched to its original starting position with a *completely straight knee* regardless of the speed of the tempo. The instep and toes are stretched throughout the movement. The bending and unbending portion of the movement must be done forcefully, clearly and with flexibility, maintaining the outline of the oval. This exercise develops lightness and accuracy in the turnout of the knee joint.

The supporting leg remains turned out and pulled up. The hips are kept equal and stable, while the head, arm and torso keep their usual position with exactness and freedom.

Rond de jambe is learned at first, facing the barre, without the circular movement and with pauses in the bent and unbent positions. The tempo is 2/4 or 4/4, each bending and unbending, and the pause takes 2/4. Later, the en dehors and en dedans circles are introduced into the exercise, at the same tempo. Still later, all the pauses are eliminated. The tempo is then increased to 1/4 to 1/8 of a measure for each circle, or the exercise is alternated between the two tempos.

The rond de jambe en l'air is done with the supporting leg flatly on the whole floor; on demi-pointe; with relevé to demi-pointe; and in demi-plié. For instance: two ronds de jambes en l'air en dehors with the standing leg on demi-pointe executed to 1/4 measure each; then three more ronds de jambes at 1/8 each ending the last rond in a demi-plié of the standing leg at the moment the working leg unbends. The beginning of the combination is again in relevé on demi-pointe.

If the rond is en dehors, the head at the time of the demi-plié turns slightly toward the arm in Second Position. When the knee of the supporting leg straightens from demi-plié, the head turns again en face. If the rond is en dedans, the head at the time of the demi-plié turns leaning slightly back as if to the movement of the leg.

When the movement has been mastered facing the barre, it is practiced with one hand on the barre. At this point, the preparation is learned: The arm rises from Preparatory Position to First Position as the head turns toward the barre. The working leg (usually the front leg from a Fifth Position) slides in tempo to the side at 45 degrees. At the same time, the arm opens from First Position to Second Position and the head straightens and turns toward the open hand. The supporting leg remains on the whole foot or rises to the demi-pointe if that is the given requirement.

In the higher levels, rond de jambe en l'air is done at 90 degrees to the side. The toes then extend to the level of the back of the knee of the supporting leg but do not touch it. The rules as described for 45 degrees apply. The rond at 90 degrees is done in a slow tempo and is not an independent exercise, but is usually in combination with battement développé to the side. It is performed no more than two to four times en dehors or en dedans. The rond at 90 degrees may be performed on demi-pointe and with demi-plié.

GRAND ROND DE JAMBE EN L'AIR

This movement outlines an arc in the air in the shape of a large half circle. (See illustration #41.) (This movement is known as grand battement arrondi in the French School.) Beginning in Fifth Position with a battement développé to 90 degrees front, the leg continues in an arc to the Second Position and Fourth Position back and lowers to the starting position, or, by means of a passé at the knee, repeats the movement from the beginning. This movement outward, away from the body, is called en dehors (clockwise). When it makes the half-circle arc in reverse from the back to the front, it is going in the en dedans direction (counterclockwise) or toward the body.

The approaches to this movement may be from battement développé as described, or from battement relevé lent, or grand battement jeté with a stop of the leg at 90 degrees. The open leg in the grand battement jeté may not make a full half circle, but only a quarter of a circle, from Fourth to Second Position or from Second to Fourth Position front or back, en dehors or en dedans.

The arm, in this movement, is usually kept in Second Position or is moved to a position held in large poses like arabesque, attitude, écarté, etc. The torso is kept straight, but during the change from Second Position to Fourth Position back, the body tilts a bit forward. It straightens when the leg moves from back to Second Position. The head turns toward the open arm when the leg moves forward or back into Fourth Position. When the leg is in the side position, the head is straight and turns toward the open arm in Second Position during the change in Second Position.

---

41   Grand rond de jambe en l'air en dehors

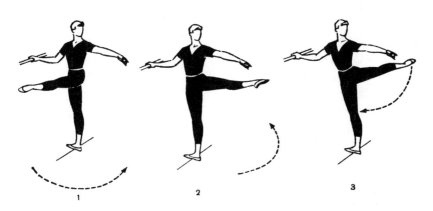

During the half circle, the working leg must maintain its turned-out position, especially from the Second to Fourth back. There should be a smooth, gradual elevation of the leg, with the knee pulled up as well as the hip of the standing leg. (The whole foot of the standing leg remains on the floor without pressure on the big toe.)

The movement is studied first at 45 degrees on the entire foot of the standing leg with a quarter circle, then a half circle and on demi-pointe. For instance: After executing a battement fondu to 45 degrees, transfer the leg en dehors to Second Position; then en croix; then both exercises en dedans.

The battement fondu and the leg transfers at 90 degrees are made evenly and studied at first in combination with battement relevé lent, and in the same sequence as above in a 4/4 tempo. After executing a battement relevé lent forward to 90 degrees, transfer the leg en dehors to Second Position using 2/4 of the measure; fix this position for 1/4; lower the leg into the starting position in 1/4. The movement is then executed en croix en dehors and then en dedans.

When the movements at 45 degrees and 90 degrees are mastered, the relevé to demi-pointe is introduced and the demi-plié. For instance: The leg is opened forward on the whole foot of the supporting leg, which rises to relevé to demi-pointe when the leg transfers to Second Position.

When combined with demi-plié, the supporting leg does a demi-plié when the leg transfers to Second Position or may bend in the forward position and straighten in Second Position. And in both of the above exercises, the demi-plié may be joined following or preceding a relevé to demi-pointe. Another form of exercise for grand rond de jambe en l'air is done in the higher levels observing all the previous rules and in the same tempos.

In this exercise the working leg moves quickly from Fourth Position front into Second Position before the measure; then without stopping it returns at the same tempo back to the Fourth Position front with the accent on the forward position followed by a stop. In the same manner, the leg may transfer from Second Position into Fourth Position and back. The movement may be also transferred in reverse from Fourth Position to Second and back and additionally from Second to Fourth Position back and return to Second. This movement is called rond de jambe en l'air balancé (rocked), and may be complicated in the usual way with demi-plié and relevé to demi-pointe.

The arm is kept in Second Position and the head in the starting position. In all forms of execution, the turnout must be strictly maintained and the legs must not become rigid.

GRAND ROND DE JAMBE JETÉ

This movement is the collecting and finishing form of the preceding forms of ronds de jambes. It adds the element, grand battement jeté. It excellently develops lightness and freedom in hip rotation.

The movement starts in First Position. The working leg, slightly bent, is thrown forward to 45 degrees. Then the knee is straightened as the leg continues to rise along an arc to Second Position at 90 degrees. The stretched leg remains elevated and, rising even a bit higher, continues to the back, lowering into Fourth Position; and finally it returns through a tendu movement, with toes on the floor, to the starting position. (The first throw to 45 degrees with the working leg in the half-bent position is in the conditional direction effacé devant—the point between direct front and direct side. The position at 45 degrees back, when the exercise is reversed, is effacé back in the conditional position—the point between direct back and direct side. This position is called "conditional" because the body is not assuming the correct effacé position but remains en face. This exercise may also begin from a tendu position in Fourth Position back for the en dehors direction of the exercise, or in Fourth Position tendu front for the en dedans direction.

42 Grand rond de jambe jeté

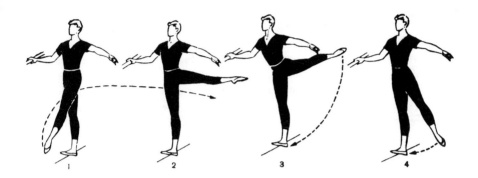

When this is the starting point, the foot passes through First Position before beginning the throw to 45 degrees. This movement has no counterpart in other schools.)

When the exercise is executed en dedans, the leg is thrown half bent to 45 degrees to the back (conditional effacé back), then unbends as it rises along an arch to 90 degrees side and is raised a bit higher as it continues to Fourth Position forward and, with toes on the floor, slides into the starting position. (See illustration #42.)

The arms are kept in Second Position, the torso and head kept straight. The movement is done in one movement, forcefully with a wide arc. The free leg goes through First Position lightly touching the floor with the entire foot, and through to a strongly stretched instep and toes. During the passage from 45 to 90 degrees, the knee is stretched to its utmost.

The turnout must be strictly maintained, especially during the en dehors direction when the working leg passes from Second Position into Fourth Position back. The supporting leg should be taut, turned out and the arm kept in Second Position and free. The supporting thigh should be well pulled up and free of the forceful movement of the working leg. The hips are even and the center of gravity is over the supporting leg. The eyes are kept looking front.

This movement is studied in four measures of 2/4 rhythm. The first stop is at the 45-degree mark of the first measure; the second stop is at 90 degrees in the Second Position; the third in the lowering of the leg to the stretched tendu position on the floor; the fourth measure is used for the return to First Position. In this manner, the movement of the leg occurs on the first 1/4 count of each measure. It is executed thus to permit a thorough understanding of the arc of the circle and all the details of the movement. This is a difficult movement and is learned in a gradual pace. Later, the movement is executed without pauses in a smooth, flowing two measures, then to one measure and, finally, in 1/4 of a measure.

TEMPS RELEVÉ

This movement has a large and a small form and is a prerequisite to the execution of large and small pirouettes. The movement is practiced at first as an elementary movement without turning and joins other exercises. The small form of temps relevé may be combined with battement fondu, battement frappé, rond de jambe en l'air, and petits battements sur le cou-de-pied. The large form may be combined with battement développé. Later, it is combined with pirouettes en dehors and en dedans.

---

43   Petit temps relevé

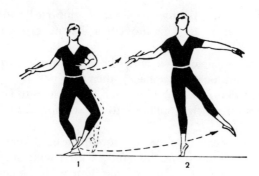

PETIT TEMPS RELEVÉ

The movement starts in Fifth Position with the front foot in sur le cou-de-pied position and the supporting leg in demi-plié. The working leg then opens from the sur le cou-de-pied position to Second Position with fully stretched instep and toes at 45 degrees, as the supporting leg rises from demi-plié to demi-pointe.

The arm moves from the Preparatory Position to First Position during the change from the starting Fifth Position to the sur le cou-de-pied. At the moment the working foot transfers to Second Position, the arm opens into Second Position. The torso and head are kept straight, en face.

The movement is then reversed. The working leg moves from Fifth Position back to sur le cou-de-pied back, then on to Second Position with fully stretched instep and toes. The arms, head and torso are added as above. (See illustration #43.)

The temps relevé is performed in a sharp rhythm, with the upper leg, knee to hip-thigh portion, kept immovable as the portion of the leg from knee to foot moves back and forth to the ankle and Second Position without bringing the hip into motion in any way. This rule is obligatory for the performance of pirouettes or tours beginning on one leg. The position supports stability and accuracy during turns.

In executing temps relevé with a small pirouette, another element is introduced. The transfer to Second Position is done in demi-plié somewhat deeper in size to practice a more clear and energetic transfer for the turn.

This form is learned at first at the barre, very slowly and without a turn. It is then practiced together with battement fondu. In that case, the temps relevé does not begin in Fifth Position, but in sur le cou-de-pied. For instance: Three battements fondus may be done and one temps relevé to 2/4. Each battement requires one measure with 1/4 falling on the demi-plié position before the temps relevé, and the next 1/4 on the transfer into Second Position. When that form is mastered, it may be combined with other movements and with small pirouettes.

---

44   Grand temps relevé

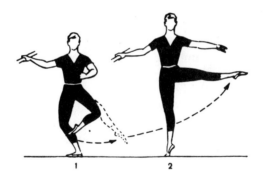

GRAND TEMPS RELEVÉ

The grand temps relevé is executed according to the same plan as the petit temps relevé, but instead of beginning in the sur le cou-de-pied position, it is kept at the knee. The supporting leg, at the same time, is in demi-plié. The working leg from the position at the knee is then thrown in an arc (made by the instep and toes of the working foot) into Second Position as the supporting leg rises to demi-pointe. This exercise must be repeated and reversed (behind the knee). The rhythm is 4/4. The first 1/4 count is for the placement of the working foot to the knee; and the next 1/4 count for the transfer to Second Position; with one count of 1/4 to remain fixed in this position; and the last 1/4 to lower into the starting position. (See illustration #44.)

When large tours are performed in Second Position by means of the grand temps relevé, no additions are introduced as in the small form.

45   Flic-flac

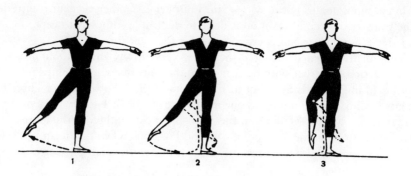

1   2   3

FLIC-FLAC

The movement is not done separately as a movement but serves as a connecting link or auxiliary movement combined with battement tendu, battement frappé, battement fondu, rond de jambe en l'air, and others.

It begins from an open Second Position at 45 degrees. The working leg then lowers, quickly brushing the floor with the toes through Fifth Position in back of the supporting leg. This is done with a light bend of the knee slightly deeper in size than usual. The working leg then moves just as quickly through sur le cou-de-pied (coupé) back and opens toward Second Position with the same brushing of the toes along the floor in front of the supporting leg, as the supporting leg does a demi-plié into relevé as the working leg moves to Second Position. This direction is called en dehors for the flic-flac movement. (The name of the movement is thought to come from the two sounds of the toes slapping against the floor in almost the same rhythm as the name is pronounced.)

Flic-flac en dedans is done in the same form except the first brush through Fifth Position is done in front of the supporting leg, the second brush, in back. (See illustration #45.)

This is the basic form of flic-flac and, as given, may begin at 90 degrees and finish in a large pose by means of a développé.

As a whole, the flic-flac is done in one tempo with a clear and light movement of the leg.

The arms may remain in Second Position, lower into Preparatory Position, or move into any given pose.

Care must be taken to see that the brush is strong, with a taut foot that is not strained. But the brush must not be made too strongly behind the supporting leg, lest the turnout be lost. Laxness in rising to demi-pointe must also be corrected.

The movement should be studied separately, first with the leg thrown to the side at 45 degrees; then a flic backward; a throw to Second; and the flac forward.

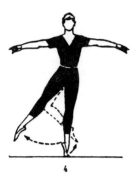

This should be repeated four times to a 2/4 count. The working leg is opened to Second Position before the measure with all other parts taking 1/4 count each.

When the movement has been mastered, including the correct passing through the sur le cou-de-pied (coupé) in Second Position, flic-flac may be done in a slower tempo without the relevé to demi-pointe. After that, the relevé may be added to demi-pointe, increasing the tempo to normal and joining the movement with different battements.

POSITIONS OF THE ARMS

There are three positions of the arms in classical dance. (See illustration #46.) (In the French School the bras au repos is the same position with only a slight repositioning of the hands as the Preparatory Position of the Russian School. The First and Second positions of the French School are the same as the Russian School. The French School has a Third, Fourth and Fifth Position, which are variations on the three basic positions of the Russian School.

(The Cecchetti Method includes a First Position which is the same as the Russian Preparatory Position and a Second Position which is the same as well. The Cecchetti Method then continues with a Demi-Second, a Third, two Fourth and three Fifth positions.)

Later, when port de bras is studied, these positions will appear in various combinations. Choreography allows for a still greater variety of arm and hand positions created by the ballet master (choreographer), but the three positions remain the basis of their movement in space.

The rules of the arm positions are as follows:

In First Position, the arms are rounded at the elbow and wrist with the fingers almost touching. The height is at the level of the diaphragm and the palms of the hands are turned toward the body.

46 Preparatory, First, Second and Third positions of the arms

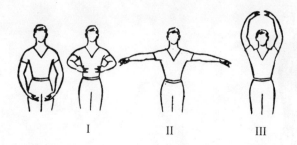

I   II   III

In Second Position, the arms are slightly rounded at the elbow and wrist and are opened to the side and slightly in front of the body. The level is somewhat lower than the line of the shoulders and the palms are turned to face forward.

In Third Position, both arms form an oval and are overhead, slightly in front of the head. The fingers almost touch and the palms face downward. The elbow and wrist are slightly rounded.

The distance between the fingers of one hand to the other in First and Third positions must be minimal.

The arms in position must retain the rounded elbow, wrist and fingers. Angularity in the elbows or flabbiness in the wrists are not permissible. The fingers must be free and unstrained, grouped softly as if following the roundness of the elbows and wrists.

At the beginning of the study, the thumb and middle fingertips lightly touch. The other fingers are less rounded and are somewhat separated from them. (See illustration #47.)

Later, the finger positions elongate with the middle and fourth fingers less rounded so the hand may achieve a more finished grouping. (See illustration #48.) The arms usually begin an exercise in Preparatory Position (see illustration #46), which is freely lowered to the thigh, not touching the body yet not too far from it. The elbow and wrist are softly rounded and the palms face upward. In the First and Second positions the arms must not go higher than the shoulder line, and in Third Position the arms must not go too far forward or backward, but remain in front of the body. The torso is pulled up when assuming these positions and the shoulders are free, lowered and open. The head is straight, en face. The eyes are forward and the neck easy and unstrained.

47-48 Position of the hand in grouped position and elongated (right)

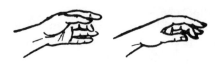

The study of the correct placement of the arms is begun in the center of the floor with the feet in a semi-turned-out First Position. First, the Preparatory Position and the grouping of the fingers are learned. Then, the First and Third positions by changing the arms from Preparatory to First then Third positions and back to the Preparatory Position. Roundness must be maintained through the transitions.

These transfers are performed slowly to eight measures of 3/4 tempo. This tempo corresponds to the character of smoothness suitable to the movement of the arms. One measure is used for the smooth transfer from Preparatory to First Position; one measure for a pause in that position; one measure to raise the arms to Third Position; pause; one measure to return to First; pause; return to Preparatory Position; pause. Repeat this exercise four times.

In the study of Second Position, the arms begin in Preparatory Position, then move into First Position; then into Second Position and lower again into the starting position. The roundness of the arms is increased in the move from the starting position to the First Position and care must be taken to see that the elbows, wrists and hands are correctly placed.

In the move from First to Second Position, the hands gradually open a little and the elbows straighten a bit. With the return to Preparatory Position, the palms turn down, the fingers straighten slightly *led by the wrist in a slight movement* to the Preparatory Position. The elbows, when the arms are lowered into the starting position, straighten a bit but not entirely, and bend again with the movement into First Position.

This exercise is also performed in eight measures of 3/4 tempo with the same pauses, but with two measures of holding the arms in Second Position. At the first of the two measures in Second Position, the hands turn smoothly to palms down and in the next measure are held in that position. The arms then continue in the pattern four times.

When this exercise has been mastered in the center of the floor, it is included with head movements as a preparation or as a component of exercises given at the barre.

When the movements are used at the barre, the head, at the start, turns from the barre to the right shoulder. The head turns, when the arms change from Preparatory to First Position, slightly bends toward the left shoulder with the eyes on the hand; when the hand moves from First to Second Position, the head rises and turns toward the right following the hand with the eyes.

At the return to the Preparatory Position, the head leans slightly forward, eyes following the hand, and takes the starting position.

All movements of the head and arms in this exercise must be closely coordinated with a clear and definite direction and focus.

When this exercise is learned at the barre, it may be transferred for use before exercises in the center of the floor. And later, when the student begins the study of port de bras, the head and arm movements must develop a more definite flexible aplomb.

PORT DE BRAS

The port de bras is an incorporated component of all movements of classical dance and, on stage, its variety is limitless. In teaching practice there are six firmly established forms of port de bras movements. The basic element of the six ports de bras is the changing of the arms in a specific sequence which includes the use of head movements and maintaining the alignment of the body. The sequence introduces the use of épaulement, combinations of different positions of the arms, bending and turning the body.

---

49 The épaulement position

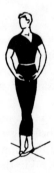

In all the port de bras movements, the head, arms and body must join smoothly in a clear, undeliberate, unstressful effect. The forms must be performed exactly, but freely and naturally. At a future time this exactness will allow the student to creatively form his dance image without mechanical gestures.

It must be remembered that all the basic rules of study and performance of the position of the arms, legs, head and trunk are to be preserved in their entirety.

The épaulement is studied before it is incorporated into the port de bras forms. The pupil stands in Fifth Position croisé, with the arms in Preparatory Position, the head turned to the shoulder directed diagonally forward. (See illustration #49. The body is facing corner 8 with the head turned toward corner 2, or facing corner 2 with the head turned toward corner 8.) The use of épaulement will give the dancer accuracy as well as aplomb. Inaccuracy in use of the shoulders, the head, or direction of the look prevents the formation of this finished image.

FIRST PORT DE BRAS

(The French and Cecchetti systems each have forms of port de bras too extensive to mention here.)

Beginning in Fifth Position with the right leg in front, épaulement croisé, the arms rise from Preparatory Position into First Position. Then they move into Third Position and open into Second Position, finally returning to Preparatory Position. The head moves from the épaulement position when the arms move to First, to face the hand and lean slightly to the left. The eyes follow the hands. When the arms change from First to Third Position, the head lifts and the eyes raise to the hands as well. When the arms move from Third to Second Position, the head turns toward the right and remains to the right when the arms return to the Preparatory Position. (See illustration #50.) In performing the first port de bras, the legs must be kept firmly in Fifth Position with the knees and hips straight and immovable. The arms move in a soft, rhythmic, exact and free manner. The body is kept straight with the shoulders freely lowered and open. The

---

50 First port de bras

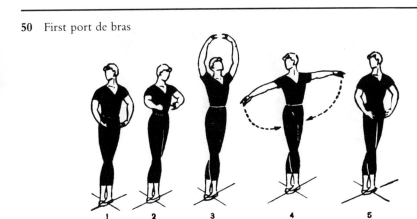

head stays, turns, and bends lightly in rhythm with the arms. The eyes look with assurance at the hands. It is inadmissible to peek in the mirror. The student must look straight and openly in the direction of the head. This first port de bras is studied to eight measures in 3/4 quiet waltz tempo. Each change of arms is done to one measure, and each pause after the position has been reached is also performed to one measure. Later, the movements are performed more flowingly to four measures of 3/4 tempo. This first port de bras as well as all the others should be repeated four times when studied.

SECOND PORT DE BRAS

The second port de bras begins in Fifth Position, épaulement croisé, right leg front. The arms rise from Preparatory Position to First Position with the head inclined slightly toward the left and the eyes directed to the hands. The left arm is raised to Third Position and the right arm to Second Position, as the head turns to the right with the eyes following the right hand. This is the preparation for the form.

The left arm opens to Second Position at the same time that the right arm is raised to Third Position. The head turns toward the left arm and the eyes follow the hand. The left arm is then lowered through the Preparatory Position and raised to First Position. At this moment the head turns to the right and the eyes look toward the right arm about elbow level. The right arm has remained in Third Position during the movement of the left arm. The right arm then lowers to meet the left in First Position and the head straightens and the eyes are transferred to the hands. The form then continues with the left arm moving to Third as the right moves to Second, etc. (See illustration #51.)

---

51   Second port de bras

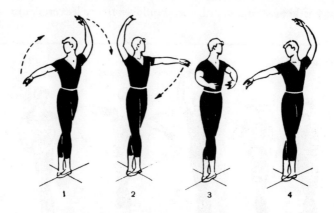

The second port de bras is ended by changing the left arm from Third Position into Second, followed by a lowering of both arms into Preparatory Position. The torso is kept straight while the head turns toward the left arm moving from Third to Second, and leans forward a bit at the Preparatory Position, finishing with a turn to the right shoulder (épaulement).

During the execution of this form, the legs must meticulously keep the Fifth Position, with stability in the knees and hips. The arms should move freely and in exact patterns according to the rules studied in the movement of the arms. The torso stays straight and unswerving during the movement of the head and arms. When one arm remains in the Preparatory Position and the other moves into Third Position, the trunk leans a bit forward, then straightens and remains erect. In general, the torso in port de bras movements cannot remain uninvolved but must "feel" the pattern of the head and arms. There must be an interaction in evidence, a connection in the body of the movement of the upper torso. Although this involvement is *barely noticeable,* it is essential in developing flexibility in dance. At this stage of learning, however, this involvement must not be permitted until an artistic nuance can be introduced into a movement which has been thoroughly mastered in form and tempo.

If too much "feel" is permitted at too early a stage, the pupil is apt to make a habit of dilettantish movement of the body and affect deliberateness, thus violating a sense of moderation. The head must move with assurance and the look should be open.

This form is studied to four measures of 3/4 tempo. The preparation is done in two measures. The first measure accompanies the left arm's move from Third into Second; the right arm's move from Second into Third uses the second measure of the music; the third measure is a rest; and during the fourth measure the arms return through First Position and on into the starting position. The movement is repeated.

---

52   Third port de bras

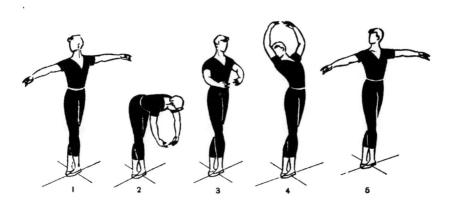

The form ends in two finishing measures. The left moves from Third into Second in the first measure; both arms lower into preparatory movement during the second measure. Later, the form is performed without pause or rest in two measures of 3/4 tempo. After these two forms are learned, the pupil may be taught the third port de bras, which includes bending the torso.

THIRD PORT DE BRAS

The third port de bras begins in Fifth Position, right foot forward, épaulement croisé. The *preparation* for this form begins by raising the arms from Preparatory Position through First Position and on into Second Position. The torso is straight and the head in First Position faces the hands. When the arms open into Second, the head turns to the right shoulder. After this preparation the third port de bras begins by lowering the arms into Preparatory Position and at the same time the torso bends forward to a right angle. Then the arms rise to First Position as the body straightens and continues to Third Position. The arms remain fixed in Third as the torso bends back. When the torso returns to its upright position, the arms open at the same time into Second. The head inclines with the body and the eyes remain on the hands overhead. When the body returns to an upright position, the head turns to the right shoulder. The head, during the inclining of the body and its return to the starting position, remains in the same ratio to the arms. (See illustration #52.) This port de bras finishes with the arm lowering into Preparation Position, the torso in an upright position and the head turned to the right. The new element in this port de bras, the bending of the body, must be done smoothly, with freely lowered and open shoulders, with the exact position of the arms and head remaining fixed. The bending forward begins in the lumbar vertebrae, not from the hips. The back must not be rounded, but remain at a right angle to the trunk and the shoulders must not be lifted. The chin should not be jutted forward nor squeezed back into the neck. (The head and neck are connected as one straight line from the back of the waist to the tip of the head.) The return should be a smooth movement of the body and head.

Bending backward should begin with an incline of the shoulders, then include all the vertebrae, not only the lumbar region, preserving the shapeliness of the body in a smooth curve. The head and neck are free, not strained (and remain in the same position until the body is erect).

When the body bends forward, the arms lower into Preparatory Position and remain fixed during the movement forward. As the body straightens, the arms rise to First and then continue without stopping to Third Position.

During the incline backward, the arms remain in the Third Position without going behind the line of the shoulders. They make a smooth transition to Second Position. During the preparation, and at the finish of the form, the arms follow the rules as prescribed.

The third port de bras is studied in a slow eight measures of 3/4 tempo. The first two measures of introduction music accompany the movement from Preparatory Position to First Position; from First to Second Position. The body bends forward during the next two measures; and returns during the next two measures. The incline backward and return is done in the same tempo using the same number of measures as the forward bending.

Later, the form is performed in four measures and in the higher levels, in two measures of 3/4 and 2/4 tempos. This form is studied first with one hand on the barre. Only the bending forward is executed and the return to the starting position. The legs are in First Position. The arm movements and the head movements from Second to Preparatory Position are followed but after continuing to the First Position the arm moves to *Second* instead of moving into Third Position. The head bends with the body, and the eyes follow the hand to Second.

The incline backward follows after the forward bending has been correctly mastered. Since it is more difficult, it is learned at first facing the barre and holding it with both hands. The tempo is 3/4 and eight measures are used as follows: two measures are used for bending backward; two for rest; two to return; and two measures to rest.

The movement is then studied with one hand on the barre with the free arm moving into the Preparatory Position during the forward bend; moving to First and rising to Third during the bend backward. When the body returns, the arm moves from Third into Second. The head turns toward the raised arm and remains until the body returns to the erect position. When the movement is mastered with the legs in First Position, it is performed with the legs in Fifth Position.

The form is then taught in reverse. Before the body bends forward, the arms rise from Second into Third. During the bend forward, they lower into Preparatory Position. At the straightening of the body, the arms move into Second and together with the backward bend, rise into Third. When the body straightens from the backward bend, the arms move through First into Second. The head turns toward the right arm and the eyes follow the hand, but during the backbend, the head turns toward the raised arms.

---

53 Fourth port de bras

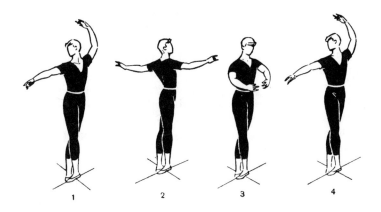

1   2   3   4

FOURTH PORT DE BRAS

The fourth port de bras begins in Fifth Position, épaulement croisé with the right foot forward. The preparation begins with the arms rising into First Position, with the left arm moving into Third and the right arm into Second Position. The torso is straight, the head turned toward the right shoulder. After this preparation, the fourth port de bras begins with the left arm moving from Third into Second as the right arm remains in Second. Both palms are down. The torso twists to the left and bends slightly back. The arms then join in First Position as the left arm goes through Preparatory Position to join the right in First Position. The left in Third, right in Second positions are assumed again to begin the form once more. The torso remains straight throughout. The head moves toward the left arm from Third into Second facing the hand. As the torso twists to the left, the head turns toward the right shoulder and leans a bit in the same direction. When the arms join in First, the head turns toward the hands and leans a bit to the left. At the move of the left arm into Third and the right into Second, the head returns to the starting position. (See illustration #53.)

The fourth port de bras is finished with a lowering of the left arm from Third Position to Second, and both arms from Second into Preparatory Position. The body is kept straight while the head turns toward the left arm. When it is lowered from Third into Second, and at the return of both arms into the Preparatory Position, the head leans slightly forward and, straightening, turns to the right shoulder.

In performing the fourth form, the Fifth Position is kept very tight with the knees and hips pulled up. The body returns at the waist and does not involve the hips. The arms turn with the body with somewhat softened elbows, the shoulders are freely lowered and open. The right and left shoulders must move evenly with the back kept shapely and flexible. The return of the upper torso to the starting position must be supple, and the release of the muscles of the legs and hips after the return to the starting position *a gradual loosening*. The form is studied in four measures of 3/4 tempo. The first two introductory measures are used for the preparation; the next two measures are used for the turn of the body to the left and the corresponding movement of the arms; the third measure is used for the joining of the arms in First and the return of the body to the starting position; in the fourth measure, the arms assume the starting position.

In order to prepare the body for the introduction of the new element—the twist of the upper torso along the vertical axis—the following exercise is recommended in eight measures of 3/4 tempo: standing in First Position, en face, in the center of the floor, the arms move from Preparatory Position into First Position during the first measure; continue to move to Third Position during the second measure; the upper torso turns to the right to its limit during the third measure; returns to the en face position during the fourth measure; turns to the limit to the left during the fifth measure; torso returns to the en face position during the sixth measure; the arms move into Second Position during the seventh measure; and during the last and eighth measure, the arms end in Preparatory Position.

The head, at each turn, moves to the shoulder moving forward and returns to en face on each return. The exercise may also begin with the first turn toward the left and be reversed in the following movements.

FIFTH PORT DE BRAS

The fifth port de bras begins in Fifth Position, épaulement croisé, with the right foot in front. The preparation for the fifth port de bras is as follows: The arms move from the Preparatory Position to First and the right arm goes into Second Position and the left into Third. The body remains straight. The head turns toward the right shoulder. The fifth port de bras is then ready to begin. The upper body leans forward at the same time as the left arm moves into First and the right, through Preparatory Position, joins the left arm. The body straightens with a light, rounded leaning to the left as the arms stay in First. Then the body, which has straightened, begins to lean back at the same time that the right arm rises into Third and the left arm opens into Second Position. The bending continues as the right arm moves to Second and the left arm to Third. Finally, the body straightens as the arms remain in the last position.

Before bending forward, the head lifts a bit, turns without strain to the left arm, eyes to the hand. During the inclining forward, the eyes follow the movement of the left hand. When the body returns to an upright position, the head is slightly inclined toward the left and moves to face the hand when the arms are in First Position. When the body inclines backward, the head turns toward the left shoulder and at the final movement of the arms—the right into Second, the left into Third— the head turns to the right shoulder and stays until the final return to the upright position. (See illustration #54.)

---

54   Fifth port de bras

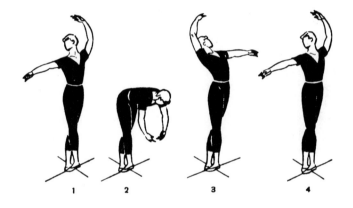

The fifth port de bras is finished by moving the left arm from Third into Second, and both arms from Second into Preparatory Position. The head leans slightly forward and ends with a turn to the right shoulder. The body is kept erect during this final movement.

During the fifth port de bras the body must be kept in a strict Fifth Position with pulled-up knees and hips. The arms must move with ease in a single consistent tempo with the head and body. The torso bends as in the third port de bras from the lumbar vertebrae, with no rounding of the back or lifting of the shoulders. The chin must not be squeezed inward or jutted forward, and the head must not lag behind in coordination with the other portions of the body. The torso must bend backward as much as possible using all the vertebrae of the upper body. In turning the torso to the side, the shoulders should move equally in the same direction and in an even tempo. The neck should show no signs of strain in any of the bending.

The fifth port de bras is studied slowly in eight measures of 3/4 tempo, then in 4/4 tempo. At first, two measures are used for each bending and returning. When the 4/4 tempo is the accompaniment, each movement is done in one measure. In the higher levels, the form may be performed even faster to two measures of 3/4 or one measure of 4/4 or 6/8 tempo.

Before the study of the fifth form, it is useful to learn additional exercises to prepare the turns to the side by the torso. As the student stands en face in the center floor with the legs in First Position, the arms move from Preparatory Position through First to Second Position. The body is held erect. As the arms rise to First, the head leans a bit to the left, eyes on the hands. When the arms open to Second, the head turns toward the right shoulder. The upper torso then twists to the right as the left arm rises into Third Position while the right arm stays in Second. All the movements are then executed to the other side. The head turns in the direction of the twist and, at the return to the erect en face position, the head turns toward the opening arm, eyes following the hand.

This port de bras is ended with a lowering of the arms from Second to Preparatory Position. The body is held straight; the head turns en face. This form is executed with taut knees and hips and a firm First Position of the legs. The twists to the side must be without a lean forward or backward, with a straight back and lowered shoulders. The arm in Second must not move lower than necessary to maintain a horizontal position with the torso. The position of the arms throughout must be preserved in relation to the body even when the torso is bending. The head, as well as the arms, must keep to the prescribed positions without deviation.

The preliminary fifth form is learned slowly, to eight measures of 3/4 tempo. Two measures for the twist to the right; two measures to return; etc. to the other side. Then this preliminary exercise to fifth port de bras is performed in four measures with each twist and return performed in two measures.

When the form is properly learned, the sixth and last port de bras should be studied.

SIXTH PORT DE BRAS

The sixth port de bras is a complicated form with a deep inclination forward. It begins with a preparation: On the first measure or introductory chord, the legs in Fifth Position, épaulement croisé, bend in demi-plié. The right leg moves forward in the direction of the croisé and slides with the toes along the floor while the left leg remains in demi-plié. The arms rise to First Position from Preparatory Position as the head inclines slightly to the left, eyes on the hands. During the second measure or chord, the center of gravity is shifted to the right leg passing through demi-plié in Fourth Position to the croisé derrière (left leg back with stretched foot, and toes on the floor). During this lunge, the left arm rises to Third and the right to Second Position as the head turns to the right and the eyes follow the right hand.

The sixth port de bras begins after this preparation on the "and" count or upbeat with a turn of the head so the eyes may focus on the left hand. The right leg lunges to its utmost point in demi-plié Fourth Position forward as the left toe and its stretched instep remain on the floor in an extended croisé back. The torso moves *in a straight line of the back,* toward the front supporting leg as the left arm remains in Third Position and the right remains in Second. The eyes follow the left hand. When the body has reached its maximum extent in the lowering to the deep demi-plié position, the left arm lowers from Third to First and the right arm moves through Preparatory Position to meet the left arm in First Position.

Then, the straight back and pulled-up center portion of the body with the help of a strong push from the supporting right leg pushes the weight back onto the whole foot of the stretched left leg as the right leg straightens. Toes of both feet remain on the floor. The right leg remains in a tendu position, croisé devant, with the instep and toes stretched. The arms remain in First as the head inclines toward the left shoulder and the eyes are focused on the hands. The torso then bends backward, slightly turning back at the left shoulder. Hips remain in a fixed position. Simultaneously, at the bending backward, the left arm moves to Second Position and the right arm is raised to Third as the head turns to the left, eyes toward the left hand. The torso continues to bend backward as far as possible as the left arm transfers to Third and the right arm opens to Second. The head turns to the right and the eyes follow the right hand.

---

55   Sixth port de bras

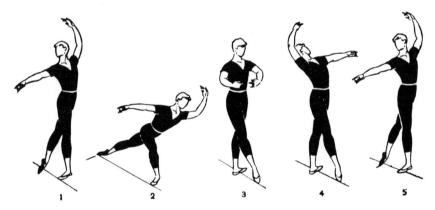

1   2   3   4   5

The sixth port de bras ends with a straightening of the body as the weight is transferred from the left leg to the right passing through a small demi-plié in Fourth Position to the tendu croisé derrière, which was the starting position. (See illustration #55.)

This form should be flowing, light and in tempo throughout. The body should show no sign of strain and move surely without striving for effect. As a whole, the sixth form is done in the character of the music and the teaching example in which it is included.

The study is, at first, to eight slow measures of 3/4 and later to 4/4 tempo. The first two measures are used for the preparation; the next two measures for the soft lunge forward; two for the return and backward bend; two for the return to the erect position; and two measures for the return to the starting position.

The sixth form ends with two final chords of music.

THE SIXTH PORT DE BRAS AS A PREPARATION FOR GRAND PIROUETTE

The sixth form is often used as a preparation for the grand pirouette. For tours en dedans, instead of the final change, a tombé forward to Fourth Position on the right leg is made. The left knee is stretched with the foot pressed strongly on the floor. The right arm moves from Third in a rounded arc through Second and Preparatory Position to First as the left arm remains in Second Position. (The turn will be clockwise, to the right, from this preparation.)

The preparation for a tour en dehors is the same except that the left arm moves from Second through Third into First as the right arm opens into Second. (The turn will be counterclockwise, or to the left from this preparation. When the legs and the arms are reversed, the turns will be en dedans or to the left, and en dehors, to the right from the preparation.)

This preparation is finished by stretching the fingers, allongé (extended), palms down.

All the forms of port de bras in various portions are used in all the teaching sections of classical dance up to the jumps. A wide, free and expressive gesture in the use of the arms depends upon the proper technical and artistic exercise of all of the forms of port de bras. The sixth form is especially important.

PART THREE

POSES
AND
DANCE STEPS

The poses in classical dance are performed in a definite, strict and established design in space and are composed with various positions of the head, arms, torso and legs.

First, it must be explained that in the poses of classical dance the turning and bending of the head is related to the movements of the other parts of the body. The movement of the head in everyday life is usually motivated by a desire to see or not see, to hear or not hear, the object that has attracted one's attention. In classical dance, each position of the head is defined by the rules for the dancer's body in space, but that does not mean that each prescribed position of the head is merely a dead rule. It is a flexible base, when mastered, upon which to create an image.

In the poses of classical dance, as in life, a leading role belongs to the use of the head, especially to the direction of looking. It is one's look that most fully bares the inner life of the stage image the dancer creates. Whether the dancer's look is turned to his partner or he seems to be looking inside himself to his thoughts, to the audience it is always the indication of the inner life of the character.

No matter how coordinated the movement of the head and body, if the look does not correspond to the position and intention of the pose, the result will not be finished and expressive.

Just as the look plays an important role in the use of the head, so the arms play as important a role in the dance gesture. In classical dance the entire arm, from shoulder to the ends of the fingers, is active. The shoulders, elbows, forearms, wrists, hands and fingers are united as a dancing gesture, especially when the allongé position is used. But it is the hand, like the look, that gives the gesture its necessary sense and supple completion.

The torso, in the poses, is active and has its own peculiarities. If it is the look that defines the movement of the head and the hands that define the movement of the arms, it is the use of the shoulders that becomes the most expressive portion of the movement of the body.

Insufficiently strong use of the arms and head added to a weak use of épaulement cannot create a properly expressive and purposeful image. In general, the use of the shoulders is involved as long as the dancer continues to express his feelings and desires through the pose.

In everyday life, man advances in a walking movement. It follows that the action of the legs in classical dance be seen as a fixed, yet passing step or walk. To look upon this movement as a technical effect and not an organic characteristic of man's movement would be an error.

In classical dance, both legs take an active part, including the hip, knee, ankle, instep and toes underlining the direction of the advancing movement of the entire figure of the dancer.

The supporting leg, in a demi-plié or relevé to demi-pointe, gives the figure the character of advancing. The most notable part of the leg belongs to the foot, which gives a supple completion to the working leg. If the foot of the dancer is not well enough "educated" in the technique of movement, the pose will not have the finesse and finish of its choreographic design. An undeveloped instep, insufficiently stretched toes and flabbiness in the use of the ankle, give the entire leg, and therefore the entire pose, technical and artistic incompleteness.

Both legs must, of course, be turned out and the knee and hip held in correct alignment. But if the foot is not disciplined in its movement, the work will be incomplete and inexpressive.

What, then, is the interdependence of movement of all parts of the body in classical dance? It is clear that the movement of the upper and lower portions of the dancer's body are different, but that they are united in direction. It is important, therefore, in teaching, to understand the correct construction of the poses, as well as the feelings inherent in dance, in order to move the figure as a whole.

The poses accepted by the school of classical dance, are divided into small, medium and large forms, which are performed arrondie or allongée.

The first form, arrondie, provides rounded lines in the arm, elbow, wrist and fingers. The second form, allongée, provides a pulled or elongated line in the arm from elbow to the tips of the fingers. While the first method seems to have a certain static and contained character, the second seems to have dash and flight. The coordination of these two methods brings to classical dance variety and contrast.

SMALL POSES

The study of small poses begins after the elementary positions of the head, arms, body and legs have been mastered. The exercises for the mastery of those movements will help in the performance of the poses.

POSES IN ARRONDIE POSITION

CROISÉE DEVANT

Begin in the Fifth Position, right foot front, épaulement croisé. The arms move from Preparatory Position to First, as the head bends slightly forward and to the left, looking at the hand. At the same time, the right leg moves to croisé forward position as the right arm opens to Second and the left arm rises to Third Position. The body is held straight and the legs are straight and taut. The head turns to the right shoulder with the eyes following the hand, and the torso inclining slightly backward. (See illustration #56.) To end the pose, the left arm opens into Second and, together with the right arm, descends into Preparatory Position. The leg moves at the same time back to Fifth Position.

---

56   Arm positions for croisé devant

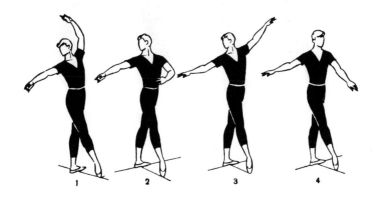

---

57   Arm positions for croisé derrière

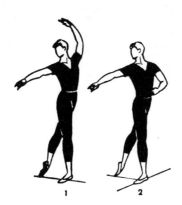

CROISÉE DERRIÈRE

The same rules apply for the movement to the back. (See illustration #57.) (In the Cecchetti method, the same position requires that the arm that is low must be on the same side as the leg that is extended. The body and head incline toward the lowered arm so the dancer looks toward the audience underneath the high arm. In the Russian School, the torso is held erect and the high arm is on the same side as the extended leg to the back. The head is turned and inclined toward the lowered arm. The French School uses the same position as the Russian.)

58   Arm positions for effacé devant (#4 in demi-plié)

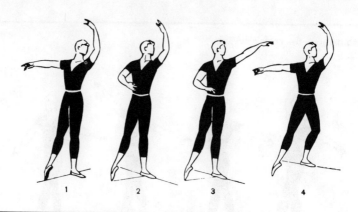

59   Arm positions for effacé derrière

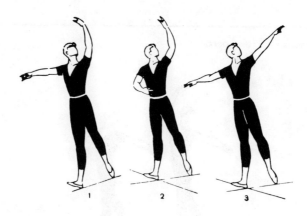

60   Arm positions for écarté devant

61   Arm position for écarté derrière

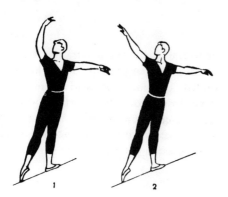

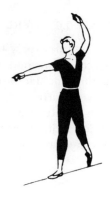

EFFACÉE DEVANT

Begin in Fifth Position, right foot front, épaulement effacé (the hips and right foot face corner 2 and the left shoulder is forward). The arms rise from Preparatory Position into First with the head slightly leaning forward to the right and the eyes on the hands. Then, at the same time, the right leg moves forward and the left arm rises to Third, and the right arm to Second. The body remains lifted but leans a bit away from the open leg. The head turns toward the left shoulder and inclines slightly with the upper torso. (See illustration #58.) (The effacée devant positions are the same in all schools.) To end the pose, the left arm which is in Third Position opens into Second and the body and head straighten. The arms close in Preparatory Position.

EFFACÉE DERRIÈRE

The pose to the back is done in the same way except that the battement tendu leg (the left leg) is opened to the back (corner 6 while the hips stay facing corner 2). The body and head lean very slightly forward over the standing leg. (See illustration #59.) (The French School uses the same pose.)

ÉCARTÉE DEVANT

Beginning in the Fifth Position, right foot front, épaulement croisé, the arms move from Preparatory Position into First. The head leans a bit forward and left, looking at the hands.

At the same time, the right leg moves to battement tendu side (corner 2), as the right arm rises to Third and the left arm rises into Second. The torso is pulled up and leans slightly toward the supporting leg. The head is turned toward the right. (See illustration #60.)

To end the pose, the right arm goes from Third to Second as the body straightens and the arms move into Preparatory Position. (The Cecchetti system uses the same pose, as well as the French School, except the latter leans backward on the supporting leg and looks under the raised arm.)

ÉCARTÉE DERRIÈRE

The pose écartée derrière is the same except the tendu leg points to corner 6 and the head turns toward the open arm in Second. (See illustration #61.) (The French School uses the same position with a pronounced lean toward the open arm in Second.)

All small poses are performed slowly and smoothly in two measures of 4/4 tempo: 1/4 for the hands to rise to First; 1/4 for the extension of the leg on the floor and the transfer of the arms to the pose position; 4/4 for the pose to be held; 1/4 to transfer the arm from Third to Second; 1/4 for the open leg and arms to return to the starting position.

When studying the poses, the working leg must retain the turnout and the body weight must stay on the supporting leg. There should be no pressure on the toes of the working leg. The body and back are pulled up and the shoulders are open and lowered. The fixing of the pose—head, arms, look—must be done boldly, clearly and with aplomb.

It is especially important in practice to maintain the rounded (arrondie) position of the arms, not permitting slackness or sharp, taut lines in elbow, wrist and fingers.

When the poses have been learned, each one separately, they may be combined by means of a dégagé. For instance: While performing the croisée devant, it may be exchanged for croisée derrière and finish in Fifth Position. All the poses may be combined in reverse or interchanged with effacée or écartée positions. The small poses may then be learned with the arms fixed in First or Second positions in this way: the arm corresponding to the moving leg will move to the Second Position; the other arm will move to First. All the other rules must be followed exactly.

POSES IN ALLONGÉE POSITION

Poses done with allongée or arrondie arm positions are the same in construction and will, therefore, not be described again. The differences are seen in the sketches. The poses in arabesque, however, differ in structure and performance and are given full description in text and sketches.

ÉCARTÉE

The pose in écartée, in which the arms are placed—one in First, the other in Second; one in First and the other in Third—are not performed allongée since the line of the arms and the working leg do not coincide or harmonize with the general structure of the given pose. These poses may be done allongée not only from a fixed position but also when the movements of the body, head and arms change position. This movement is the link between the arrondie and the allongée poses and must be done freely, simply and without unnecessary movement of the hands, nor should they be too lax or too elongated at the elbows and fingers. Movements of the head and body must be done with containment, with no superfluous bendings and turns.

The fixing of the pose itself must be strictly academic, exact in design, with a perfect performing technique.

Of course, in stage interpretations, allongée acquires a style and character that is varied according to the directions of the choreographer or performer. But in teaching, depending upon the age and ability of the student, one must undeviatingly maintain the style.

ARABESQUES

FIRST ARABESQUE (PAR TERRE—WITH THE FOOT ON THE FLOOR)

Beginning in Fifth Position, right foot forward in épaulement effacé, the arms rise from Preparatory Position into First. The head bends forward and to the right, the eyes look at the hand. At the same time, the left leg moves to tendu back while the right arm stays in First. The left arm moves into Second as the head straightens and looks to the right hand. At the same time, the elbows smoothly elongate but do not entirely straighten out. The hands turn palms down and the fingers freely elongate. This is the position for the first arabesque. (See illustration #62.) (It is also the first arabesque in the Cecchetti School and arabesque ouverte in the French School.)

The arms then lower into Preparatory Position as the head returns to the starting position. The leg lowers and returns to Fifth Position.

SECOND ARABESQUE (PAR TERRE)

The second arabesque is done according to the same plan except that the First Position is assumed by the left arm and the Second Position by the right arm. The right shoulder moves back as the head turns slightly toward the left shoulder. The eyes follow. (See illustration #63.) The pose closes as in the first arabesque. (The second arabesque is the same in the Cecchetti School. The French School has only one other arabesque, the arabesque croisée, which is the same as the Russian fourth arabesque.)

THIRD ARABESQUE (PAR TERRE)

The third arabesque is done from an épaulement croisé position as in the first arabesque. However, in the third arabesque, both shoulders are kept even and the head and eyes turn toward the left hand. (See illustration #64.) (The Cecchetti School at this point has third, fourth and fifth arabesques which do not resemble the Russian School in any way.)

FOURTH ARABESQUE (PAR TERRE)

The fourth arabesque is done from an épaulement croisé in the manner of the first arabesque with the left shoulder moved back and the body leaning somewhat backward. The head is turned toward the right shoulder and the eyes focus on the hand. (See illustration #65.) The pose closes as the others closed.

When the small poses have been well learned, they may be studied in demi-plié, increasing the degree of the lift of the working leg to 45 degrees. In combining relevé to demi-pointe in these poses, the working leg increases the angle of the leg movement to 25 degrees. (See illustrations #58, #62.)

62   First arabesque par terre and on demi-pointe

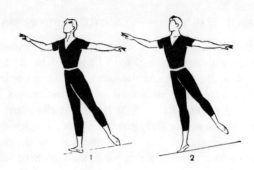

63   Second arabesque par terre and #2 as a big pose on demi-pointe, #3 and #4 approaches to first and second arabesques, #5, an approach from demi-pointe to third and fourth arabesques

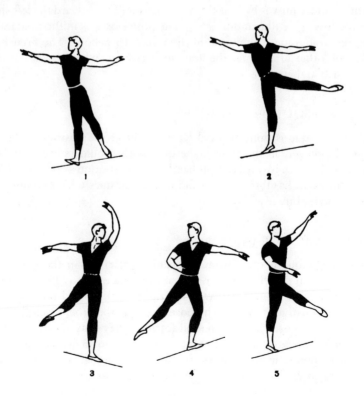

64 Third arabesque par terre

65 Fourth arabesque par terre

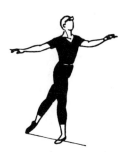

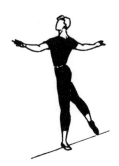

It is recommended that the small poses be studied in the order they have been described. If they have been well learned and impressed emotionally on the student, one may hope that the large poses will also receive a good basis for artistic perfection. Strength and vivid feelings in dance poses arise not from a highly raised leg (45 or 90 degrees or higher) but from the ability to perceive the composition and character of its performance. Therefore, before continuing the study of large poses, it is necessary in all small poses to strengthen the feeling of aplomb and freedom.

MEDIUM POSES

The structure of medium poses differs from small poses in the working leg, which rises to 45 degrees. The entire figure, with this change, acquires a raised and daring character.

The description of medium poses is not given because of their similarity to the small poses. However, several examples illustrating the rules of their performance are given. These too should be studied on the basis of well-mastered elements and not before the small poses have been properly learned.

The raising of the working leg to 45 degrees for the study of medium poses is recommended to begin with the battement relevé lent, then the battement fondu, etc.

All medium poses are studied together with demi-plié at a later time and with relevé to demi-pointe at the barre, then at the center. In performing medium poses, the arms are placed in First and Second positions or in First and Third positions like the small poses. All medium as well as small poses are done with the arms in arrondie and allongée positions. (See illustrations #55, #56, #58, #60, #63.)

BIG POSES

Big poses differ from small and medium poses in the height of the working leg, which is raised to 90 degrees by means of a battement relevé lent or a battement développé jeté. They are performed with more dance and a larger design. A description of the structure of each large pose in arabesque is not described but may be seen in illustrations #66–75. One must remember that the study of large poses cannot be done without the previous elementary work.

The study of big poses with weak legs and an inexact technique is senseless. Because the big poses will be executed at a later time with a turn, in a turn or in jumps, the teacher must prepare the student thoroughly for the study of big poses. Big poses are studied in a similar rhythm to battement relevé lent. The arms rise from Preparatory Position to First, the leg at the same time is moved with the toes along the floor. Then the arm, head and body take positions that correspond to the pose. The leg at the same time rises to 90 degrees and is fixed in a pose. The arms lower into Preparatory Position and the leg lowers and slides along the floor with the toes returning to Fifth Position. The study is begun to two slow measures of 4/4 tempo. One quarter is used to raise the arms to First and for the tendu along the floor to begin; 1/4 is used to transfer the arms into the pose and for the raising of the leg to 90 degrees; 4/4's are used to fix the pose; 1/4 is used to lower the leg and toes to the floor; 1/4 to close the arms and the leg into Fifth Position.

The big poses are then studied by means of the battement développé. All are performed smoothly to two measures of 4/4 from Fifth Position. One quarter is used for the transfer of the working leg from Fifth Position to the sur le cou-de-pied (coupé); 1/4 for the transfer of the leg to the knee position and the raising of the arms to First; 2/4's for the opening of the arms and leg into the big pose; 2/4's to fix the pose; and 2/4's to return the leg and arms to the starting position. Next, the attitude—a large pose with the movement of the partially bent leg in the forward or back position at 90 degrees in croisé or effacé—is studied.

ATTITUDE CROISÉE

Beginning in the Fifth Position, right foot front in épaulement croisé, the arms rise to First Position from the Preparatory Position. The head moves slightly forward and to the left and the eyes are focused on the hands. *At the same time,* the left leg rises from Fifth in back to the sur le cou-de-pied position and transfers to the back of the knee. The right arm then goes to Second, and the left to Third. The head turns to the right shoulder, and the eyes follow the right hand. The leg, together with the movement of the arms, rises to 90 degrees at a right angle to the body. (See illustration #76.) (The thigh is kept turned out and the knee and toes are in horizontal alignment, and the position from hip to toes is a right angle.)

66 Grand battement croisé devant with arm positions

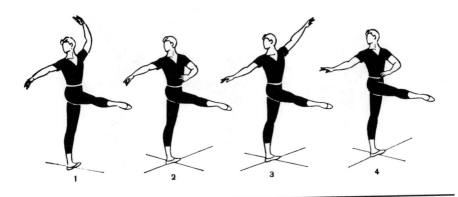

67 Grand battement croisé derrière with arm positions

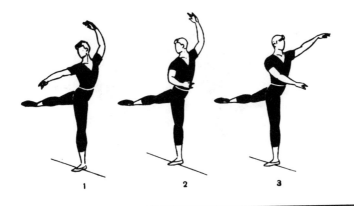

68 Grand battement effacé devant with arm positions, #3 in demi-plié

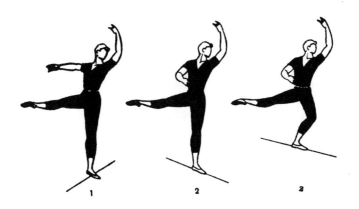

69 Grand battement effacé derrière with arm positions

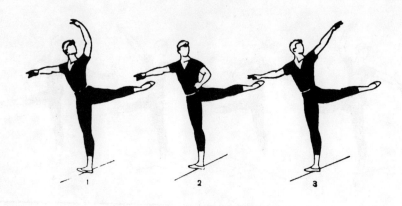

70 Grand battement écarté with rounded and allongé arms

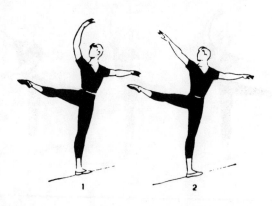

71 Grand battement écarté derrière

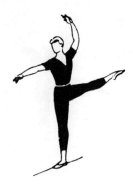

The left arm moves from Third to Second, the raised left leg is stretched at the height of 90 degrees to the back and finally both arms and leg return to the starting position. (The Cecchetti system requires that the head and body remain erect with the eyes focused on corner 8 and is called attitude croisée derrière.)

The study of attitude is done to two measures of 4/4: 1/4 for the transfer of the arms into First and the raising of the leg in back to the knee; 2/4's for the transfer of the left arm into Second and the right to Third as the leg rises to 90 degrees; 3/4's for the fixing of the attitude position; 1/4 for the left arm to move to Second as the working leg straightens at 90 degrees back; 1/4 for the arms and leg to return to the starting position.

ATTITUDE EFFACÉE

Attitude effacée is learned in the same manner except that the Fifth Position begins in épaulement effacé (facing corner 2) and the leg raised to 90 degrees is less bent. In its final position, it should form an angle more obtuse than the attitude croisée position. The head, at the same time as the opening of the arms, turns to the left with the eyes focused slightly higher than the left elbow, and the torso leans slightly forward. (See illustration #77.) (In the Cecchetti system, the torso leans slightly backward.)

ATTITUDE CROISÉE DEVANT AND ATTITUDE EFFACÉE DEVANT

These two attitude positions to the front are performed using the same rules, except the partially bent leg is raised forward. (See illustrations #78 and #79.) In view of the difficulties in the performance of these poses, they must be studied first to the back with both hands on the barre. From this position, the working leg rises in back in a relevé lent (tendu raised slowly) until it reaches 90 degrees. Then it bends a little to the obtuse angle. The teacher must see to it that the knee of the working leg is not lowered or moved away from the line of the hip, and that the instep and toes are fully stretched. When this exercise has been learned, the leg may rise to 90 degrees bent at the wide angle, then to a straighter angle. The body moves very slightly forward but does not turn, so the hips remain immovable and fixed. The next exercise in this study is the performance of the movement with one hand on the barre with the free arm moving to Third and the head turning in the same direction. The study is then taken to the center of the floor where attitude croisée in the proper épaulement and attitude effacée in profile position, then diagonal position, are added. Attitude devant is also first studied at the barre with one hand holding and the other in Third Position. The head turns away from the barre slightly forward and the eyes look from underneath the arm.

When the big poses have been mastered, they must be studied with demi-plié and relevé to demi-pointe incorporating the use of pas dégagé and pas tombé. The turnout must be maintained and the body held in the proper position with the shoulder open and lowered (the center portion of the body is pulled in and

72 First arabesque

73 Second arabesque

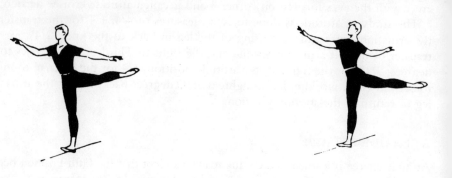

74 Third arabesque

75 Fourth arabesque

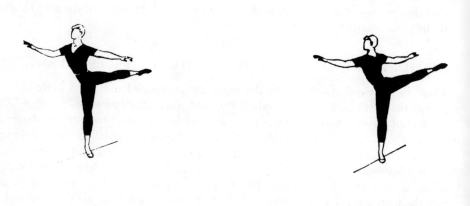

76 Attitude croisée derrière

77 Attitude effacée, #2 on demi-pointe

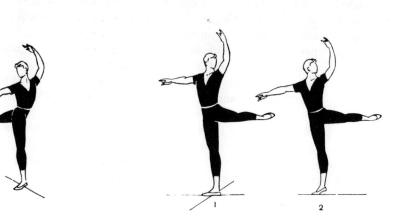

78   Attitude croisée devant

79   Attitude effacée devant

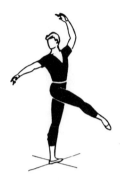

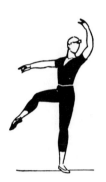

80   Grand battement croisé with same arm and leg raised

81   Attitude croisée derrière with arms in Third Position

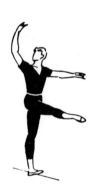

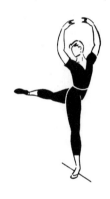

82   Attitude croisée derrière with arms in Third and head inclined to diagonal corner upstage

83   Grand battement croisé in Fourth with arms allongé

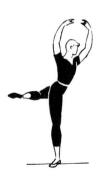

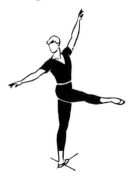

84   Pose in écarté at 90 degrees with arms in second allongé

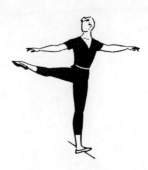

up). The head movement and the fixed position must be assumed clearly and with aplomb, combined with a lively look in the eyes. The elements are brought together in a rhythmic flow with a feeling that ties all the components into the formation of a big pose. As the large, medium and small poses are studied, the basic rules for the positions may be altered for variety. In the basic pose, croisée devant and croisée derrière, the arms in Third and Second might be exchanged. Then the body and head should bend a bit forward and the eyes look underneath the arm, which is in Third. (See illustration #80.) Another variation might be in the use of the arms in First or Third Position with the head and body retaining the same position. (See illustration #81.)

In the poses écartée devant and écartée derrière and the poses effacée devant and effacée derrière, both arms may also be held in the positions described above, keeping the head and body in the same positions. In the écartée position, both arms may be in Third with the body and head in the same position.

In arabesque, both arms may be extended forward, one a bit higher than the other (the Cecchetti third arabesque). The head and shoulders turn slightly to the open leg.

In attitude croisée, effacée devant and effacée derrière, the head and body may also vary from the basic rules. (See illustration #72.)

In addition, all poses and their variations may be done reversed and facing corner 5, upstage, or viewed from the back of the dancer. The use of the pose with its variations must be incorporated with restraint. Do not forget that the rules are the foundation that must be meticulously exercised in classic purity and strictness. (See illustrations #83 and #84.)

DANCE STEPS THAT CONNECT

These steps tie, connect or are considered approaches to other steps. At the same time, they are not secondary. The better the steps in this group are mastered, the better the entire quality of the movement in which these steps will be combined.

PAS DÉGAGÉ

The pas dégagé is from Second or Fourth Position and may start or be included in approaches to small and big poses. The dégagé exists in all movements concerned in the transfer of gravity to the working leg or from both legs to one leg. (Note that the dégagé or pointe tendue is not a transfer of weight but a pointing of the foot in the open position. Tarasov, however, uses the term in its literal sense, to disengage the weight from one center to another.) A description of possible forms of dégagé are as follows:

As the leg moves from Fifth Position into Second or Fourth through the use of a battement tendu, it is followed by a demi-plié with a transfer of the weight to the tendu leg. The battement tendu must be executed according to the rules and the transfer of weight to the opening leg must be a smooth sequence from the toes to the whole foot. The passage through demi-plié must be even, supple and using both legs in a soft movement, and straightening both at the same time.

The arms are clearly fixed in a starting and finishing position. They move softly and together during the demi-plié from one position to the other. The body in demi-plié is supported evenly on both legs and moves in the correct tempo in a stable and pulled-up position. The head turns clearly in rhythm with the change of arms. On the whole, the dégagé is done freely, in one continuous rhythm with no harsh or rough points in the transfer of weight.

The movement must be studied with a pause or a fixing of the demi-plié position to better comprehend the need for it to be even, turned out and flexible.

The dégagé (or transfer) may start from an open leg at 45 or 90 degrees. In this case, the demi-plié is done by the supporting leg. The rise from the demi-plié is done with a wide advance at the moment of transfer to the open leg. The transfer is completed when the open leg accepts the weight by moving through the stretched toes to the whole foot. The use of the arms, head and trunk depends upon the starting and finishing pose. Suppleness in the transfer, a turned-out position and a correct building of the pose must be strictly maintained.

The study of pas dégagé in the center of the floor combines with battement fondu to 45 degrees. The battement fondu is done on demi-pointe in Second Position and the demi-plié is executed by the open leg after it descends. In this study, the pause or fixed position should be when the dégagé is to the side at 45 degrees and the supporting leg in demi-pointe. The same exercise may be performed in croisé devant, in croisé derrière, to the side and reversed.

The tempo is 2/4. In one measure, the battement fondu is begun; in 1/4, the demi-plié is performed on the supporting leg; in 1/4, the pas dégagé is performed (the weight is transferred to the extended foot after it descends to the floor).

The study of pas dégagé may then begin at 90 degrees in adagio movements finishing on the whole foot. For instance: From a large pose at 90 degrees in effacé devant, and by means of a wide step, the dégagé moves the position into a first arabesque at 90 degrees. (See illustration #85).

---

85   Pas dégagé

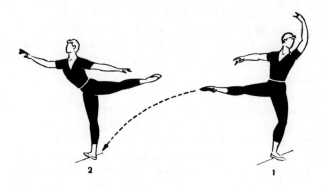

2   1

The study of the dégagé with battement fondu at 90 degrees may then begin as an exercise which was described above at 45 degrees. The pas dégagé begun at 45 degrees may end at 90 degrees, or begin at 90 and end at 45 degrees.

PAS TOMBÉ

The pas tombé is a fall onto the open leg in demi-plié to the Second or Fourth Position. The leg may begin with a battement fondu or battement développé. The tombé is the fall onto the open or working leg which then does a demi-plié as the other leg rises to 45 or 90 degrees or even a quick pull into sur le cou-de-pied. The transfer from one pose to another by means of pas tombé is generally preceded by a relevé to demi-plié on the supporting leg.

The position of the head, body and arms varies at the beginning and end of the movement depending upon the structure of the pose. (See illustration #86.)

In performing pas tombé, the working leg must not be lowered too soon, as the line of advance and its push onto the leg will be shortened. Tombé means fallen, and a shortened movement always gives the transfer an unfinished and flabby look. An exaggerated advance breaks the softness and harmony of the step. The finish on demi-plié should be done softly, lightly and flexibly from the toes to the whole foot. The freed leg rises at the same time as the working foot does the demi-plié. The body, in proper time, leans toward the leg in demi-plié and remains taut and shapely (held in pulled-up manner). The arms and head keep the position of the pose strictly and act in harmony with the transfer of the weight.

The fall and demi-plié portion of the step must be well practiced and felt by the pupils. It may be done slowly or faster, but always in accord with the given tempo.

---

86 Pas tombé from demi-pointe

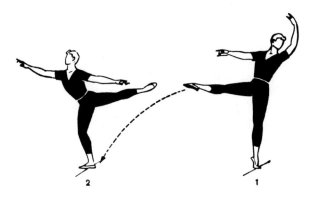

2   1

The study of pas tombé begins at the barre in combination with battement fondu and then with battement relevé lent and finally with battement développé tombé.

It should be noted that many jumps in classical dance—sissonne tombée, temps levé tombé, cabriole tombée—are finished with the pas tombé. Consequently, this movement should be practiced in the center of the floor and only then brought into jump combinations.

Another form of pas tombé may be performed from Fifth Position as an exchange without an advance in space. In this case, the supporting demi-plié rises to demi-pointe as the working leg assumes the sur le cou-de-pied position and opens into 45 degrees energetically. Here too one must strive for suppleness and lightness in the transfer to demi-plié and a clear pose in the starting and finishing positions. The arms, head and body act in this form of pas tombé according to the structure of the beginning and ending pose. The movement just described is studied in combination with pas de bourrée simple and then in combination with battement fondu, battement frappé, rond de jambe en l'air and petit battement sur le cou-de-pied.

87 Pas coupé

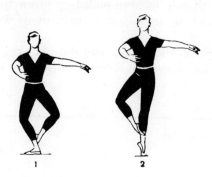

PAS COUPÉ

The pas coupé is done in place (en place) in a quick exchange of weight through the Fifth Position. The starting position is demi-plié on the right foot with the left foot in sur le cou-de-pied position back. At the moment of the exchange, the left foot lifts to a high demi-pointe as the right straightens from demi-plié into a quick rise to sur le cou-de-pied forward. Or, the right leg may straighten as it opens to 45 degrees in Second or Fourth Position. (See illustration #87.) In this way, through the use of pas coupé, the free leg seems to dislodge the supporting leg and stand in its place through the Fifth Position.

The pas coupé may start from an open position of the leg in 45 degrees. It will end in that case with a sur le cou-de-pied in front or in back.

The pas coupé may be done repeatedly without the demi-plié from a high demi-pointe position transferring the free leg to the cou-de-pied position in front or in back. The arms, head and body act in strict accord with the composition of the starting and the finishing pose.

The pas coupé, like the pas tombé, is studied by means of the pas de bourrée, then, as a small addition, is combined with battement frappé, rond de jambe en l'air, petit battement sur le cou-de-pied.

The turnout, a supple demi-plié, resilience in the high demi-pointe and exact position of the sur le cou-de-pied must be clearly maintained as the transfer is made. This applies to all forms of pas coupé. (Coupé is called dessous, or under, when one foot cuts under the heel of the supporting foot, and coupé dessus when it cuts over the toe of the support.)

PAS GLISSÉ (GLIDED)

This step is based upon the pas tombé and consists of an advancing glide in Fourth or Fifth Position. For instance, the pas glissé croisé devant is performed in this way: Demi-plié begins in Fifth Position followed by a relevé to demi-pointe. The working leg moves along the floor with a light gliding movement forward

88 Pas glissé into Fourth

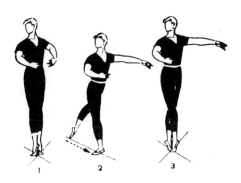

into croisé and smoothly falls into a demi-plié on the whole foot. The leg left in demi-pointe moves with the same light, gliding movement up to the starting leg and onto demi-pointe. The step may be repeated or finished in a demi-plié in Fifth Position.

The arms at the time of the first relevé move from Preparatory Position into a lowered First Position; at the gliding change into demi-plié the arms stay in First, but the arm corresponding to the forward moving leg remains in First and the other arm opens into Second somewhat lowered. The arms remain in the same position if the next movement is the relevé, but if the next movement is the end of the·movement, the arms descend into Preparatory Position.

The body during the first and second relevé is erect and at the glide into demi-plié moves a bit forward to the forward leg. The head turns to the forward elbow. (See illustration #88). In this way, the pas glissé may be performed in all directions and end in small poses.

The pas glissé may be performed only in its first part, the first glide and demi-plié, which ends in an exchange into a large pose in relevé to demi-pointe.

The pas glissé also serves as an approach to small jumps that start from one leg. The arms, head and body are in the corresponding position to the starting leg. In any variation of pas glissé, lightness in the glide, softness in the demi-plié and clarity in the use of the arms, head and body are required. Not to be permitted are a poor turnout, too wide a transfer in demi-plié and a weak, flabby finish pose. The movements must be studied in the center floor, first en face, then in croisé and effacé together with battement tendu.

PAS FAILLI (TO JUST MISS)

This movement is based upon the pas tombé but is done only in Fourth Position. Starting in a small or big pose with the open leg in Fourth front, back, in croisé or effacé, the supporting leg rises to a high demi-pointe. Both legs descend into

89 Pas failli

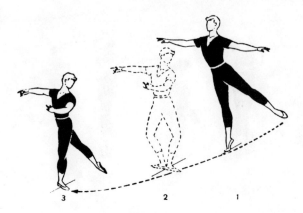

a First Position in demi-plié and on into a Fourth Position forward or backward. The freed leg may remain on the floor or rise to 45 or 90 degrees in any pose in Fourth Position. (See illustration #89.) The transfer of the leg through First is done with a light, gliding movement of the whole foot at the same time as the demi-plié of the starting leg. The pas failli is ended softly with an even deepening of the demi-plié and not too wide a Fourth Position. The head and arms and body must be plastic and move strictly in accord with the pose.

The pas failli may be studied at first forward, back, in the center floor and used as a tie of one pose to another. It may also serve as an approach to large and small pirouettes. (The pas failli with the soaring or quick jump, as it is commonly known, will appear in the section on jumps. This version is an auxiliary step useful in teaching advancing moves.)

PAS DE BOURRÉE

There are a number of varieties of pas de bourrée all based upon a shift from one leg to another by means of a pas coupé or a pas tombé.

Each pas de bourrée must be done on turned-out legs, a clear high demi-pointe and with resiliently stretched legs. The free leg must be just as turned out as the supporting leg and move clearly in sur le cou-de-pied with well-stretched instep and toes and finish in a demi-plié that is soft and elastic.

The study is practiced in a medium tempo with each step and sur le cou-de-pied fixed clearly. In a faster tempo, the pas de bourrée is done together and uninterruptedly.

The use of the head, body and arms will be described in each separate form, but they all should be executed with lightness, exactness and in harmony with the movement of the legs.

90   Pas de bourrée with change of legs

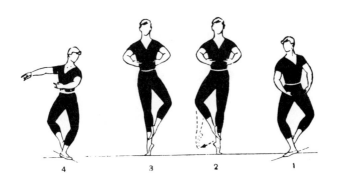

All forms should be studied to a 2/4 or 4/4 tempo. At first, all stepovers are done to each 1/4, then on each 1/8.

PAS DE BOURRÉE WITH A CHANGE OF LEGS (THE LEG WHICH BEGINS FORWARD ENDS IN BACK)

Beginning in Fifth Position in épaulement croisé, raise the back leg into sur le cou-de-pied position, at the same time executing a demi-plié on the supporting leg. Then, en face, the back leg rising onto a high demi-pointe through Fifth Position, frees the front leg to move at the same time into sur le cou-de-pied front. The free leg in the front cou-de-pied position now steps half the distance of a Second Position onto a high demi-pointe as the other leg moves into sur le cou-de-pied forward.

The body is changed from en face to épaulement croisé and the legs execute a pas tombé through Fifth Position into demi-plié on the front leg, as the back leg rises to sur le cou-de-pied in back. From this position, this form of pas de bourrée may be repeated to the other side.

The arms begin at first demi-plié in Preparatory Position; at the first stepover they rise into a lowered First; and at the second stepover, they stay in the same position but end in the final demi-plié with the corresponding supporting leg in First, and with the other arm opened to Second. The body at both stepovers is straight during the first and second demi-plié but bends lightly toward the advanced shoulder at the final pose.

The head during the first demi-plié remains in épaulement, but in both stepovers turns en face and ends at the last demi-plié toward the advanced shoulder. (See illustration #90.)

This pas de bourrée must be studied facing the barre in a simplified version.

Beginning as usual from the demi-plié on one leg, the other moves to sur le cou-de-pied in back. Then two stepovers are done in high demi-pointe with the transfer of the free leg through Fifth Position into cou-de-pied forward and back. The movement ends in demi-plié tombé, but with the sur le cou-de-pied forward. This exercise may be done in reverse and from the other leg.

Then the study of pas de bourrée with the change of legs may begin facing the barre. Later it is continued in the center of the floor.

PAS DE BOURRÉE WITHOUT A CHANGE OF LEGS (THE SAME LEG THAT BEGAN THE PAS DE BOURRÉE ENDS IN FRONT)

Beginning in the Fifth Position, with the body en face, the leg in front does a demi-plié as the other leg opens through sur le cou-de-pied position into Second at 45 degrees. The open leg then exchanges through a coupé back into a high demi-pointe. At the same time, the front leg rises into sur le cou-de-pied forward. This same leg then steps over into a high demi-pointe in the direction of a shortened Second Position. The freed leg at the same time moves to sur le cou-de-pied back and does a tombé onto that foot, thus freeing the front foot once more to move through sur le cou-de-pied along Second Position into 45 degrees.

---

91 Pas de bourrée without a change of legs

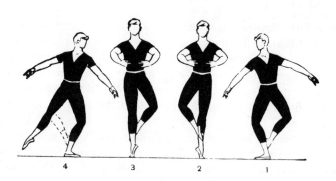

4   3   2   1

From this position the pas de bourrée may be continued going to the opposite side or may end by lowering the open leg into the starting Fifth Position.

The arms during the first opening of the leg into Second rise from the Preparatory Position into the direction of the Second Position lowered. At the first stepover, they are moved through Preparatory into a lowered First and stay in that position during the second stepover. At the finish of the movement, in demi-plié, the arms open into a lowered Second Position.

The body, during the stepovers, stays en face, but on demi-plié turns in the same direction as the demi-plié. (See illustration #91.) This pas is studied without a preparatory exercise in the center floor. It is then studied in écarté and with small poses in Fourth with stepovers forward and back. The leg opens softly. The arms, head and body act freely and clearly in the proper positions.

PAS DE BOURRÉE DESSUS (OVER—THE FIRST STEPOVER IS IN FRONT, OR OVER THE SUPPORTING LEG)

Beginning in Fifth Position, épaulement croisé, the front leg does a demi-plié as the body turns en face and the other leg opens through sur le cou-de-pied into Second at 45 degrees.

Then the open leg does the first stepover to demi-pointe *in front of the supporting leg* (dessus), exchanging it for the leg in demi-plié which rises at the same time to sur le cou-de-pied back. The free leg then does the second stepover to a high demi-pointe in the direction of a shortened Second Position at the same time the other moves into sur le cou-de-pied back. Finally, the leg in cou-de-pied back falls into a demi-plié (tombé) with the free leg now opening through the sur le cou-de-pied in the direction of Second Position to 45 degrees. (See illustration #92.)

---

92   Pas de bourrée dessus

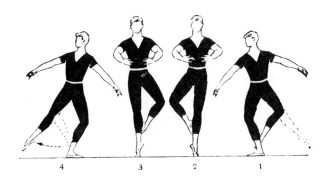

The arms during the first opening of the leg rise from Preparatory Position through a lowered First into a lowered Second. At the stepovers they gradually lower into Preparatory Position.

The body, during the stepovers, is straight and in demi-plié bends lightly in the direction opposite the open leg.

The head at the first opening turns and bends slightly with the body in the opposite direction.

93   Pas de bourrée dessous

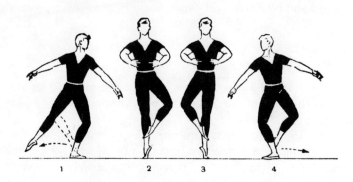

PAS DE BOURRÉE DESSOUS (UNDER—THE STEPOVERS ARE BEHIND OR UNDER THE SUPPORTING LEG)

This movement is done in the same way as the above pas de bourrée, only in reverse. First the demi-plié is on the supporting back leg of a Fifth Position with the other leg opening at the same time through sur le cou-de-pied front into 45 degrees to the side. The first stepover onto demi-pointe is done in back of the supporting leg as the free leg rises to sur le cou-de-pied front. The second stepover onto demi-pointe in the direction of a shortened Second Position is an exchange for the freed leg to move into sur le cou-de-pied front. Finally, the demi-plié tombé is made with the supporting leg as the other leg opens through sur le cou-de-pied in the direction of Second to 45 degrees. The head, arms and body follow the rules of the bourrée dessus. (See illustration #93.)

PAS DE BOURRÉE DESSUS-DESSOUS (OVER-UNDER)

This form consists of the combination of the two previously described exercises performed one after the other.

After the pas de bourrée dessus (over), the leg opens to 45 degrees in Second and moves to demi-pointe in back of the supporting leg. It then continues into a pas de bourrée dessous. The movement is performed uninterruptedly. When it is performed in a quick tempo, the legs open into Second Position, rising only slightly from the floor, which gives the entire movement a compact and together look. The arm, body and head take alternating positions for the first and second forms of this pas.

In the study of pas de bourrée dessus-dessous, the leg opening along Second Position must be straight, not an arched line but directly underneath the leg, changing legs, and the toes should glide lightly over the floor.

94 Pas balancé

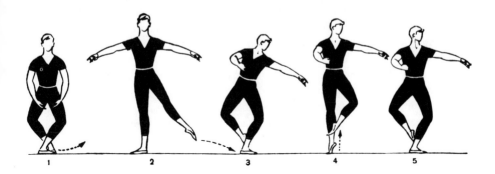

PAS BALANCÉ (ROCKED)

This movement consists of even stepovers and a small rocking movement of the body, head and arms. The movement begins in Fifth Position in demi-plié. The front leg slides to the Second as the supporting leg straightens. The free leg then falls onto the Second Position as the back leg places itself in sur le cou-de-pied back. Then the stepover is made by the back foot, which takes the weight from the front foot on a high demi-pointe as the front foot moves into sur le cou-de-pied front. The front foot falls from that position into another demi-plié and the back leg once more moves into sur le cou-de-pied front. The front foot falls from that position into another demi-plié and the back leg once more moves into sur le cou-de-pied.

The movement from this point may be performed to the other side, not from the Fifth Position but from the sur le cou-de-pied back position in which it ended. The back foot then falls to the side in Second Position and the movement continues. In this way the balancé combines a tombé into Second, a pas coupé and a tombé through Fifth.

The arms in pas balancé are low. As the leg moves to the side, the arms rise from Preparatory to Second. As the leg opens, the corresponding arm remains in Second as the body leans in the direction of the tombé and the other arm moves into First. If the balancé is performed in the reverse direction, the arms smoothly move in the same direction—one from the First into Second and one from Second into First. Additionally, the arms may move from Second into Third and back.

The body at the change onto the leg in demi-plié leans in the same direction. During the next step, it returns to a straight position where it remains to the end of the step. The head turns in the direction of the lean and stays until the end of the movement. (See illustration #94.)

In performing pas balancé, the leg must open lightly and very exactly to the

Second with a smoothly stretched knee, instep and toes. The stepover movement to demi-pointe must be performed with the same stretched knee. The first move to Second is done with an advance in space not wider than a Second Position. It must be executed softly from the toes to the whole foot and the transfer to sur le cou-de-pied must be done exactly and softly with a stretched foot. The stepover is a supple movement which requires a smooth transfer into sur le cou-de-pied. And the finish, as well, in demi-plié, must be done softly, lightly and connected to the other movements.

The arms move freely, which in their turn must move clearly and together with the leg movements.

As a whole, pas balancé is done with restraint, with no exaggerated turning of the head or body, without rough accents and with a turnout maintained throughout.

It is studied at first without using the arms and in a slow tempo of 3/4. All three stepovers are done to 1/4 of the measure. When the basic form has been learned, the balancé may be complicated by first moving the leg to the side from a high demi-pointe position before the tombé and with the body leaning a little more than usual with the opposite arm in Third instead of First Position. The other arm may be in Third as well. At the repeat of the step the opposite side is performed. The arms are simply moved into defined position but not by going through First Position. (The pas balancé may be performed advancing front, back or en tournant—with half turns—as well.)

---

95   Pas couru

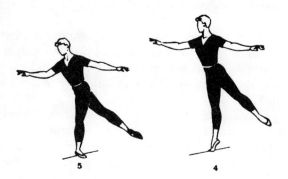

5   4

PAS COURU (RUNNING)

This movement is an energetic run performed as an advance forward or an approach for a big jump such as a grand jeté, etc.

It consists of four small stepovers in Fourth Position begun from a small pose, tendu croisé forward. The first movement is a tombé onto the leg in croisé and two steps advancing forward on demi-pointe by means of the dégagé. The movement comes to an end with no interruption in the advance in a pas tombé forward from which a short, forceful, jumping push creates a preparation for the large jump to follow.

The four steps (runs) are done with a dash at the same tempo and an energetic propulsion of the entire body forward to the approaching jumping push.

The arms are in Second, palms down, and at the push are transferred energetically through Preparatory into First and then into the pose position, thus helping in the trajectory of the high jump. The body, at the start of the couru, is energetically sent forward and actively participates in the jumping push, preserving the shapeliness and tautness. It also leans a bit toward the advancing shoulder. The center of gravity at the moment of the jump is exactly over the supporting leg so that the jump may be high and stable. (See illustrations #95, #96.) The head during the pas couru is turned away from the advanced shoulder and, at the moment of the push, turns energetically toward that shoulder. (See illustration #95.) As a whole, the movement is a light and free run to the jump which follows.

Pas couru may also be performed in three steps. In that case, the first pose with the tendu on the floor is fixed in a small pose with the working leg in croisé derrière. This leg does the tombé forward, followed by one step forward from pas dégagé onto high demi-pointe and the final pas tombé on the freed foot. The

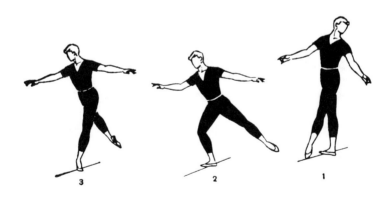

use of the arms, head and body are the same. This step should be studied when all forms of pas de bourrée and the methods of big jumps without an advance have been well mastered. (This is not the same form of pas couru performed by female students.)

96   Temps levé passé

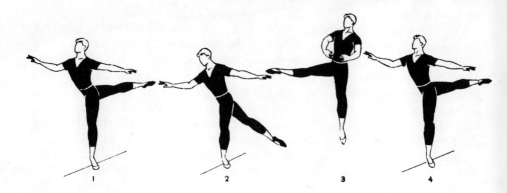

TEMPS LIÉ (CONNECTED)

This is an exercise to develop a smooth flow of transfers from one position to another by means of dégagé and demi-plié. It is constructed in two forms and is performed on two levels. It contains a fixed pose par terre in the first form, and in the second, a pose at 90 degrees.

TEMPS LIÉ PAR TERRE (FIRST FORM)

In the first level and first form, the temps lié par terre begins in Fifth Position with the right leg forward, épaulement croisé. Both legs execute a demi-plié and the right leg glides, stretches forward, as the left leg remains in demi-plié. And, through a pas dégagé (transfer of weight in Fourth Position croisé), the front leg passes through a demi-plié as the left leg stretches out in croisé derrière. Then the same leg slides into Fifth Position again in back and both legs do a demi-plié en face.

98   Temps lié par terre through Second Position

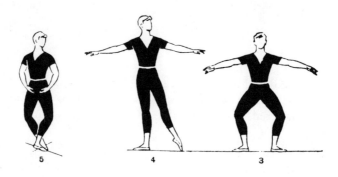

97 Temps lié par terre through Fourth Position

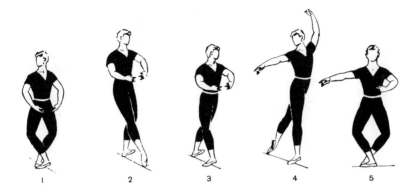

The arms at the movement of the right leg forward rise from Preparatory into First Position. At the dégagé, the left goes into Third, the right into Second. At the end of the movement, when the legs close in Fifth, the left arm goes from Third to First. The body, during the move of the right leg, stays over the supporting leg and during the transfer moves from the back leg to the forward leg.

The head moves with the arms into First, with the eyes on the hands. At the movement of the right arm from First into Third, the head turns at the same time in the same direction. When the left arm moves from Third into First, the head turns toward the hand of the same arm. (See illustration #97.)

TEMPS LIÉ PAR TERRE ALONG SECOND POSITION

The right leg moves from the demi-plié which ended the previous form, gliding and stretching to the Second Position. The pas dégagé (transfer of weight now

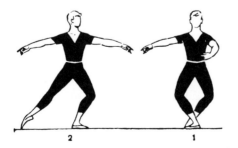

99　Temps lié at 90 degrees through Fourth Position

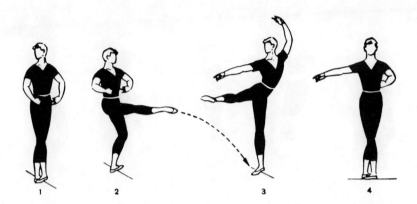

in the Second Position) is done through demi-plié. Then, the left leg stretches, straightens and closes forward in demi-plié at the same time the body turns into épaulement croisé (left shoulder forward).

When the right leg moves to the side, the left arm goes from First into Second. At the dégagé, the arms stay in Second and descend into Preparatory Position as the left leg closes in Fifth.

The body, during the dégagé, changes from left to right and the head at the movement of the left arm from First into Second turns in the same direction. The head keeps this position at the final demi-plié. (See illustration #98.)

The entire movement is repeated from the other leg. Temps lié par terre to the back is done after the same pattern but in the first form, the dégagé is done from the back leg and in the second form, the leg which goes to the side, in the Fifth Position in back.

The temps lié must be studied slowly, both in two measures of 2/4: 1/4 for the demi-plié on both feet; 1/4 for the move front or side; 1/4 for the pas dégagé or transfer of weight; and 1/4 to the next fixed pose; etc.

Once the movement is learned, it may be done with a bending of the body at the fixing of the pose in croisé derrière and in tendu in Second.

In the first form, the body bends backward during the tendu croisé derrière. The arms and head keep their described positions. In the second form the body bends toward the side opposite the open legs in Second Position.

In the performance of the second form, backward, the body bends away from the open leg. Arms will keep their pose, until the right arm moves into Third and then to Second.

All the rules for port de bras with a bending body are to be observed. Temps lié with the bending body is done in two measures of 4/4 for both sections.

In performing temps lié par terre with or without the bending of the body backward or sideways, all the rules for the head, body and arms described by

100 Temps lié at 90 degrees through Second Position

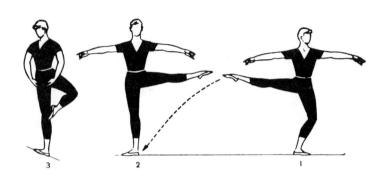

classical dance are in full force here. The basic role of this exercise is to develop a smooth, soft and flowing connection of all the elements of the temps lié.

Later, the movement without the bending may be done to two measures of 3/4 tempo with each pose performed to 1/3 of the measure. Here, especially, there must be an uninterrupted flow of demi-plié, pas dégagé, port de bras and the fixing of the pose.

TEMPS LIÉ AT 90 DEGREES (SECOND FORM)

This form differs from the par terre form in the first movement. It is no longer a glide along the floor but a battement développé from demi-plié.

First, begin in Fifth Position with the right leg forward, épaulement croisé. The right leg does a battement développé croisé forward, with a demi-plié at the same time on the left leg. Then, a dégagé is done with a wide advance in space forward on the whole foot through the stretched demi-pointe and the fixed pose. This is an attitude croisée derrière. The left leg stretches at the knee, and is then lowered back to Fifth Position with a turn of the body en face.

The arms at the time of the battement rise into First and at the dégagé the right moves to Second, the left into Third. At the return of the left leg to Fifth, the right stays in Second and the left moves into First. The body and head, as in temps lié par terre, move in the same directions. (See illustration #99.)

In the second section of the temps lié, the right leg does a battement développé to the side at the same time the left does a demi-plié. Then there is a dégagé with a wide advance sideward onto the whole foot through stretched toes. The fixed pose at this point is à la seconde at 90 degrees. Finally, the left leg bends into a passé position with an épaulement. The movement is then ready to be performed beginning with the other leg.

The head, body and arms function as in the second section of the temps lié par terre. (See illustration #100.)

This movement is done to the back according to the same pattern, but in the first section the battement développé and the pas dégagé are done to the back in croisé.

The study of this movement is in a slow tempo of two measures of 4/4. The first section: 1/4 for the bending of the leg to the passé or knee position; 1/4 for the battement développé; 1/4 for the dégagé; and 1/4 for the fixing of the attitude pose. In the second section: 1/4 for the movement to Fifth and the right to the knee; 1/4 for the battement développé; 1/4 for the pas dégagé; 1/4 for the fixing of the pose in à la seconde, etc.

Once the movement has been learned slowly, the tempo may be increased. In the study of temps lié at 90 degrees, there must be a flowing exactness and aplomb. It develops the feeling of cantilena, which, at a later time, will be revealed in more difficult and complex forms of movement.

Later, the temps lié at 90 degrees may become more complicated with demi-pointe added. In that instance, everything except the demi-plié and the battement développé are done on a high demi-pointe.

PART FOUR

JUMPS
AND
BEATS

JUMPS

The most difficult and technically complicated movements in classical dance are jumps.

Jumps are a means of diversified and rushing flights of movement, which, however, must not become an end in themselves. The problem consists not in having the dancer jump as high as possible while doing a complicated form of turn or a tour de force step, but in doing that jump with the utmost lightness, flexibility and musicality, depicting the emotional state of the character he is re-creating on stage. Then the jump becomes an expressive component of acting.

Jumps are composed of the previously learned elements of the exercise and adagio portions of the class. It is therefore extremely important that those elements have been mastered thoroughly and with comprehension before being used in jumps.

At the same time, the technique of jumps has its own performing methods. One of these methods is called elevation, which allows the dancer to jump softly, high, lightly and exactly with stability. Elevation requires a proper push for height, an advance of the body in the right direction, correct tempo and correct rhythm. But elevation alone does not fulfill the perfect technique necessary for the jump. The dancer must be able in certain big jumps to fix the culmination of the flight. In classical dance, this fixing method is called ballon.

Ballon consists of a push by the legs which sends the body on a shorter yet stronger trajectory, by which the jump acquires a greater degree of airiness and the dancer seems to be held up in the air. The position in the air must be clear, fixing the movement and pose exactly. Otherwise, the jump loses its accuracy and virtuosity, and the dancer, in that case, is said to have no ballon.

One of the most difficult and complicated elements of the jump is the demi-plié, which is needed for the push from the floor, for the flight and for the finish of the movement. In performing the jump, it is necessary that the whole foot in the demi-plié be pressed to the floor tightly, especially the heels. The foot leaves the floor in a consecutive pattern from heel to toes, ankle and hip—all taking an active part in the push and the entire leg parting from the floor with stretched and resilient knees, insteps and toes. Without this consecutive use of the several parts, the jump will look weak, unstable, low and stiff.

The jump must end in a soft, light and supple demi-plié, accepting the body weight into taut leg muscles and toes and onto heels which hug the floor noiselessly but firmly. The ankle and hip must also take an active part in the supple and soft finish of the jump according to all the rules of demi-plié.

If there is no consecutive use of the parts of the foot, leg and hip, thus causing an interrupted flow of the movement, the ending will be heavy and rough (and the possibility of injury will increase). Therefore, in classwork, developing and strengthening the demi-plié within the jump exercises must be given the strictest attention. In learning the technique of connecting jumps, one must see that the finishing demi-plié and the following push are done together, using the force of inertia within the body as a trampoline for flight. This is the same in jumps of various heights, done in a variety of rhythms and tempos, from the contained softly coiled jumps to the rushing and energetic.

Additionally, during the push, flight and finish of a jump, the movements of the head, arms, body and legs must be coordinated properly. If the pupil cannot create the proper design in the jump or sustain the entire dance phrase, then he has not yet acquired full elevation and ballon. Theatrical performances without these two elements in jumping portions do not reflect masters of virtuoso technique.

Good elevation and ballon depend upon sufficient strength, endurance and resoluteness in the pupil. Therefore the exercises for various jumps must be performed in the classroom to their limit. Small and insufficient repetitions in each teaching portion cannot establish a sufficient measure of good elevation and ballon. One must have good sense and consideration in the increase of physical demands, in order not to hurt the natural abilities of the pupil. It is not permissible to allow the performance of jumps when the legs are "cold" or the breathing is not prepared for the additional taxing. This lack of consideration would interfere with the development of elevation and lead to trauma (injuries) which would interfere with the acquiring of a technique for jumps at a later time.

All jumps must be studied at first separately with pauses, for a more thorough development of the technique of the push, the flight and the finish in demi-plié. Then one may go on to the uninterrupted performance of two or three jumps, depending upon the given task.

The elementary jumps, without an advance in space, performed in one place, ought to be performed facing the barre in the lower classes. While studying these jumps at the barre, the pupil must place his hands lightly on it, without hanging or pressing. The hands must lie upon the barre at the width of the shoulders, with the elbows slightly bent and lowered.

Each jump must first be learned thoroughly by itself, alone, and then introduced into combinations.

The jumps in classical dance are divided into five groups:
1. jumps from two legs to two legs
2. jumps from two legs to one leg
3. jumps from one leg to two legs
4. jumps from one leg to the other leg
5. jumps from one leg to the same leg

Following are descriptions of all jumps in the five groups which are combined by means of a push and a finish.

JUMPS FROM TWO LEGS TO TWO LEGS

TEMPS SAUTÉ (JUMPED, JUMPING)

This exercise provides the pupil with the elementary basis for jumps. From this exercise, the technique for jumps begins in the elasticity of the demi-plié, the resiliences of the push from the floor, in the light flight and soft finish.

Temps sauté is done in First, Second or Fifth Position and is divided, like all jumps, into petit (small) or grand (large or high) movements.

PETIT TEMPS SAUTÉ

The petit temps sauté principle consists of starting in the First, Second or Fifth Position and in a small flight, maintaining the position until the jump finishes in a demi-plié in the same position. (See illustration #101.) (When the movement is performed in First Position it is called sauté en première by the French School.)

101   Petit temps sauté in First Position

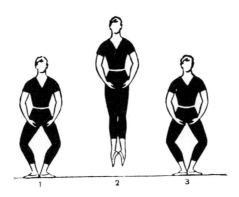

In the performance of this movement, the elasticity of the demi-plié before and after the jump must be preserved. There must be a lightness in the push and flight. The legs must be kept in the turned-out position and, during the jump, the knees, instep and toes must be well stretched. The entire jump must be done with pulled-up thighs and the preservation of exact leg positions. The body must be straight, the muscles of the back assembled to support the return to the floor, the shoulders open and lowered, the waist kept stable and the head kept straight without tension in the neck.

This jump is first studied facing the barre in First Position, then in Second and Fifth positions, to 4/4 count: 1/4 is used for the demi-plié; 1/4 for the pause; 1/4 for the jump and landing; 1/4 for the straightening of the legs from the landing in demi-plié.

Later, one may study the temps sauté combined with two jumps: 1/4 for demi-plié; 1/4 for a jump; 1/4 for the second jump; 1/4 for the straightening of the legs from the demi-plié landing.

This exercise may be done afterward, with the demi-plié before the measure, a few times in succession.

When the jump has been well learned at the barre, it may be studied in the center of the floor. The arms during all exercises are held correctly but freely throughout the movement in Preparatory Position.

GRAND TEMPS SAUTÉ

The grand temps sauté is executed from a deepened demi-plié and goes as high as the pupil can manage *with all the rules strictly observed.*

If performed in the center of the floor, the tempo is to a 4/4 measure: 1/4 for the demi-plié; 1/4 for the jump and the landing in demi-plié; 1/4 to straighten from the demi-plié; and 1/4 for the rest. Later, the exercise may be done with the jump before the measure to 2/4: 1/2 for the finish of the jump in demi-plié; 1/4 for the straightening from demi-plié landing. Finally, the exercise is performed in sequence with 1/4 for each jump. (See illustration #102.)

Later still, the exercise may be performed with épaulement croisé and en volé (flying). In the latter form, the jump is preceded by a push given by the whole body with the arms forcefully raised at the same time as the push or thrust from Preparatory Position into Third Position.

102   Grand temps sauté in Fifth Position

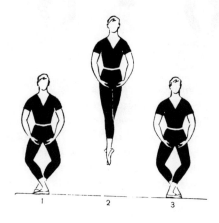

1   2   3

CHANGEMENT DE PIED

This exercise is done from Fifth Position into Fifth Position. At the crest of the jump, the legs exchange positions. (If the right leg is in front at the start, it ends at the finish in back.) The change is not counted (as the changes in batterie are counted). The technique for the changement de pied is the same as the principles used in temps sauté.

PETIT CHANGEMENT DE PIED

During the demi-plié preparation in Fifth Position, the thrust is made. Then in a small flight, the legs separate slightly (in First Position) and cross again at the finish in demi-plié. (See illustration #103.)

The beginning and the finish in demi-plié must be done turned out, with flexibility and evenly from both feet. The legs separate at the crest of the jump only enough to avoid the heels touching at the exchange of the feet. At that moment, the legs must be stretched at the knee, instep and toes while keeping the turned-out position. The body is kept straight and the shoulders open and lowered with the head straight.

The study of this jump must be progressive and in the same pattern of rhythm as the study of petit temps sauté, first at the barre and then in the center of the floor. The arms in the performance of petit changement de pied in the center floor are in Preparatory Position.

In the middle and higher classes, the exercise may be performed at a faster tempo, almost without a plié, separating from the floor only by an elastic and resiliently stretched instep and toes and in very small jumps.

---

103   Petit changement de pied

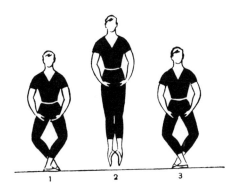

The feet at the finish of these small jumps must bound off the floor with a spring and join the floor again in the same springy quality.

This exercise is done to a 2/4 count: 1/8 for each jump. Petit changement de pied is useful to do in a slower tempo as well. The feet must join the floor very smoothly and almost without the demi-plié, and bounce with resiliency from it.

The execution of the next exercise is quite difficult, but it develops force, resilience, stability in the ankle and shin and especially develops the toes. It is done slowly to 2/4 with 1/4 for each jump.

---

104   Grand changement de pied

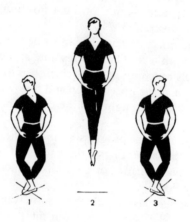

GRAND CHANGEMENT DE PIED

This movement is done according to the same rules as the petit changement de pied, except that the force of the thrust and the height of the jump must be increased to the limit. In addition, the legs before the crest of the jump is reached must be tightly joined in Fifth Position, and at the moment the jump is about to end, the legs exchange places. This exercise may be done in épaulement croisé and with an advance in space—en volé (flying), keeping to the rules previously described. (See illustration #104.) This exercise is done to the same rhythmic pattern as the grand temps sauté.

(In the French and Cecchetti schools the grand changement de pied is performed with the knees bent in the air and the feet drawn up so that the flat of the toes of both feet meet.)

SOUBRESAUT

The soubresaut is begun in demi-plié Fifth Position and moves along a diagonal forward. At the moment it is in full flight, the legs are tightly pressed together in the region of the shin and are thrown back, then return to the Fifth Position, in demi-plié. (The tightly held legs in flight are said to be collé, glued.)

The body, at the beginning of the demi-plié, moves slightly forward and at the crest of the jump, together with the legs, is arched backward. At the same time, the entire body, at the time of the demi-plié is given a light push forward in space so that the finish of the step is a little farther than the start. At the finish of the step, the body is erect.

The arms in demi-plié are in Preparatory Position and when the jump is at its

---

105 Soubresaut

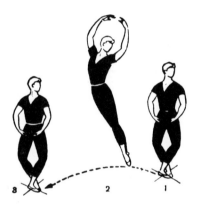

crest the arms have been raised energetically to Third Position, or any other position given as a variation.

The head at the demi-plié moves slightly forward to the advanced shoulder. (See illustration #105.) The study of soubresaut begins with a gentle jump without the forceful throw of the body or legs. The jump is increased gradually to the limit as all the details are included. It must be practiced beginning before the count to a 2/4 tempo; 1/4 for the jump; 1/4 for the rest. Then, later, without a rest or pause.

(Steps that begin before the count are classified as contretemps. They begin on the "and" or upbeat of the count.)

PAS ÉCHAPPÉ

This movement, in the category of a jump from two feet to two feet, is a step which transfers one position to another. The technique does not differ from previous exercises. The turnout must be preserved exactly, the position must be held with flexibility, and there must be softness in the demi-plié. The torso must be held and pulled up and the step requires a clear action of the arms and the head.

PETIT PAS ÉCHAPPÉ

This smaller version begins in Fifth Position, épaulement croisé. The first small jump is used to separate the legs and transfer to Second Position en face. At the second small jump (échappé consists of two jumps), the legs return to the Fifth Position, épaulement croisé. Each small jump begins in demi-plié and ends in demi-plié. The beginning and ending position is Fifth with a change of legs, meaning that the foot that began in front ends in back. At each jump the legs are stretched at the knee, instep and toes.

At the first jump, the arms move from Preparatory Position through lowered First, into a lowered Second. At the second jump the arms return to Preparatory Position. The body is kept straight and the head, at the performance of the épaulement, turns toward the advanced shoulder. (See illustration #106.)

---

106   Petit pas échappé

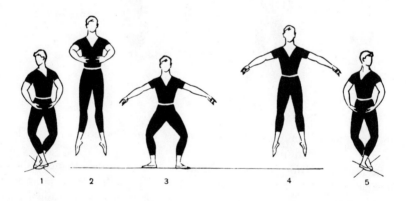

1   2   3   4   5

The petit pas échappé is studied facing the barre in four measures of 2/4: 1/4 for the demi-plié; 1/4 for the first jump into Second Position; 1/4 for the knees to straighten from demi-plié; 1/4 rest. The second jump is done in the same pattern.

Later, the movement is studied on the floor to two measures of 2/4, keeping the pauses after both jumps, and finally without the pauses.

The arms at the beginning of the study stay in the Preparatory Position but when the two jumps are done without interruption they open as described above.

The petit pas échappé may be done from Fifth Position into Fourth Position croisé. The arms in that movement open during the first jump into the lower

Second, but at the second jump return to the Preparatory Position. Or, at the first jump one arm may rise into First and the other into Second. The head turns toward the advanced shoulder. At the second jump, the arms remain in their position or lower into the Preparatory Position.

This exercise must be kept to the established size of Fourth Position and all the rules pertaining to the performance of jumps.

At a later time, when the sissonne simple has been learned, the petit pas échappé into Second and Fourth ending on one leg will be studied. This form of pas échappé would be more correctly encountered as sissonne, but established terminology presents this movement as pas échappé.

The second jump in Second to Fourth ends on one leg as the other is moved through sur le cou-de-pied forward or sur le cou-de-pied back.

The arm corresponding to the leg Fourth Position moves to First from Second, as the other arm remains in Second Position. The body leans toward the supporting leg, keeping the shape and pulling up the legs. The head turns toward the advanced shoulder.

Another form would be to begin the first jump from the sur le cou-de-pied

---

107 Grand pas échappé

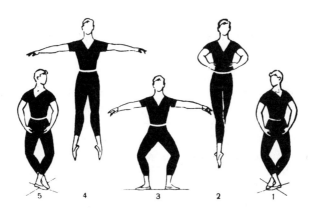

position instead of the Fifth Position and end on the same leg. The body, arms and head would follow the same described pattern.

The petit pas échappé from Second as well as from Fourth may serve as a preparation for small pirouettes. The turn is then done from the demi-plié after the first jump.

GRAND PAS ÉCHAPPÉ

The grand pas échappé is performed with a deepened demi-plié and with the utmost height. The legs remain in Fifth Position (collé) during the first flight until the crest of the jump has been reached and opened to Second or Fourth Position only at the landing. At the second jump, the legs remain in Second Position until the last possible moment before ending in Fifth in demi-plié. (See illustration #107.) At the first jump, the leg must not be held so long that the jump looks sharp or rough in the demi-plié.

The body, arms and head follow the description for petit pas échappé but are used more energetically and actively.

This movement is studied in two measures of 2/4: 1/4 for the first jump; 1/4 for the second jump; 1/4 for the straightening of the knees from demi-plié; 1/4 for a pause. Then the exercise is done uninterruptedly in one measure of 2/4.

In addition, this grand pas échappé may end in sur le cou-de-pied or in a pose at 90 degrees.

In the first instance, the movement is performed as for petit pas échappé. In the second, during the jump from Second to Fourth, the grande pose is assumed. The jump for the grande pose is done advancing toward the supporting leg. This jump is performed on the principle of sissonne ouverte, although not from Fifth Position, but from Second or Fourth.

The arm, head and body perform according to the rules described. The grand pas échappé onto one leg is studied first from Second, finishing in sur le cou-de-pied, then in poses at 90 degrees with and without interruption.

JUMPS FROM TWO LEGS TO ONE LEG

SISSONNE SIMPLE

The sissonne simple begins in Fifth Position, épaulement croisé. The jump is performed with the legs together. At the finish of the jump, only one leg performs the demi-plié landing while the other takes a sur le cou-de-pied position in back or in front. The arms are fixed in a Preparatory Position and the head and body are kept in épaulement. (See illustration #108.)

The push for this movement is done forcefully and evenly from both legs and they are, during the flight, kept tightly together with stretched knees, insteps and toes. The jump ends softly and with stability with an exact and clear change into sur le cou-de-pied at the landing without any sign of overexertion. The arms are kept free without tension and the body is pulled up. The shoulders are lowered slightly and are open. The head turns toward the advanced shoulder.

This sissonne should be studied facing the barre with a carefully maintained turned-out position and with a soft landing in demi-plié. The sissonne simple sur le cou-de-pied is performed first to the front, then to the back. Then, from Second to Fifth landing in the sur le cou-de-pied, which opens into battement tendu, closes in Fifth and is ready to begin again. The entire exercise is repeated four times and reversed.

In the center floor, the sissonne simple sur le cou-de-pied is studied like the exercises described above, then combined with petit pas assemblé and other jumps,

108 Sissonne simple

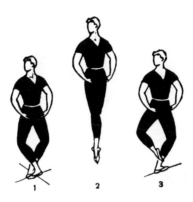

beginning from the sur le cou-de-pied. The tempo recommended is 2/4 or 4/4 with the jump begun before the measure. The exercise is done at first with pauses, then without pauses. (This step is termed temps levé—a hop from any position on one leg. In the Cecchetti method the spring from Fifth raising one foot into sur le cou-de-pied is termed temps levé while the same step in the Russian and French schools is termed sissonne simple.)

SISSONNE TOMBÉE

This movement is similar to the sissonne simple except that it ends in Second or Fourth Position by means of a tombé.

Beginning in Fifth Position, épaulement croisé, the flight is done, legs together in Fifth, with the jump ending in sur le cou-de-pied but continuing without interruption by gliding the toes on the floor, into croisé front in demi-plié. The other leg at the landing in tombé croisé stretches out in back with the toes touching the floor. Finally, a pas assemblé to the back with a little advance in space or a small pas de basque complete the movement.

The arms during the flight change from Preparatory Position into First at the performance of the tombé and take the position of third arabesque. During the second jump, they descend into Preparatory Position.

The body at the time of the crest of the movement is kept straight but at the finish moves slightly forward toward the leg changing into the tombé position. At the second jump, it straightens out.

The head during the flight turns toward the tombé and, during the second jump, returns to the starting position. (See illustration #109.)

In the same manner, this jump may be performed backward, incorporating small poses which are learned with the sissonne ouverte and other small jumps. But whatever poses are performed, all the rules must be kept for sissonne simple,

109   Sissonne tombée into Fourth Position

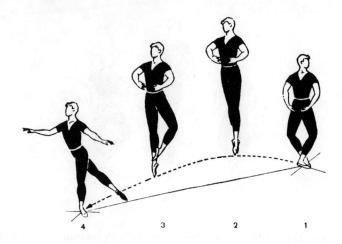

pas tombé and petit pas assemblé, including transferring the arms and fixing the positions of the head and body.

On the whole, this jump must be done with no interruption, flowingly, so that the tombé flows from finishing demi-plié. The flight must be ended in a light, easy change from one leg to the other. The actions of the arms, head and body must be clear in design and sure in character.

The sissonne tombée should be studied at first en face, in the form of the following exercise: sissonne tombée forward into Fourth Position, assemblé backward. Then, sissonne tombée in Second in both directions, then backward. The arms in tombé open to Second. The tempo is 2/4 with all jumps done each to 1/4.

Then, one may begin the study of this jump in poses croisées, effacées and écartées. Because this movement is often used as an approach for big jumps, the movement of the arms, the head and body may be varied depending upon the force, form and character of the preceding flight. All these things must be considered in the teaching and must be worked thoroughly.

PETITE SISSONNE OUVERTE

The petite sissonne ouverte is performed in all poses at 45 degrees. Beginning in Fifth Position, the position is maintained during the jump but at the moment of landing the supporting leg does a demi-plié and the other opens at the same time through the sur le cou-de-pied position into développé.

The arms at the first demi-plié are moved from Preparatory Position into First and remain there during the jump. At the moment of the landing, the body and head simultaneously assume the position for the pose being performed.

110 Petite sissonne ouverte to Second Position

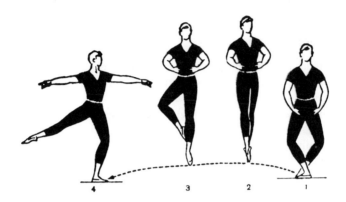

4   3   2   1

The performance of the petite sissonne ouverte starts from a flexible demi-plié. The knees, instep and toes are stretched during the jump. The jump must be finished smoothly, with a soft and clear opening of the leg through the sur le cou-de-pied. The body, head and arms coordinate with the rules of the performing pose.

Petite sissonne ouverte must be studied en face, first to the side, then forward and backward opening the leg with toes on the floor. The arms stay in Preparatory Position, the head and body remain straight. Each opening of the leg is ended in pas assemblé. That means, from this position, that the open leg should be pulled back into Fifth Position in a jump which is executed forcefully by the supporting leg. The closing ends in demi-plié.

Both jumps are done to one measure of 4/4: first jump before the beat; 1/4 for the opening of the leg, toes to the floor; 1/4 for rest; 1/4 to finish the pas assemblé; 1/4 pause in demi-plié.

Later, the leg may be opened to 45 degrees with the arms and head participating and keeping the pattern of study.

If, in the Fifth Position, the right leg is forward and opens to the side, the arms move from Preparatory to Second and the head turns toward the supporting leg. (See illustration #110.) If the leg to the back opens to the side from Fifth Position, the arms are the same but the head turns away from the standing leg. When the leg opens to the front or to the back, the arms open to Second and the head turns away from the standing leg.

At the closing of the leg into Fifth, with a pas assemblé, the arms lower into Preparatory Position. During the demi-plié, the head turns en face.

When the petite sissonne ouverte en face has been mastered, the study of the croisée, effacée and écartée may begin. The arms, in these positions, open from

Preparatory into First, then one arm opens together with the opening leg into Second as the other remains in First Position.

The head and body follow the rules for the ending poses, including the poses of arabesque.

At first, each jump is made with a pause in demi-plié, then, later, smoothly without any pauses.

GRANDE SISSONNE OUVERTE

The grande sissonne ouverte is performed with the greatest height in the capacity of the student and ends in a pose at 90 degrees. During the jump, the opening leg passes through the sur le cou-de-pied and rises to the knee position, stretching out at the demi-plié landing into the given direction.

The arm, head and body correspond to the rules for the poses at 90 degrees and for big jumps. (See illustration #111.)

---

111   Grande sissonne ouverte opening into effacée

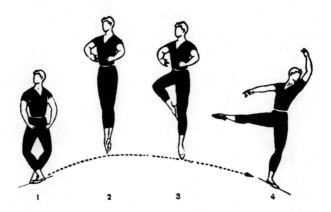

The starting and finishing demi-pliés are deepened with suppleness and lightness. The opening leg stretches out at the knee with the instep and toes maintaining the height and direction. (This is a very important point. The portion of the knee from the knee through the toes must not lower the height of the pose but continue the line of the leg in a straight line or higher.) Loss of the turnout in the pose is inadmissible.

The movements of the arms and head must be performed in one rhythm with the movement of the legs.

The entire jump is performed with a slight advance begun with the opening leg. It must be smooth, soft, but with sufficient energy and clarity.

The study of the grande sissonne ouverte starts en face in Second and Fourth, then continues in croisée, effacée and écartée. The jump is followed by a pause and performed in a 2/4 or 4/4 tempo. Each grande sissonne ouverte is finished by a pas assemblé followed by a pause. Then both jumps must be done smoothly without pauses.

GRANDE SISSONNE OUVERTE PAR JETÉ INTO ARABESQUE

The sissonne ouverte par jeté is a variety of sissonne ouverte which incorporates a jeté. In this movement, the leg opens not with the développé, but is thrown to 45 or 90 degrees directly from the Fifth Position in flight. The other leg rushes to the advance, which is done energetically and in a protracted manner but must not be excessive. In this way, the pose at the crest of the jump is fixed and is kept in the finishing demi-plié. (See illustration #112.)

In teaching the sissonne ouverte par jeté, all the small and big poses should be included.

---

112 Grand sissonne par jeté into first arabesque

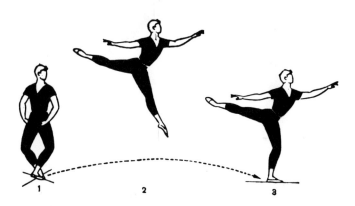

The teacher must see that the pupil pushes away from the floor evenly, and with flexibility, with both legs. In the flight the knees, instep and toes must be fully stretched. At the finishing plié, the open leg must be kept at the given height and in the given direction. The turnout must be maintained throughout the jump.

The arms, head and body follow the rules of the petite sissonne ouverte. At the start in demi-plié, the body is sent somewhat in the direction of the advance with the arms moving from Preparatory Position into First and the head and eyes turned toward the hands.

At the crest of the flight the entire body must be in one rhythm, rushed along in the trajectory. The given ending pose must be kept in the demi-plié.

It must be remembered that some pupils may need help in breathing during these big movements. The teacher must take into consideration that, even with help, not every student has the endurance and strength needed to master these movements on a soloist level.

The study of sissonne ouverte par jeté is recommended to begin with the small poses; then include the large poses. After each sissonne, a pas assemblé into Fifth Position should be performed. At first, the movement is studied with pauses, then without pauses to a 2/4 or 4/4 tempo.

Like the smaller sissonnes, the legs in this version must be tightly joined in Fifth Position and separated after the crest of the jump has been reached. The open leg must be kept at 90 degrees at the finishing demi-plié. The body, head and arms follow the rules for the performance of big poses. (See illustration #113.)

113   Sissonne ouverte soubresaut into first arabesque

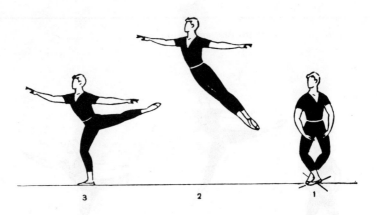

The entire jump must be clear, flexible and with sufficient height and advancement, with special attention paid to a soft landing at the finishing demi-plié.

The element of soubresaut (maintaining the legs in a tight position—collé) may be incorporated in the study only after the pupil has acquired a good technique and strength to add this element to the jump.

The study of sissonne ouverte soubresaut must begin in first arabesque as the ending pose. Later, the second and fourth arabesques may be studied. The jump is done before the measure and studied at first with a pause, then without the pause to a 2/4 tempo or a 3/4 valse.

SISSONNE FERMÉE (CLOSED)

This version of the sissonne is a development of the sissonne ouverte pas jeté finishing in the closed Fifth Position. The opening leg does not remain in the 45-

or 90-degree position. All the rules for sissonne are followed. (See illustration #114.)

The leg which closes in Fifth Position must be kept turned out and, during the demi-plié, must glide lightly and softly with the toes along the floor into its final Fifth Position.

The position of the head, body and arms are as in sissonne ouverte, depending upon the given final pose. All movement must be performed flowingly, with sufficiently clear and energetic advancement.

The study of sissonne fermée must begin as the sissonne ouverte, en face. It is then studied in small poses at 45 degrees, and finally in big poses at 90 degrees. The tempo is 2/4 or 3/4.

---

114 Sissonne fermée through first arabesque

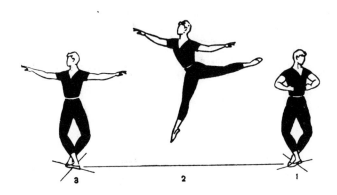

The sissonne fermée may end in sur le cou-de-pied as well. This version should, however, be the last one for study.

The sissonne fermée form may be the finish in the performance of sissonne simple as well. In this form, the jump is begun in the sur le cou-de-pied position, not the Fifth Position. The leg begins to close at the crest of the jump after the in-flight pose, and the landing is simultaneous on both legs from toes through the foot to a soft demi-plié in Fifth Position.

This form is not widely used but is seen in sharp, vivid color for grotesque and semiclassical roles. The higher the jump, the higher the leg should rise along the shin of the supporting leg to 90 degrees. This form may end in Fifth with the same leg front as began the jump; or with a change of legs; or it may be done in a sequence with different leg patterns.

The arms in this movement may take any position from Third; Second and Third; or First and Third. The body, as a rule, is kept en face or épaulement, but under stage conditions the body may bend or turn various angles. The head, however, follows the rules of coordination with the arms and body. In stage compositions, according to the direction of the choreographer, the positions may be different from those given. This form is studied only as the last form of sissonne fermée. The turnout must be maintained, as well as the exactness of the Fifth Position, the flexibility of the demi-plié, and the plasticity of the arms, body and head.

PAS FAILLI (GIVING WAY)

This movement belongs to the sissonne fermée with a landing in Fourth, not a Fifth Position. The pas failli is usually done as a small jump forward and, rarely, as a jump backward. (See illustration #115.)

Beginning in Fifth Position, épaulement croisé, the jump is done with a turn of the body at the crest of the jump to the effacé position, with a simultaneous opening of the leg to 45 degrees back.

At the landing in demi-plié, the open leg moves with a glide along the floor through First Position forward into croisé as the weight is transferred onto the moving foot. The movement ends on one leg in demi-plié while the other remains stretched out in back, with the toes touching the floor. Finally, the back leg pulls up into Fifth Position through a pas assemblé.

---

115   Pas failli par sissonne

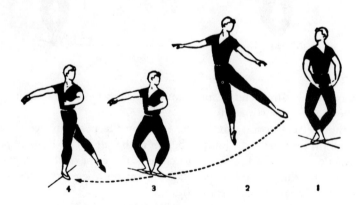

During the jump, the arms move from Preparatory into a lowered Second and the arm which corresponds to the open leg is led with it into a lowered First Position. The pas failli may, however, end in a third or fourth arabesque. The body at the time of the transfer of the leg through First moves with the leg with a slight bend forward.

The head, during the first demi-plié and during the jump, turns toward the advanced shoulder and remains in that position until the end of the movement or follows the rules for third or fourth arabesque if either of those are the ending pose. At the finish of the pas assemblé into Fifth Position, the entire body assumes the starting Fifth Position.

The entire movement must be flowing and light especially if it is an approach to a big jump or a pirouette. The pas failli must be joined to small jumps and later to big jumps.

The pas failli is performed before the measure and is at first learned with rests after each jump, but later without pauses. The tempo is 2/4 or 3/4.

ROND DE JAMBE EN L'AIR SAUTÉ

This rond de jambe is done on the structure of the sissonne ouverte par jeté in a Second Position with the addition of one or two ronds de jambes en l'air at 45 degrees during the flight. (See illustration #116.)

Beginning in the Fifth Position with the right leg in front, épaulement croisé, both legs perform a demi-plié. The jump is in place, en face, with the right leg thrown to the side at 45 degrees. At the crest of the jump, the open leg performs a rond de jambe en l'air en dehors which ends at the same time as the landing in demi-plié on the supporting leg. The entire movement is ended with a pas assemblé

---

116 Rond de jambe en l'air sauté

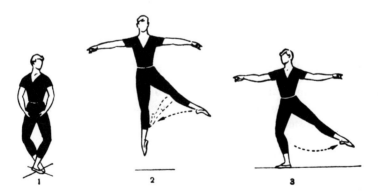

into Fifth Position with the right leg ending in back and in the épaulement croisé position.

The arms during the first demi-plié are in Preparatory Position and move to the First Position during the jump when they are open to Second.

The body is kept straight during the jump but at the finish in demi-plié it leans slightly away from the open leg, then straightens again at the pas assemblé.

The head during the jump is kept en face, and at the finish in demi-plié it turns away from the open leg. The pas assemblé finds the head turned toward the left shoulder.

Rond de jambe en l'air sauté en dedans is performed according to the same rules, but the open or working leg comes from behind in the Fifth Position and the rond de jambe is, of course, en dedans and the leg ends in front. All the details required in the performance of the rond de jambe en l'air without the sauté (jump) are obligatory here. During the jump the right leg must be clearly stretched out after each rond and the left leg must not bend in reflex to the movement of the right leg. It too must be stretched at the crest of the jump with the knee, instep and toes in one line.

The entire jump must be done at a good height with energy, but softly and freely.

This movement must be studied at first en dehors, then en dedans with pauses after each jump to a 2/4 tempo.

The double rond de jambe en l'air sauté may be studied only after the technique of a forceful big jump has been mastered, since this movement demands maximum height that has been properly prepared from the ballon movement previously described.

JUMPS FROM ONE LEG TO TWO LEGS

PAS ASSEMBLÉ

Pas assemblé is done petit and grand with a throw of a leg in Second or Fourth Position.

PETIT PAS ASSEMBLÉ

The petit pas assemblé in Second begins in the Fifth Position, right foot front, épaulement croisé. Before the jump, and during the demi-plié, the weight of the body must be transferred onto the right leg. The right leg is then the source of the push. At the same time, the left leg glides from the Fifth Position and is thrown to the side in 45 degrees. The right leg after the push from the floor straightens forcibly, maintaining a perpendicular position. At the crest of the jump the working left leg is clearly in 45 degrees to the side and the supporting right leg stretched completely from knee through toes. At the moment the jump is about to descend, the left leg returns to the Fifth Position in front of the right leg, and both legs perform the supporting demi-plié finish (assemblé dessus—over).

The arms are kept in Preparatory Position or, at the crest of the jump, rise slightly to a lowered Second Position. At the end of the jump, the arm corresponding to the closing leg is transferred into a lowered First while the other arm remains in lowered Second. From this position comes the next pas assemblé, the arm in First moving into Second and, at the end of the jump, the other arm moving from Second into First, etc., in subsequent repetitions.

The body changes during the jump from épaulement and remains straight until the descent into épaulement with the opposite shoulder forward. The head before and after the jump turns toward the advanced shoulder. During the crest of the jump, the head is en face. (See illustration #117.) (This assemblé is called demi-positioned in the Cecchetti and in demi-hauteur by the French School.)

During the pas assemblé, the arms move back into Preparatory Position.

---

117 Petit pas assemblé in Second Position

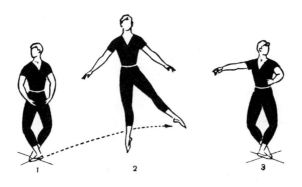

The reverse of the pas assemblé is begun after the demi-plié by the foot in front. The same foot closes in back in Fifth Position at the final demi-plié (assemblé dessous—under).

The arms are retained in Preparatory Position or the arm contrary to the closing leg is moved from Second into First. The body and head follow the same pattern as previously described.

Petit pas assemblé in Fourth Position is done in the same manner as the en face described except that the working leg is in the croisé or effacé position. (The hips face the diagonal corners of the room, #2 or #8 for these movements.) All the other details remain the same. The arms remain in the Preparatory Position or assume the position for small poses or arabesques. The body and head take positions which harmonize with the given poses.

DOUBLE ASSEMBLÉ

Another variation of this movement is the double assemblé, which has two jumps performed twice by the same leg in Second or Fourth Position. The leg in the first jump closes in Fifth Position in its starting place and changes after the second assemblé to the front position. The reverse double assemblé follows the same rules. When the double assemblé is performed in Fourth (effacé and croisé), both jumps return the working leg to the starting position. The head, body and arms keep the positions described above.

Each petit pas assemblé must begin and end with a turned-out and supple demi-plié. The supporting leg must join the floor tightly with the heel on the floor. Care must be taken not to permit the pupil to "ride off" during the push. (The demi-plié and pushoff must be in the same place on the floor.)

The other leg must open exactly and in a straight line along the Second and Fourth position with the glide, a light movement along the floor by the entire foot and the turnout maintained throughout. At the crest of the jump, both legs must be totally straight from the knee through the instep and toes. The jump is done in place without advancement and ends simultaneously on both legs in a correct Fifth Position.

On the whole, the petit pas assemblé must be done flowingly without pauses, but without overstating the movement of the leg or overworking the body. The arms and head are kept free and used with aplomb.

The study of petit pas assemblé should begin facing the barre with the working leg moving to Second Position in this simpler form: After the demi-plié in Fifth Position, the leg in back moves with an even glide into Second with the toes along the floor. Then the small jump is executed and the open leg is pulled forward into Fifth Position in demi-plié.

The tempo is 4/4: 1/4 for the first demi-plié; 1/4 for the opening of the leg; 1/4 for the jump into Fifth; 1/4 to straighten from the demi-plié. The movement should be repeated four times forward, then four times backward. When this is mastered, the student may begin to throw the leg from Fifth Position in one measure of 4/4: 1/4 for the demi-plié; 1/4 for the jump; 1/4 to straighten from demi-plié; and 1/4 for a pause.

When this has been correctly mastered, the petit pas assemblé may be performed on the center of the floor with the arms in Preparatory Position and the head en face.

Subsequently the pas assemblé may be studied with the jump executed before the measure with a stop or pause in the demi-plié to 1/4 count. At this point in the study, the use of the head may be introduced with a turn toward the opening leg which ends forward in Fifth Position and which turns away from the closing leg when that leg closes in back in Fifth Position (when the pas assemblé moves backward). Finally, the épaulement is added in the Second Position version. Two or three jumps are joined consecutively, changing the arms from First to Second, and the other, from Second into First as previously described along with the proper head movements.

As the last study, the petit pas assemblé double in Second Position must be mastered. Both jumps must be joined in a flowing manner in one measure of 2/4 with the pause an entire measure between double jumps. Then, the double assemblé is done with stops.

The arms at first should be kept in the Preparatory Position, but later moved from First into Second at the second jump, with a turn of the head and body, according to the rules for épaulement.

Then, the study of petit pas assemblé in Fourth Position should begin with the first exercise in croisé forward and croisé back. The movement then should be mastered in effacé. These assemblés in the croisé and effacé positions should be performed before the measure with the stop pattern of demi-plié to 1/4 measure and later should be performed without the pauses.

The arms at first should be kept in Preparatory Position, then moved to small pose positions varying to the movement of the head and the body. Later, the double assemblé should be mastered in these diagonal positions. Here too, the arms remain at first in the Preparatory Position and then the exercises are performed with the arms in small poses with the corresponding movement of the head and body.

(It seems a strange omission not to mention the assemblé derrière—beginning and closing in Fifth Position back—and the assemblé en avant—beginning and closing in Fifth Position front. Both of these assemblés are frequently used and may be performed with or without the advance. It is possible that these forms are not favored in Soviet choreography, but it would seem logical to teach them.)

GRAND PAS ASSEMBLÉ

The grand pas assemblé is similar to the petit version except that the leg is thrown to 90 degrees with an advance along a diagonal line and requires the utmost height within the capacity of the student. During the flight in this version, the legs are joined tightly in Fifth Position and are kept joined until the finish in demi-plié. The arms, head and body are fixed in the position of the large poses.

In order to achieve height and ballon, there is usually an approach—pas tombé, pas glissade, pas de bourrée, pas failli, sissonne tombée, etc.—before the grand pas assemblé. These steps prior to the execution of the grand pas assemblé permit the push from the floor to be with considerably more force and greater trajectory when the leg is thrown from Fourth Position instead of Fifth Position. This approach lengthens the jump in space and strengthens the flying push. The movement of the arms, body and head must be more active in this more forceful version and partake in the greater advancement in space.

All approaches to the grand pas assemblé should be done energetically with a rush, but not with artifice or deliberation, to achieve the required greater height. Each approach must be free and exact and with a light use of technique which does not stress its difficulty but, on the contrary, brings to it the element of surprise and easy virtuosity. Too great a rushing sendoff by the body, however, will interfere with the full force of the demi-plié. The flight in that case becomes a long, drawn-out movement insufficiently high, unstable when completed.

In the performance of the grand pas assemblé, the leg must be thrown with a rush and with exactness through First, but no higher than 70 degrees. Both legs must be joined in the air so that the end in demi-plié is done evenly on both legs in a soft and correct Fifth Position. The body, head and arms simultaneously move along the flight pattern without lagging or moving ahead of the leg. The position in the crest of the jump must be clear and fixed until the landing.

It is important for the body, during the approach, to bend toward the supporting leg and together with the push, move energetically in the direction of the flight. The position in the air must be pulled up during the flight, with the shoulders free and open. The arms, too, make a contribution to the movement for height and advancement by opening forcefully with the throw of the leg from the Preparatory Position to Second in concert with the fixed position in the air. The head is joined in coordination with the other parts of the body to project the body with force by the proper coordination of all its parts in the given pose.

In general, the approaches and grands pas assemblés are done in a fluid manner, in one tempo and with a swoop into flight. The rules for the performance of the grand pas assemblé require that, in the Second Position form, the crest of the movement is fixed in écarté, in its usual use, or in an allongé position. (See illustration #118.) Performed in Fourth, the pose is usually fixed in croisé position with both arms in Third Position during the crest of the jump. But these positions may vary. (See illustration #119.)

---

118   Grand pas assemblé in Second Position

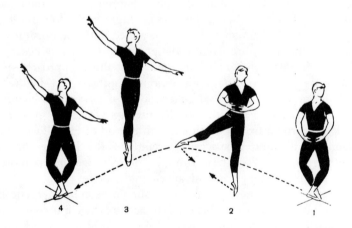

The grand pas assemblé in Fourth with an advancement backward is usually not done in consecutive assemblés. This form provides insufficient push or progressive gathering of momentum for a high jump and ballon.

The grand pas assemblé should be studied in place in écarté forward to 4/4 measures. Beginning in the Fifth Position, épaulement croisé and before the measure, the forward leg is moved into the sur le cou-de-pied position in front at the same time as the demi-plié on the standing leg. On the 1/4 count, the pas coupé moves into Fifth for the push; 1/4 is used for the pas assemblé; 1/4 to straighten from demi-plié; 1/4 for the transfer into sur le cou-de-pied forward, etc. During the straightening movement, the arms move from Third into Second and at the change of the leg into sur le cou-de-pied, both arms lower into Preparatory Position. The body during the coupé turns, clearly changing the épaulement and actively leaning toward the direction of the advancing leg. During the flight, the body is pulled up and collected so the jump may end evenly on both legs. The head, during the pas coupé, leans slightly toward the hands, which are in First and which during the crest of the jump rise and swoopingly turn in the direction of the advancement, remaining there until the end of the exercise.

In the beginning of the study of grand pas assemblé, special attention must be given to the details in the use of pas coupé. The leg which performs the push must join the floor resiliently from toes through the entire foot into a deepened demi-plié with a strong passing rest of the heel and thigh. The following push for the assemblé must be done with energy, without delay and through the foot from heel through the instep and toes to the knee.

The study may include the approach of a pas glissade to the side from Fifth to

---

119 Grand pas assemblé in Fourth Position croisé

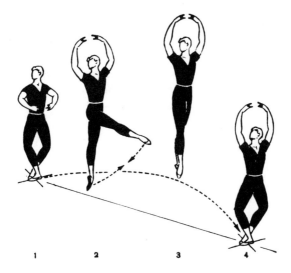

1   2   3   4

Fifth Position without a change of legs (the foot which begins in back for a glissade which moves to the right, ends in back).

The pas glissade begins in Fifth with the right leg in back. The glissade must end in an exact Fifth Position for the grand pas assemblé to have correct and sufficient push. The body is en face and the arms immediately and energetically pick up the momentum by moving into a pose allongée. The head follows the pattern described previously. The final change to épaulement is done in flight in a soft and stable manner.

The entire exercise is done to two measures of 2/4. The glissade is begun before the measure: 1/4 for the push and jump; 1/4 for the finish in demi-plié; 1/4 to straighten from the landing; 1/4 for a demi-plié, etc. (This exercise moves first to the right, then to the left.)

The exercise is then practiced in reverse in the same pattern. Later, the exercise is performed without stops and, finally, practiced in Fourth Position with a pas tombé, pas chassé, sissonne tombée or pas failli approach.

When these approaches are used, the throw of the leg must pass through First Position in écarté forward practicing constantly for a pliable, light push and for ballon in the flight. There must be a soft and stable landing. The arms, legs, head and body follow the same rules as described.

The grand pas assemblé in croisé forward should be studied at first from the pas tombé approach, then from the sissonne tombée and pas de bourrée approaches.

For instance: Beginning in Fourth Position with the right leg in tendu forward, épaulement croisé, the left executes a pas tombé forward in effacé. The right is then free to do the pas assemblé croisé forward. *Both movements* are done through the First Position. During the flight, the left leg is pulled energetically to the right leg and in flight must be tightly joined to it in Fifth Position. The entire jump ends softly and flexibly in demi-plié.

The arms in pas tombé move from the Preparatory Position into a lowered Second, palms down, (allongé) and during the push energetically perform the "pickup" through Preparatory into First, then swoop into Third and remain there until the end of the movement. The body is sent with force into the pushing leg and during the flight it swoops along the trajectory of the movement. At the completion of the movement, it is kept even and shapely on both legs. The head in pas tombé leans slightly forward and in flight clearly straightens out and turns toward the advancing shoulder, fixing the pose to the end of the jump.

It must be remembered that it is very important to develop a light and elastic push for the jump which will, at a later date, become an obligatory element in more complicated allegros, such as the grand pas jeté, the grande cabriole, etc.

The study of this form of grand pas assemblé should be started with the usual pauses, then without them and gradually introducing more complicated approaches, various positions of the arms and combined auxiliary movements.

After the grand pas assemblé croisé forward has been mastered, it is useful to introduce the position for the head, arms and body of the third arabesque. This position in flight with the legs joined in Fifth aids the forward movement and adds to the performance of this assemblé greater ballon and dynamics.

JUMPS FROM ONE LEG TO THE OTHER LEG

PAS JETÉ

This movement as well is divided into small and large jumps.

PETIT PAS JETÉ

The petit pas jeté is done with a throw of the leg into Second as in petit pas assemblé, but the movement ends in the sur le cou-de-pied position. Begun like the pas assemblé, the petit pas jeté beginning in Fifth Position demi-plié glides the leg in back along the floor to a throw in Second at 45 degrees. The other leg at the same time moves with force into a push. At the crest of the movement, both legs are stretched out, fixing with clarity the pose and finish of the movement. At the finish of the jump, the leg that was thrown returns softly into the place of the leg that made the push. That leg is then free to move into the sur le cou-de-pied back. This jump ends exactly where it started with no advancement.

---

120 Petit pas jeté

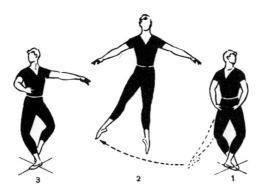

In reverse, the petit pas jeté starts with the leg in front in the Fifth Position and ends with the other leg in sur le cou-de-pied front.

The arms, head and body in both jumps move in the pattern of the petit pas assemblé. (See illustration #120.)

In the performance of the petit pas jeté without stops, the leg is led into the Second Position directly from the sur le cou-de-pied and in the opening the toes lightly graze the floor.

The entire movement, beginning with a supple demi-plié, must be turned out.

The supporting leg must slide tightly and evenly with the heel on the floor during the push. The leg must move lightly and exactly to Second Position and, at the crest of the movement, both legs must clearly and simultaneously stretch out at the knees, insteps and toes. The sur le cou-de-pied position must be assumed at the soft and supple demi-plié landing.

The arms, head and body, as previously described, work in the pattern for petit pas assemblé with as much freedom and shapely fixing of the small poses.

The petit pas jeté must be studied at first facing the barre, and with a stop after each jump to a measure of 4/4. Jumping before the measure, 1/4 for the finish in demi-plié; 1/4 for the pause; 1/4 for the straightening from demi-plié; 1/4, the leg in sur le cou-de-pied position is placed into Fifth Position in demi-plié, etc. The exercise must be repeated four times, first with the leg beginning in Fifth Position in back, then reversed.

When the student has mastered this movement, the exercise may be transferred to the floor in the same learning pattern.

The arms at the start of the study of pas jeté must be kept in Preparatory Position and the body en face. The use of the head should be introduced as in the petit pas assemblé. Later, the épaulement and the combined positions of the arm are studied and the movements executed two or three jumps in a row.

Petit pas jeté is similar to petit pas assemblé, so the study of this movement must not be prolonged but must nonetheless be given thorough and detailed attention until it is exact and stable.

Petit pas jeté with advancement is done in Second or Fourth as a small jump and with small poses. In the ordinary pas jeté the pushing leg stays perpendicular during the flight and the working leg is fixed to an angle of about 45 degrees. Then the step may be performed at 60 or 70 degrees. All other rules are followed.

Performed with an advance, the body is projected in the direction of the toe of the open leg, to the front, side or back depending upon the direction of the movement and in which direction the advance has been given. The finish of this jump, therefore, will be in another place from its start.

The description of the pas jeté with an advance in Second need not be given in detail except to remark that in flight the opened leg must be fixed in a clear position with the knees, instep and toes forcefully stretched. The body, together with the arms and head, must help the swoop of the flight, which should end in a stable and soft demi-plié.

This form of pas jeté is studied on the floor with pauses after each jump and in conjunction with petit pas assemblé croisé forward and backward. The arm, head and body follow the pas jeté and pas assemblé pattern. The small pose is fixed during the flight and to its end. In a 4/4 measure: pas jeté before the measure; 1/4 is used for the finish; 1/4 for rest and demi-plié; 1/4 for pas assemblé; 1/4 for pause in demi-plié, etc. This is then performed without stops and joined with other small jumps.

Petit pas jeté in Fourth with advance forward or backward is studied in the following manner:

Beginning in the Fifth Position, épaulement croisé, the forward leg glides from the demi-plié with a light brush and is thrown croisé forward to 45 degrees at the same time that the supporting leg forcefully makes a supple push. The entire body at the crest of the jump swoops forward with the legs fixed in open 60 to 70 degrees. The completion of the movement should be stable and soft and in a correct sur le cou-de-pied in back (left leg). The arms during the jump rise from Preparatory to a lowered Second and at the finishing demi-plié correspond to the thrown leg in a lowered First while the other remains in Second.

The body keeps the épaulement at the finishing demi-plié and leans a little toward the supporting leg while the shoulders lean slightly back. The head stays in the starting position until the finishing demi-plié complementing the leaning body.

After this movement a petit pas assemblé to the side (leg to corner #6) ends in Fifth Position forward. During this assemblé, the arm at the crest of the movement moves from First to Second. The body and head turn en face and, at the finish of the jump, the arms return to the Preparatory Position. The body returns to épaulement and the head turns forward to the advanced shoulder.

To a 4/4 measure and with the first jump executed before the count: 1/4 is used for the completion of the petit pas jeté; 1/4 for a pause; 1/4 for the pas assemblé; 1/4 for rest or pause.

The same exercise is reversed in the study and performed without stops. The arms, head and body must work without changes. Those may be introduced at a later time when the pas jeté is combined with other elements.

There is no point in exercising the pas jeté with advancement along Second or Fourth Position without stops in an uninterrupted series between two points along the same line of space. That does not progressively strengthen the aplomb of the performance of this jump. Joining the pas jeté, however, with advance varying the jumps along Second and Fourth, does. For instance, it is useful to do a pas jeté with advance sideways (end with the right foot in sur le cou-de-pied in front), then pas jeté croisé forward finishing with a petit pas assemblé backward (left foot back). This exercise is then studied on the other leg and reversed in direction.

As a general rule, the pas jeté with an advance in Second is done with a change of leg. The leg in Fifth Position back will end, after the throw to the side, as the supporting leg in front, with the other in sur le cou-de-pied back. But there is an exception to this rule when there is no change of legs. The épaulement in that case is kept and not changed either.

The pas jeté is executed not only in the croisé position but in the effacé position as well. The épaulement is changed in this case and the movements of the head, body and arms follow the pattern as previously given. These forms must be used in combination with other steps. (Petit pas jeté may be executed to the front and to the back as well.)

GRAND PAS JETÉ

The grand pas jeté is done with an advance and a high jump during which the fixed pose is in Second or in Fourth Position. The leg must reach 90 degrees and the pushing leg 60 degrees. At the crest of the jump, both legs fix the step in relation to the floor's surface at 150 degrees. At the completion, the leg thrown to 90 degrees lowers into a demi-plié through 45 degrees while the other remains in 90 degrees at the finish of the jump. (See illustration #121.)

The impulse of the pupil at the crest of the jump to fix the movement at 180 degrees or more must not be permitted. This effect would be in the character of an acrobatic eccentricity. In addition, an execution of this step which is too big, as in the form of a split, does not place the body in the correct alignment to descend through the toes, heels and into a supported demi-plié ending. Nor is a smaller size desirable, since it does not increase the dynamics or the ballon in flight, which must always be sufficiently high and swooping in its advance. The fixing of the arms, body and head in flight and afterward must be in strict harmony with the rules of performance of classical dance.

---

121   Grand pas jeté

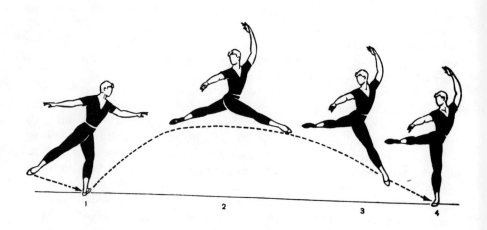

The grand pas jeté, as a rule, is begun from an approach which will prepare a takeoff of the greatest force in order to fix the pose clearly in the air and facilitate a soft and stable demi-plié ending. The approaches may be the pas tombé, the pas glissade, pas failli, pas de bourrée, sissonne tombée, etc.

Whichever form of approach is used, it must be executed energetically and prudently for a trampoline-like sendoff of the entire body in the direction of the trajectory of the flight. At the same time, an approach that is too strong will elongate but lower the crest of the jump and give it a stock, squat development and an unstable ending.

In performing the grand pas jeté, the student must place the pushing foot on the floor from the tips of the toes through the foot to the heel. Care must be taken to see that the heel is firmly placed. The demi-plié must be resilient with the image of a *swooping* push. The thrown leg must be energetically timed with the supporting push increasing the force by this coordination of movements. At the crest of the jump, the legs must be totally straightened from knees to toes (unless the jump is in attitude) and the direction properly aimed along the Fourth or Second Position. The landing of the jumps must be soft, stable and in demi-plié with an almost imperceptible lift of the open leg. And all these details must be maintained in a turned-out position.

The arms at the sendoff, in their rise from Preparatory to First, must actively lift off, involving the arms in the strength and clarity of the fixed flight position. The body, too, must be in a fixed and freely suitable position during the crest of the jump. The weight is pulled up, and the shoulders lowered and open. The spine is held but not with excessive strain, while the weight of the body during the approach for the push must, in the proper time and exactly, transfer the weight over the thigh of the supporting leg. This permits a stable and supple ending.

The head, when the arms lift off, leans a bit toward the hands but turns at the crest of the jump to coordinate with the performing pose. The look is directed resolutely in the same direction. On the whole, each grand jeté must be performed freely with clear ballon in flight without an excessively sharp, tense or carried-away image. It must be in harmony with the character of the given example and to the given musical form.

The study of the grand pas jeté should be done in place without the approach. Beginning in Fifth Position, épaulement croisé, the demi-plié starts the movement; then the forward leg glides along the floor through the whole foot and is thrown forward in croisé as the other leg simultaneously pushes from the floor. The jump with an advance is in the form of an arc during which the leg that pushed off bends in the fixed pose into attitude croisée back and the thrown leg stretches forward. The jump is completed with a flexible demi-plié and the half-bent leg in attitude back is kept in that position.

The arms at the first demi-plié rise from Preparatory Position to First and, during the crest of the jump, move energetically into Second and remain fixed until the ending demi-plié. The body, in the first demi-plié, and at the time of the throw of the leg, leans slightly toward the hands in the Preparatory Position. At the crest of the jump, the head turns toward the open arm and is fixed there until the end of the jump.

After the landing, a pas assemblé croisé backward is done as the arms lower into Preparatory Position and the body becomes straight while the head remains in the same position.

The entire exercise is repeated four times, then performed on the other leg. The measure is 4/4 with the pas jeté before the measure; 1/4 ends the jump; 1/4 for the rest in demi-plié; 1/4 for the pas assemblé; 1/4 for the rest, etc.

Then the study with the pas tombé approach should begin. Here, the exercise begins in Fourth, épaulement croisé. The body is supported by the leg in Fourth front. The leg in back is stretched out through the knee, instep and toes, with the toes lightly touching the floor. The arms are in a lowered Second and the head is turned toward the advanced shoulder (downstage). From this beginning pose, the free leg in back moves through the First Position in a battement tendu into a pas tombé in effacé forward while the other leg, at the same time, is thrown forward through First into Fourth. The pose in flight ends as previously described (in attitude back).

During the execution of the pas tombé, the body energetically and exactly leans toward the pushing leg but in flight it swoops along the forward trajectory. At the finish, it is stable and pulled up. The arms in pas tombé softly turn palms down and at the push energetically pick up or lift off through Preparatory Position into First and attitude position and remain until the finishing demi-plié. The head in the pas tombé leans slightly forward and turns to the opposite shoulder. During the flight, it resumes the starting position until the finish.

At the finish of this jump, the open leg (in attitude) is stretched out at the knee and the leg lowers the toes to the floor as the supporting leg straightens from the demi-plié. The arm in Third (attitude position) moves into Second as the head remains steadily in the same position. The position is then ready to be the starting position from which to repeat the exercise four times consecutively, and reversed. The tempo is again 4/4 with the pas tombé before the measure: 1/4 for the pas jeté; 1/4 for the rest; 1/4 to lower the open leg to the floor in tendu; 1/4 to move the leg to the next pas tombé, etc.

Later, this approach to pas jeté may be performed without lowering the leg with the toe on the floor in the middle of the movement, by keeping the end of the jump in attitude for 1/4 instead of lowering the leg and, finally, by performing the entire exercise with 1/4 for each tombé and jeté.

To strengthen the flight before the pas tombé, the exercise may begin with a pas chassé forward in Fourth Position; or with a pas failli, or a sissonne tombée or even a simple pas de bourrée forward consisting of three rushing steps in Fourth Position. The arm, body and head at the moment of the push and flight follow the same pattern as described above. The approaches given are not used in reverse because it would be extremely difficult and inadvisable, even in a teaching context.

One may start the study of the grand pas jeté from the attitude effacée or in first or second arabesque. The approaches may be pas tombé in croisé forward; sissonne tombée en croisé forward; pas failli, pas glissade forward from Fourth Position croisé. The approach to third arabesque is the same as the attitude croisée, beginning from a pas tombé forward.

All the described forms of grand pas jeté are to a certain measure a law or principle which must be learned sufficiently well in combination with other jumps. Later, one may perform the grand pas jeté in poses in Fourth croisé and effacé to the back, in attitude allongée and in fourth arabesque.

In the poses in Fourth Position backward, the arms may be arranged in a combination of Second and Third; First and Third; First and Second; or both in Third Position. The head and body in every case must be fixed in the coordinating position suitable to the teaching task.

In attitude allongée in fourth arabesque arms, head and body fit the generally accepted teaching forms of grand pas jeté in Second but is performed rarely onstage or in teaching. The reason is that the approach may only be a pas coupé or a pas glissade ending in Fifth along the line of the jump, which lessens the force and spring of the push and, therefore, its height and ballon. However, students in the more advanced classes must master all the forms of grand pas jeté no matter the difficulty of form, tempo, rhythm or character.

The pas jeté is learned in Second Position after it has been mastered from the Fourth Position approach and executed in place without an approach.

The starting pose is Fifth, épaulement croisé. The forward leg glides along the floor with the whole foot until it is thrown to the side in Second Position. The other leg at the same time makes a forceful push from the demi-plié. At the crest of the jump, which is done with an advance to the side, both legs stretch out from the knees, insteps and toes. The jump is finished with a soft, stable demi-plié and the open leg remains *without hesitation* in the same position. The arms in demi-plié rise from Preparatory Position into First, and in the flight move energetically into Second and remain until the finish in demi-plié. The body during the demi-plié leans slightly in the direction of the leg, which is thrown into Second, and in flight turns en face, where it remains until the end.

The head in the first demi-plié turns and bends slightly toward the hand in Preparatory Position. At the crest of the jump, the head is lifted and turned en face and, at the end, turns slightly away from the open leg.

This movement ends in a pause, followed by a pas assemblé forward into Fifth Position. The arms, which are in Second Position, descend at the same time into Preparatory Position. The body straightens out and the épaulement position is assumed as the head turns to the advanced shoulder. The entire exercise is repeated backward to a measure of 4/4: the jump before the measure; 1/4 for the finish of the jump; 1/4 for rest; 1/4 for the pas assemblé; 1/4 for rest, etc.

Later, the exercise may be performed without the pauses, using 1/4 for each jump.

Afterward, the grand pas jeté may be studied with the pas coupé and pas glissade approach.

In the pas coupé approach, the leg behind in the Fifth Position assumes the sur le cou-de-pied position as the supporting leg makes the first demi-plié. The jump from this position must be uninterrupted and energetic along Second and the finish must be in the same open leg position in demi-plié support.

Thereafter, the pas assemblé into Fifth behind makes the movement ready to be repeated on the other leg, four times forward and four times in reverse. The arms, head and body follow the described pattern.

The pas coupé and the pas jeté are executed before the measure: 1/4 is used for the rest in the open position; 1/4 for the pas assemblé; 1/4 for the transfer of the leg to sur le cou-de-pied, etc.

In the pas glissade approach, the movement is from Fifth Position into Fifth in the direction of the jump and without a change of legs. The pas jeté follows without interruption and energetically into Second Position and finishes with a pas assemblé forward or backward as given. The arms, head and body follow the previously described patterns.

The pas glissade is done before the measure: 2/4 pas jeté; 1/4 for the rest; 1/4 for the pas assemblé, etc. (The upbeat or count before the measure is frequently accompanied by a bellowing "EEEEEEEEE"—"and" in the Russian language.)

During the performance of the pas coupé and pas glissade, the leg making the push from the floor must be placed exactly and forcefully in Fifth Position underneath the body weight over the supporting leg. At the same time, the body must be placed in the trajectory of the flight with sufficient energy or the advance will be insufficient.

There is a variation in the performance of the grand pas jeté along the Second Position which consists of not leaving the leg fixed in 90 degrees at the finish but moving it into Fifth or into sur le cou-de-pied as in sissonne fermée or petit pas jeté with an advance. The arms, head and body follow the rules while the start of the jump follows the rules of the grand pas jeté.

The movement, therefore, does not demand special study, as all the elements were prepared in previous exercises. It must be remembered, however, that this jump like all the others must be flowing in the approach, have sufficient advance, be high and soft especially at the finish. This movement is called grand pas jeté fermé if it ends in Fifth Position, and grand pas jeté fondu if it ends in sur le cou-de-pied.

The suggested plan of study may be enriched with the addition of movement of gradual complexity in the approach to the jump. Force and elasticity in the pushing leg develop normally under these conditions. The leg that is thrown must gradually learn to accept the weight of the body softly and lightly.

When the plan of study has been mastered, a variety of arm movements may be introduced with economy and as an exception to the rules.

The grand pas jeté may be performed along the Second and Fourth positions without the described approach from the sur le cou-de-pied position or from a previously opened step such as the sissonne ouverte, temps levé, etc. In this way, the jump may be performed from a pose on the floor along Second or Fourth. The arms, head and body follow the performance rules as given.

The same method of grand pas jeté may be done twice, for instance, as from pose effacée forward into first arabesque and back without stopping. Or two or three movements may be performed forward with each jump going through the first arabesque. These jumps must be done with clarity and lightness. The push must be impetuous and trampoline-like, the advance prolonged, and the pose fixed in flight. The arms, head and body are kept in the given design during the flight.

All these jumps must be done along one line. At the same time, it is permissible to gradually increase the height of the jump with a smooth raising of the head and arms. The image may be an imaginary line flowing over the floor in a horizontal advance that guides the student.

It must be remembered that in flight the legs must be stretched out energetically to the tips of the toes and that every throw of the leg must be done exactly and through the First Position and *simultaneously with the push.*

Finally, it must be observed that the forms of the performance of the grand pas jeté should vary and that the larger jumps are learned only after all the facets of the movements have been thoroughly learned.

(An aid to remembering the rules for the head during big jumps might be in knowing that the Russian School, with few exceptions, seldom requires the body to be en face. Épaulement is largely used and the head is always turned in the direction of the forward shoulder.)

---

122   Pas jeté passé

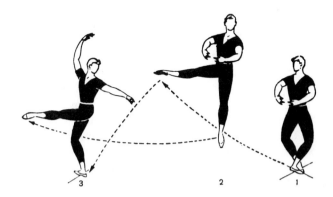

PAS JETÉ PASSÉ

The pas jeté passé is a movement done as a big jump in a large pose along Fourth croisé, effacé, in arabesque or attitude. The leg performs two throws as a grand battement jeté forward or back. The first throw is from Fifth Position at the same time as the push; and the second throw is in flight. After reaching the crest of the jump, the leg that made the first throw begins to lower into demi-plié as the other continues to rise to 90 degrees.

In this way, the legs pass each other approximately at the height of 60 degrees. This moment of passing is the peculiarity of this movement and as a component enters into other big jumps, such as the pas ciseaux, jeté entrelacé, and others.

During the flight, and together with the first throw, the arms move from Preparatory Position into First; at the second throw, they move into the given performing pose. The head and body at the same time may assume the pose in illustration #122.

The pose in this movement is fixed at the end of the jump, not in flight, as in the grand pas jeté.

Combined with other movements, it may begin not only in Fifth Position, but also in any pose along Fourth, or from pas tombé, pas chassé, pas failli or pas de bourrée or pas couru.

Finally, the second throw of the leg in this movement may be done through the position at the knee as a développé (temps de flèche).

The first demi-plié is done energetically and the final demi-plié, softer, deeper but as supple as the first demi-plié. During the jump the legs must pass as close as possible to each other.

The open leg position at the end of the jump must be fixed, stable and light. The arms during the jump move exactly and actively, holding their position at the end of the jump in the performing position.

The head moves clearly and in coordination with the arm movements. The body at the time of the push from the floor is pulled up and sent in the direction of the advance. During the flight, it participates as actively as the arms and head. At the finish, the body is over the supporting leg, preserving the harmony and correctness of the position.

During the jump, the shoulders are kept freely open, lowered and the upper back and waist are pulled up. The advance must be done by opening the legs with sufficient sendoff, underscoring the lightness and impetus of the flight.

As a whole, the pas jeté passé is a soft, slowing movement clear in design, especially in its final pose. The study of this movement should begin from the Fifth Position in the following manner: with the legs in Fifth Position, épaulement croisé, the first throw is done to the back in croisé by the back leg; the second throw is done by the other leg in effacé to the back.

The arms move at the first throw from Preparatory Position into First, and, at the second, open to first arabesque. The body and head coordinate to the first arabesque.

Then a second jump is performed as the supporting leg makes a throw backward and the open leg lowers into demi-plié. The arms, head and body and the back leg assume the positions for attitude croisée. The exercise ends in pas de bourrée with a change of leg in Fifth and is then done from the other leg and repeated four times, then four times in reverse. The tempo is 2/4 with the first jump before the measure; 1/4 to finish the jump in its pose; 1/4 for the second jump; 2/4 for the pas de bourrée. Later, this movement may be varied with different approaches and different poses.

The pas jeté passé may be introduced into complex combinations with an advance in the given direction of the combination. In combining big jumps, this movement is usually used as a connecting and transferring element as it is not remarkable in any special ballon or virtuosity. At the same time, it demands a true feeling for dance phrasing, musical coloring, and it must be exercised by the students.

PAS GLISSADE

The pas glissade is a minimal gliding jump that moves sideways with an advance, forward or backward. The starting post is Fifth, épaulement croisé. It begins with a demi-plié during which the forward leg moves with a sliding movement into the Second Position as the other leg, at the same time, does a slight push. At the crest of the movement, both legs are stretched out with a minimal separation from the floor. At the finish, the leg which began the movement does a demi-plié without any further advance as the other, gliding along the floor, is pulled up into its starting Fifth Position.

At the crest of the movement, the arms move from Preparatory Position into a somewhat lowered Second and at the finish of the demi-plié they return to the Preparatory Position. The body and head stay in épaulement.

This form of pas glissade may be done with a change of épaulement. If the legs exchange places at the finish of the pas glissade in Fifth Position, the head turns toward the opposite shoulder. The arms and body keep the same position. Or, the pas glissade may begin with the leg in back in Fifth Position, with or without an exchange at the final Fifth Position. The rules in any case, for the head, arms and body, follow the given rules. (See illustration #123.)

---

123 Pas glissade

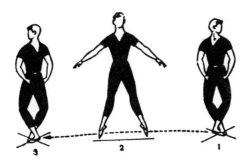

The pas glissade is also performed with an advance forward and backward and with small poses in croisé and effacé. The legs in the croisé and effacé positions move along Fourth in the same way as described above. The body maintains the épaulement. The arms at the demi-plié move from Preparatory Position into First and, at the crest of the movement, one arm opens into a lowered Second. At the finishing demi-plié, both arms return to Preparatory Position. The head, during the arm movements, assumes the position that corresponds to the ending pose.

Each pas glissade must begin and end in a supple demi-plié. The glide forward with a slight rise is executed lightly and softly. At the crest of the movement, the legs must be clearly stretched at the knees, instep and toes. On the whole, the movement must be flowing, in one tempo, without walking along the floor or raising the jump into a pas jeté fermé. The arms and head must act freely and accurately, but without sharp movements.

The study of pas glissade must begin to the side from Fifth Position to 2/4 tempo. The first 1/4 is used to open the leg into Second; 1/4 for the slide and final demi-plié into Fifth. In this pattern, the exercise is repeated four times from the same leg without changing the leg in Fifth Position. Then it is repeated four times from the other leg. The arms remain in Preparatory and the body and head remain en face. Later, one may study pas glissade without pauses and exchanging the legs into Fifth Position; from side to side; along Fourth Position forward and backward; and into small poses.

If pas glissade along Fourth Position is used as an approach to a big jump such as the pas jeté forward, grande cabriole forward or other big movement, it is somewhat altered and performed through First in the same pattern and with minimal height. For instance: beginning in a small pose croisée backward, the back leg, which is in a tendu pose with the toes on the floor, moves through First into Fourth; then the other leg does a slide through First, minus the minimal height, into Fourth and into a strong demi-plié, which forms the basis for the energetic push for the forthcoming big jump.

The arms during this glissade are in Second, with the palms down. During the push for the jump, they move energetically through Preparatory Position into First and into the given pose. The body is pulled up and leans forward onto the pushing leg. The head and arms assume the position suitable to the given pose. This form of pas glissade must have a light character and a short sendoff, and not be lengthened in tempo or size, nor be squat with half-bent legs.

The legs, during this glissade, must move clearly with stretched knees, instep and toes and must not be in too wide a Fourth. The actions of the arms, head and body must also project the resolute and clear approach needed.

This form of pas glissade is studied in the higher levels, where the pupils have already mastered complicated virtuoso jumps.

PAS CHASSÉ (CHASED)

The pas chassé is done along the line of Second or Fourth while remaining in Fifth Position. (See illustration #124.)

This movement may begin from jumps that end on one leg, but in classroom practice it is studied from sissonne tombée and is usually performed several times in a row: beginning in Fifth Position, épaulement croisé, a sissonne tombée forward effacé starts the movement. The jump with an advance is in a pose like a hanging Fifth as the back leg pulls up to push the forward leg as they join together in the crest of the jump (the back leg chases the front leg out of position). The descent is in Fourth Position as in sissonne tombée and the pas chassé is ready to be repeated. The series of single steps is finished with a petit pas assemblé forward. The exercise is then done from the other leg.

The arms at the sissonne rise from the Preparatory Position into First Position. At the tombée, the arm corresponding to the advanced shoulder remains in First and the other arm moves into Second. During the following pas chassés, they remain in the same position but at the pas assemblé descend into Preparatory Position. The body in sissonne tombée changes épaulement and keeps straight, sent by the pushing leg (facing #2 or #6). The subsequent chassés continue with the same sendoff, in the same direction and an advance in pas assemblé. The head at the change of the épaulement turns toward the opposite shoulder and remains in that position until the end of the exercise.

Later, pas chassé is studied in croisé forward and along Second in the following exercise: beginning in the same sissonne tombée pose from Fifth, épaulement croisé, two chassés in the same direction should be completed followed by a pas assemblé back into Fifth Position.

The arms follow the same rules, but the body does not change épaulement and the head stays in the starting position.

Then the sissonne tombée en face and to the side along Second is executed with two chassés in the same direction pulling the free leg back into Fifth and ending the exercise with a pas assemblé forward. The arms in the first jump move from Preparatory through First and open into Second, where they are kept during the two pas chassés. At the pas assemblé they return to Preparatory Position. The body during the sissonne tombée turns en face; at the two chassés, it remains en face, and at the pas assemblé, it turns épaulement. The head at the first jump is en face and at the second and third jump is still in the same position. At the pas assemblé, it turns toward the forward shoulder. Then the exercise is repeated on the other leg and in reverse. The reverse exercise is done the same number of times and in the same order with the same poses.

---

124   Pas chassé along Fourth Position

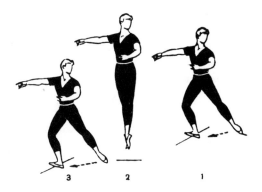

3   2   1

All pas chassés may be performed with varied arms, positions of the body and head that are used in big poses. The pas chassé along Second may be done in écarté forward or back with the head turned toward the advanced or forward shoulder.

In combinations, the pas chassé along Second is often a most powerful and trampoline-like approach to a big jump such as saut de basque, jeté entrelacé, grand fouetté sauté, etc. At the same time, this movement may be done as a medium or small jump. In whatever tempo or size, the jump must be done in a soft and elastic manner.

Beginning with demi-plié, the jump, which is not too energetic or sluggish, and the joining of the stretching legs in Fifth must be a flowing and clear exit into the following jump. Softly, and with an increased advance, the legs must be turned out and the knees, instep and toes correctly stretched. The arms must act freely, exactly and softly with no unnecessary strain. The body must be carried uninterruptedly in the direction of the advance, if there is a succession of jumps. The center of gravity must be "caught up" by the pushes for each jump and properly transferred to the supporting leg. The body must be pulled up and the shoulders freely lowered. The turns and inclinations of the head must be done easily and in one rhythm with the movement of the body.

The pas chassé should be studied as a medium jump in small poses and in a somewhat slower tempo, but united, with no pauses.

The tempo is 2/4. Later, the force of the jump may be increased as well as the advance with the legs kept tightly together in Fifth. Later, pas chassé is studied as a minimal jump and with lowered arms.

The pas chassé is a complicated movement in its progressing dynamics and should therefore be studied with no haste in a strictly progressing way (as described).

It must be noted that some dancers perform the pas chassé as a free and easy run in their approach to big virtuoso jumps. Those elements do not enter into the teaching of the subject. One must not make use of such free translations during the lessons of classical dance as it destroys discipline, harmony and clarity in future performances.

PAS DE CHAT (CAT'S STEP)

The pas de chat is found, for the most part, in choreography performed by women, but boys must study this step since it is found in several styles of stagework.

Of course, in performing any of the pas de chat forms, strictness and simplicity must be demanded. But the gracefulness expected in the pas de chat as performed by girls is not acceptable in a class for boys.

This movement has several variations but all are done with two throws of the leg with bent knees along Fifth, closing forward of back. The degree of advance and the leading of the legs away from the vertical line of the body correspond to the height required, which may be from 30 to 90 degrees.

The pas de chat, with movement of the legs forward, starts in Fifth Position, épaulement croisé. From a demi-plié the back leg, pausing in sur le cou-de-pied, opens somewhat along a Fourth Position as the other leg does a push from the floor. In flight, the leg that pushed rises to the level of sur le cou-de-pied, then, slightly delayed, it lowers into Fifth forward in demi-plié.

The arms during the jump rise into First, and at the finish of the jump the arm corresponding to the advanced shoulder opens into Second as the other arm stays in First. The head turns during the jump in the direction of the jump and stays there until the end. The body is pulled up during the crest of the jump and is bent slightly forward.

A variation for the arms, body and head occurs when the pas de chat is finished.

The arm in First opens into Second, the head assumes the starting position, and the body leans slightly backward.

Both variations must be used alternately changing positions of the head, body and arms. The entire movement must be done lightly and softly. For a better study of the pas de chat for female performers, I refer you to the textbooks of Vaganova and Kostrovitskaya. (The descriptions are similar to the Cecchetti system for the execution of pas de chat except that the above description would be termed petit. The grand pas de chat Cecchetti system would require the throw of the half-bent legs to be at knee level. The female form of pas de chat in the Soviet system requires the second leg to be thrown back in a half-bent position in effacé.)

GRAND PAS DE CHAT

Later this movement may be done as grand pas de chat—a big jump. The legs bend at the level of the knee and the jump requires a more energetic push and impetuous character. The arms may rise into Third.

The grand pas de chat must be studied from Fifth into Fifth Position at first, with pauses and then without pauses and, finally, along Fourth Position. Later, the pas de chat may emerge from an approach such as the pas chassé or pas failli, etc.

In the higher classes, this form of pas de chat may be done in a very fast tempo with a minimal jump. The same form may be performed along a diagonal gradually increasing the height of the jump. The arms, head and body take the position suited in the previously described variations.

The tempo for small and medium jumps might be 2/4 and for the large jumps, 3/4.

In performing any form of the movement in any tempo, the legs must be turned out. There must be resilience in the shape of the movement, with the instep and toes fully stretched. The flight must be light and the finish, soft. The arms, head and body must act clearly but with a flow.

It bears repeating that softness in the performance of the pas de chat in these classes must not become excessive grace.

The pas de chat with a throw of the legs back is done with two throws back with half-bent legs at the height of 45 degrees. It is done in the following manner: in the demi-plié in Fifth, the back leg is thrown back into croisé. At the same time, the other leg pushes away from the floor and, in flight, follows the first into effacé back. At the finish, the open leg opens backward, descending to close into Fifth forward or to pass through First into Fourth croisé.

The arm corresponding to the advanced shoulder moves from Preparatory into a lowered First as the other moves into a lowered Second. The body at the first throw leans slightly forward but at the crest of the jump is thrown somewhat back but not too sharply or too far. At the finish, the body becomes erect. The head at the first throw leans slightly toward the forward arm and then turns toward the advanced shoulder.

This jump must be done at first from Fifth to Fifth and then in Fourth with small and medium jumps. This form, as well as the preceding form, may be done as a big jump with the throw raised to 60 degrees. The arms, body and head take the position of the first arabesque.

An approach to this movement just described may be a pas chassé, a pas failli, or a pas couru, etc. The performance of this form must be flowing and soft without deliberateness in the action of the head, body or arms.

GRAND PAS DE CHAT WITH ONE BENT LEG

This form of pas de chat incorporates the special features of the two previously described jumps. The first throw is in effacé forward, beginning with bending the leg to the knee as in the first description. The second throw is done backward (in effacé) as described in the preceding large jump. It is finished by leading the open leg through First and into Fifth forward at the finish of the demi-plié. The head and body assume the position of arabesque (First or Second).

This movement is done only in a big jump with an approach along Fourth such as pas glissade, pas faille, pas chassé. The jump must have sufficient advance and end in a soft demi-plié.

---

125   Pas de chat with one bent leg

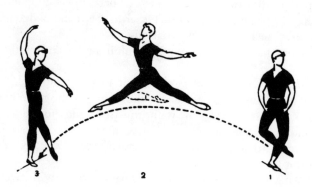

GRAND PAS DE CHAT WITHOUT A BENT LEG OPENING THE JUMP

This form of pas de chat is performed like the preceding forms except that the leg which makes the first throw is forcefully straightened at the crest of the flight. In this way, the pose in the jump along Fourth is a grand jeté effacé forward. The arms in this movement are raised in allongé in first arabesque. The body is pulled up with a slight lean forward. The head at the crest of the jump turns to face the direction of the jump. (See illustration #125.) The forward leg in the jump should be stretched without a sharp accent. The step must not be extended like a string, however, but arch and finish in a stable, soft transfer into demi-plié. The entire movement ought to carry the character of resolute impetuosity with a high jump and a large advance. (It is currently dubbed "stag leap.")

PAS DE BASQUE

The pas de basque is one of the most complicated movements in classical dance and is divided into a small and a large form.

PETIT PAS DE BASQUE

The petit pas de basque is done with two minimal jumps from the starting pose in Fifth, épaulement croisé. From both legs bending in demi-plié, the front foot glides and stretches out into a croisé forward. It describes with the toes on the floor, a semi-circle en dehors into Second Position. The other leg remains in demi-plié during this movement. A jump is made onto the leg making the semi-circle in demi-plié. The free leg then glides through First to croisé Fourth, as the supporting leg remains in demi-plié. Then a transfer is made to the forward leg and with a small gliding advance the movement is completed with a pas assemblé into Fifth backward.

The arm at the time of the semi-circle transfers into Second, rising from Preparatory Position through First and into Second. At the moment the leg passes through First, the arms lower into Preparatory and together with the pas assemblé, open into Second or take a position required for the next movement. The body, at the time the leg moves into croisé forward, leans a bit toward the leg. At the time of the transfer of the leg into Second, it turns en face. At the transfer of the leg through First, the épaulement is changed. At the First and Second jump, the body leans toward the leg.

The head, before the movement starts, is turned to the advanced shoulder. At the demi-plié, it turns toward the hands. At the semi-circle and transfer to Second and the jump onto the open leg, the head turns in the same direction. In the pass in demi-plié along First, it bends a bit forward in the direction of the opening leg and, as pas assemblé, assumes the starting position. (See illustration #126.)

The body is kept pulled up in all the progressing movements. It must be sent lightly and exactly after the opening leg has moved. The transfer to the supporting leg must be in time and with stability.

The arms go through all the positions uninterruptedly in one tempo with the movement of the leg and strictly observing all the rules of port de bras. The head must move in one rhythm with the arms, with no deliberate accents. The eyes look in the direction of the inclination and turn of the head, giving the movement a finished and assured look.

On the whole, the petit pas de basque is done from beginning to end, in a clear flow of movement. All the leg movements must be turned out and light. The start, passing and finish in demi-plié must be elastic and soft. When each leg is leading into another position or is in flight, it must be well stretched at the

126 Petit pas de basque

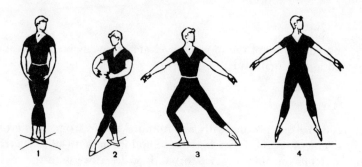

knee, instep and toes. The semi-circular leading into Second must be done in a full design and in one tempo. The passing of the leg through First into Fourth as well as the finish in pas assemblé must be done with light, gliding movements. In the first instance, in the First Position the entire foot is on the floor; in the Fourth, the toes of the back leg are on the floor.

In reverse, the petit pas de basque is done with an advance backward in the same pattern and following the same rules.

The movement must be studied with pauses in a 2/4 tempo: 1/4 for the first jump; 1/4 pause; 1/4 demi-plié in First; 1/4 rest; 1/4 transfer of leg forward; pas assemblé and straightening from demi-plié; 1/4 demi-plié as preparation to begin the step from the other leg. The movements must be studied without the rests but in a slow tempo of 3/4 mazurka: 1/4 for the first jump; 1/4 transfer of the leg through First into Fourth; 1/4 for pas assemblé backward, etc.

Finally, the study of this movement in the correct tempo should begin. The exercise should be a repeat four times of the movement forward and four times in reverse. In combinations, the pas de basque may end in the Fourth (without the finishing pas assemblé) as a preparation for turns.

GRAND PAS DE BASQUE

The composition of this form is similar to the small form. It includes one big and one small jump with two throws of the leg to 90 degrees and is executed in the following manner: from demi-plié in Fifth, the forward leg does a rond de jambe jeté as a large semi-circle en dehors to Second at 90 degrees. At the same time, a jump with an advance onto the open leg is executed as the other leg, bending into the position of passé (at the knee), opens into croisé at 90 degrees forward. The transfer forward to croisé and pas assemblé is the same as in the petit pas de basque.

The arms at the first throw of the leg and in the flight transfer from Preparatory through First and into Third. At the moment the leg opens into croisé forward,

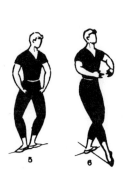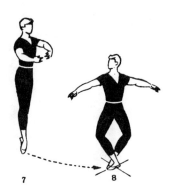

they open into Second, and, at the pas assemblé, return into Preparatory Position.

The body during the first demi-plié leans a bit forward. It straightens during the flight and changes épaulement. During the pas assemblé it returns to the starting position.

The head, before the start of the movement, turns toward the advanced shoulder and during the demi-plié straightens and leans a bit forward. During the flight, the head is en face and, at the finish, turns toward the advanced shoulder and leans a bit forward. At the pas assemblé, the head straightens but keeps the same position. (See illustration #127.)

The entire movement must be smooth, clear and with great lightness during the flight. The first demi-plié must be done with a strong and resilient push, and the second and third demi-plié with more softness but with the same elastic and light quality. The position at the knee in passé must be high and supple, and the stretching out of the leg into croisé forward and its lowering, a soft movement followed by a gliding transfer into pas assemblé.

All leg movements must be turned out and both throws kept flexible with well-stretched knees, insteps and toes.

The body must be pulled up and kept pliable throughout all the movements. It must show aplomb and be included in the transfers to the supporting leg. The arms move from Preparatory with energy and in one tempo simultaneously with the push from the floor and the throw of the leg. The arms must be light and clearly fixed in Third. They open from Third into Second and return to Preparatory softly and freely. The head must move strictly and surely along its proper course, including the exact direction of the look.

In reverse, this movement includes a semi-circular throw of the leg en dedans and a second throw croisé backward. The actions of the arms, head and body are the same as in the forward form. It is studied without pauses and in a somewhat slowed tempo, 3/4: with the first jump before the measure, 1/4 is for the finish of the first jump and the throw of the leg into croisé forward; 1/4 for the exit to the open leg; 1/4 for the pas assemblé.

127 Grand pas de basque

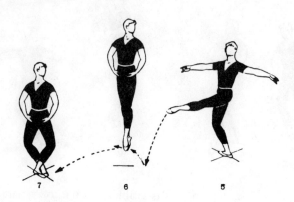

The tempo may be increased, but not before the movement is well learned in all its details. Then it may be introduced into combinations.

The pas de basque must be studied forward and, at a much later time, backward, because of the complexity of the movement and its difficult coordination. In studying and exercise of four repetitions in one direction, four repetitions in the other would be useful.

PAS DE CISEAUX (SCISSORS)

This step is a big jump which ends, after a scissor-like movement, in first arabesque. The legs make three succeeding throws in grand battement jeté: one forward in effacé with the starting leg; one forward in croisé by the leg that pushes off the floor; one backward through First Position in effacé by the leg that made the first throw.

The first two throws are done forward as in pas jeté, and the third, backward, which is the peculiarity of this movement. The arms, in flight, move from Preparatory into First and at the third throw open into the positions for first arabesque. The body at the first throw leans backward to about 45 degrees and at the end of the second throw begins to move forward. At the third throw, while the leg moves through First, it becomes vertical. At the throw of the leg backward into first arabesque, it leans forward energetically.

The head is turned toward the advanced shoulder during the change into First, but at the performance of the arabesque, it assumes its position for that pose. (See illustration #128.) The position is fixed at the final demi-plié.

The jump includes an advance forward and is usually preceded by an approach such as pas tombé, pas chassé, pas failli, etc.

The first demi-plié must be done with energy for a trampoline-like sendoff.

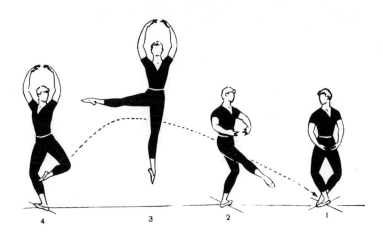

128 Pas de ciseaux

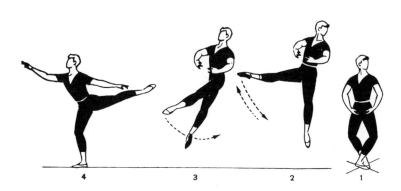

All three throws are done with increasing force and in one tempo and even height, especially the last throw. The first and second throws are performed a little faster in order to begin the third throw in time. At the performance of the third throw, the leg opening forward must move immediately to the back exactly through First Position, with a light and fast gliding movement.

The final demi-plié starts when the leg passes through First and ends softly and with suppleness. The open leg is fixed with stability and stretched knee, instep and toes.

The arms, in flight, are transferred actively but without sharpness and continue the line of the arabesque from the impetuous jump. The body is collected and has energy but acts without haste, nor does it lag behind. The counterbalance of the position in relation to all three throws of the leg is kept exactly and freely without exaggeration and without strain.

At the moment of the push from the floor, the body is sent forward with the advance in spite of the fact that it will be thrown back during the flight. The degree of advance must be proportionate to the performance of the first throw, so that the jump will be along a trajectory and not under itself. Together with the start of the third throw, the body, clearly and energetically, is placed over the forward leg that is the support and will finish in demi-plié. At the moment the leg passes through First into arabesque, the body is vertical.

The bend back, which is necessary for the performance of the first arabesque, is done without a lag in time. (See illustration #128.)

At the end of the movement, the body is kept correctly and with stability over the supporting leg.

The shoulders are open and lowered and are fixed freely but without weakness. The head, together with the transferring arms, acts resolutely and clearly, thereby increasing the strength of the final portion of the jump.

The movement is studied with a small advance at first and with pauses after each jump. Easy approaches are pas tombé; later, sissonne tombée and pas failli, etc. The tempo is 2/4 or 4/4. The approach is done before the measure: 1/4 for the flight; 1/4 for the finish of the jump; 2/4 for pas de bourrée with a change of legs. This exercise is repeated four times from one leg and then four times from the other. It is not performed in reverse. The first arabesque is traditional, but the movement may also be ended in second arabesque.

GARGOUILLADE (RUMBLING STEP)

This is a complicated movement studied by female students but useful to boys, since it develops clarity, speed and coordination throughout the whole body. The basis of the gargouillade is the pas jeté fermé along Second and rond de jambe en l'air.

Starting in Fifth Position, épaulement croisé, the movement begins with a demi-plié as the forward leg does a rond de jambe en l'air en dehors and, with no interruption, a pas jeté along Second. At the end of the pas jeté, and at the moment of the final demi-plié, the other leg does rond de jambe en l'air en dehors and closes in front in Fifth. (See illustration #129.)

The arms during the first rond de jambe en l'air move from Preparatory through First into Second. At the jump, they stay in that position until the leg closes into Fifth, when they return to the Preparatory Position.

The body, during the jump, changes épaulement. The head, during the jump, turns en face and then toward the advanced shoulder.

This movement may also be done in reverse. The leg standing in back in the Fifth Position begins the movement and both ronds de jambe en l'air are en dedans.

At first, the gargouillade is studied in separate sections to 2/4: 1/4 for the first

129 Gargouillade

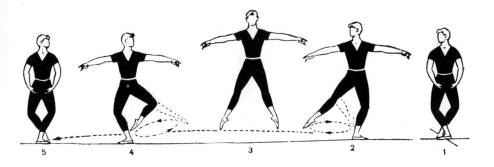

rond de jambe; 1/4 for the jump; 1/4 for the second rond de jambe and closing of the leg into Fifth; 1/4 rest in demi-plié. Then the same is done on the other leg. This is repeated four times forward and four times in reverse.

Now the gargouillade may be done more smoothly without the stops, but in a slower tempo.

The student must strive for lightness and supple connections in the leg movements. The rond de jambe is done with well-stretched knees, insteps and toes and is turned out. The start and the finish in demi-plié must be sufficiently deep but free of unnecessary strain and effort.

The advance in flight must have sufficient length so that the design of the movement opens freely as it progresses.

The body is pulled up and is over the supporting leg before and after the jump. The change of épaulement in flight must be done clearly and in time, without the slightest lag. The opening of the arms into Second ends together and in the same tempo as the first rond de jambe. The return to Preparatory Position is simultaneous with the second rond de jambe and the final demi-plié.

During the flight, the head together with the lean of the body and the change of épaulement end the jump.

This movement must be performed as a whole, without being fragmented in any way and with a clear design and impetuous advance in flight.

PAS EMBOÎTÉ (BOXED)

The pas emboîté is performed in place with a minimal jump in the sur le cou-de-pied position forward or back. It begins in Fifth Position, épaulement croisé. The back leg rises to sur le cou-de-pied at the ankle of the supporting foot in demi-plié. Then a small jump is made in which both legs stretch out and exchange places through First Position. (The legs stretched out make this version different from the former Russian and Cecchetti forms, which do not include this position and contain an advance forward or backward. The French School calls this move-

130   Pas emboîté

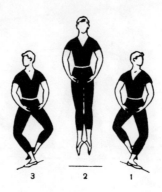

ment petit jeté, reserving the term pas emboîté for a movement sur la pointe.)
The jump is completed in demi-plié on the leg which was in back, and the leg
which did the push from the floor has moved to sur le cou-de-pied in back. The
movement may then be repeated, beginning each time from the sur le cou-de-
pied position. (See illustration #130.)

The arms are usually held in Preparatory Position or one arm may move in
flight into First and the other into Second and remain until the end of the jump.
The body is held erect but changes épaulement during the flight. The head at the
change turns toward the advanced shoulder.

In reverse, this movement is performed in the same way, but the free leg is
moved to sur le cou-de-pied front.

The movement must always be turned out, be soft and supple and contain a
somewhat shortened demi-plié. The legs in the jump must be stretched to the
utmost at the knees, insteps and toes. The transfer of the pushing leg into sur le
cou-de-pied must be done close to the other leg but not touching it.

131   Pas ballotté in two jumps

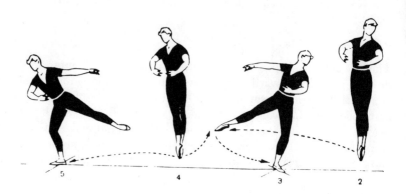

The arms remain free in the lowered position. The head at the turn to épaulement is a light move to the advanced shoulder and bends a bit in the same direction.

The pas emboîté is usually done in a fast tempo and consecutively to 1/8 or a 2/4 measure. Therefore, the change of épaulement, the transfer of the arms and the turn of the head are done not at each jump, but at the first or third jump, as given. The movement must be studied in a somewhat slower tempo to 2/4; the first jump is before the measure and ends on 1/8; the second jump is 1/8; and the third jump to 2/8 with a deepened demi-plié. Repeat this four times and in reverse.

The arms are kept at first in Preparatory Position, then transferred into positions at the change of the épaulement. The head and body act in accordance with the changes.

Later, the tempo may be brought to its normal speed and the movement may be introduced into combinations.

There is a variety of pas emboîté in which the half-bent leg is led to a 45- or 90-degree angle in front or in back. This is usually performed by female dancers and is not described here.

PAS BALLOTTÉ (ROCKED OR TOSSED)

The peculiarity of the pas ballotté consists in the counterbalancing of the body against the opening forward or opening backward leg. There are two forms of the movement: in one jump; in two jumps.

PAS BALLOTTÉ IN TWO JUMPS

Beginning in first arabesque, the open leg in back along Fourth lowers as the other leg does a demi-plié and pushes off. In flight, both legs stretch out and join in Fifth, advancing on a diagonal to effacé forward. The back leg then makes a demi-plié as the other leg is thrown forward to 45 degrees with a stretched knee. Without interruption, the second push from the floor is made and the legs reverse the movement, in the opposite direction.

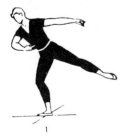

1

The arms rise from Preparatory Position into First, and at the finish of the jump the arm opposite to the thrown leg stays in First as the other moves to Second. At the second jump, the arms change positions. The body at the first jump changes épaulement and at the moment the leg is thrown forward, it leans backward to 45 degrees. During the second jump, it straightens and at the moment the leg is thrown back, it leans forward to 45 degrees.

The head, during the first jump, turns to the advanced shoulder; when the body moves back, it remains in the same position. During the second jump, the head turns in the same direction as the body. In this way, the counterbalancing movement of the upper part of the body against the opening leg after each jump creates the impression of a smooth rocking. (The French School sees this rocking as jeté bateau, a tossed boat.) (See illustration #131.)

The push in demi-plié must be done very energetically, considering the need of advance and flight with tightly joined legs in Fifth and the sendoff required to move them forward. The finishing demi-plié and the throw of the leg must be done with suppleness and stability, beginning softly and gradually with force, deepening for the following energetic push from the floor.

The arms in flight are moved with vitality and with aplomb, softly fixing the final pose. The body is pulled up and the shoulders held lightly open and lowered.

At the moment of the push from the floor, the body's weight is sent along the trajectory of the flight and begins to lean toward the opposite direction. With the finishing demi-plié and the throw of the leg, the body lightly finishes the bend and with the next push passes vertically through to the next position. The head turns and bends to the same degree as the body. All movements are made in a flowing, supple, soft, smooth and wave-like rocking.

The movement must be studied in sections from Fifth, then with a pas assemblé at the end of each opening of the leg. In this way, the movement may be practiced from both legs at once: 2/4; 1/4 for the first part of the pas ballotté; 1/4 for pas assemblé forward. Repeat this exercise four times. Then repeat backward with pas assemblé back.

At the first assemblé, the arms and head keep their position and the body straightens perpendicularly. At the second pas assemblé, the arms change position.

---

132   Pas ballotté with développé

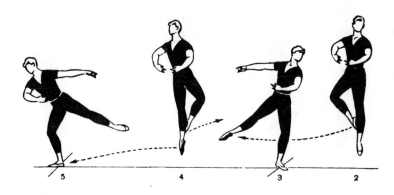

5   4   3   2

The head turns toward the advanced shoulder and the entire exercise is repeated from the other leg. Then the movement must be studied from sissonne ouverte as an approach with the pas assemblé closing in front accompanied with suitable movements of the arms, head and body.

The exercise is repeated from the other leg and in reverse.

PAS BALLOTTÉ WITH DÉVELOPPÉ

This form of pas ballotté may be done opening the leg through développé to 45 degrees. After the push from the floor, the supporting leg moves with a soft movement through sur le cou-de-pied and opens forward to effacé. In this version the legs are not kept in Fifth during the flight. The head, body and arms act as previously described, but the advance is shortened somewhat. (See illustration #132.)

This pas ballotté must be studied without separating the sections into two separate jumps. It must be a seamless flow of movement.

Both forms of pas ballotté may be performed with the opening leg in tendu position, toes on the floor. This requires a small spring, with the movements of the head and body imparting a softer and more constrained character to the movement.

PAS BALLOTTÉ IN ONE JUMP

The pas ballotté in one jump is with an approach like the pas tombé croisé forward, the pas failli or other approaches. The first opening of the leg is done through First into Fourth to effacé forward as a grand battement jeté, then the same leg is bent to passé position and begins to straighten perpendicularly, permitting the other leg, at the same time, to rise through the sur le cou-de-pied to the level of the knee open backward in effacé. Both movements are at 90 degrees.

The body follows the same rules as in the first form of pas ballotté but with less bending. The arms, at the throw of the leg forward, rise into First or Third and, at the finish of the jump, assume the position for first arabesque. The head,

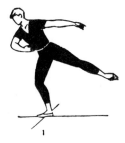

1

in flight, turns toward the advanced shoulder and, at the moment of the finish of the movement, turns into the first arabesque position.

This form of ballotté is difficult, but it must be studied in the higher classes striving for clarity, softness and togetherness in its performance.

PAS COUPÉ (CUT—ONE FOOT CUTS THE OTHER FOR ITS PLACE)

The pas coupé is a step that links other steps and is in the form of a short exchange of legs for a jump which follows. Beginning in Fifth Position, épaulement croisé, the back leg moves into sur le cou-de-pied as the supporting leg does a demi-plié at the same time. The free leg is then lowered into Fifth as a tombé to perform a jump. The other leg at the same time and in the same tempo acts according to the rules for the performance of the following jump: pas assemblé, pas jeté, pas ballonné, etc. But the pas coupé itself ends at the moment of the transferring push from one leg to the other, which is the peculiarity of this movement.

The head, body and arms take the position dictated by the preceding and the following movement. (See illustration #133.)

The pas coupé in combinations may begin not only from the sur le cou-de-pied position but also from an open position of the leg in Second or Fourth. They may be sissonne ouverte, grand pas jeté, cabriole, etc. If that is the case, the opening leg moves directly into Fifth and, as if pushing into its place, quickly, lightly and with resilience, takes its place on the floor. Turnout and elasticity in the legs are obligatory.

The depth of the demi-plié and the force of the push depend upon the jump that follows. But no matter how easy or difficult the change of leg to leg might be, the move must be soft and flowing, without roughness. The arms act freely without constraint at the pushoff. The body clearly and at the proper time is sent in the direction of the advance if the following jump requires it. In addition, the body may keep or change the épaulement, depending upon the following move-

---

133 Pas coupé

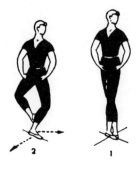

ments. The upper back must always be held and the shoulders lowered and freely open. The head in the performance of the pas coupé acts clearly, without superfluous marking of its turning or bending.

The pas coupé, as a rule, is done before the measure in the same tempo as the following jump. The movement ought to be studied in an easier form, as a normal jump from one leg to another, transferring the sur le cou-de-pied forward or backward. Later, the pas coupé must be studied in combination with pas ballonné, making each jump to 1/4 of a 2/4 measure.

The same form may then be studied as 1/8 of the measure. In both cases, the legs in flight must be kept in Fifth Position clearly with stretched knees, instep and toes. Finally, the pas coupé may be studied combining various jumps and striving for the utmost lightness, clarity and flexibility. Later, the easier form may be used in combinations.

JUMPS FROM ONE LEG

TEMPS LEVÉ (TIME RAISED)

The jumps in this group are difficult but develop excellent force and elasticity in the legs.

Temps levé simple is a jump on one leg which is stretched out vertically and with the other in sur le cou-de-pied forward or backward. The arms are fixed in Preparatory Position, or one arm may be in First and the other in Second. The body is pulled up directly over the supporting leg in épaulement. The head is turned toward the advanced shoulder. (See illustration #134.) This movement should be repeated a few times in succession to work on the force of the push and the lightness of the flight. The push must be done energetically, stretching

---

134 Temps levé simple

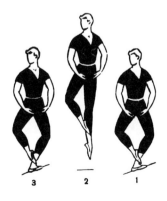

3 2 1

out the supporting knee to its utmost and stretching the instep and toes as well. The leg in sur le cou-de-pied must be fixed, not rising higher or lower and not released by the push from the floor.

The finish of the jump must be supple, with a short transfer into the next push still keeping the sur le cou-de-pied correctly.

The arms are kept quiet, without reflecting the movement of the legs. The body is pulled up and presses exactly onto the pushing leg. There must be no excessive strain in the neck. On the whole, these jumps are done with height, turned out, flowingly, lightly and not with too much bounce, but not too softly. (Care must be taken that the heel hugs the floor and is not released before the push from the floor.)

As a study, facing the barre after a sissonne simple back, two temps levés may follow and one petit pas assemblé forward. The tempo is 2/4. All jumps are performed to 1/4. The same exercise with the leg sur le cou-de-pied forward may be done to the same rules.

Then the study is continued in the center floor, gradually increasing the number of temps levés in the combination.

When the temps levé is well learned to 1/4 counts, it is useful to practice the movement in 1/8 as a minimal jump but with the same accuracy in the knee and foot. The demi-plié in this case is reduced to a minimum, but the force of the action of the instep and the toes must be kept all the same. Especially, it is useful to perform this exercise at the end of the lesson after the big jumps for the final strengthening of the feet and the feeling of flight.

---

135 Temps levé tombé

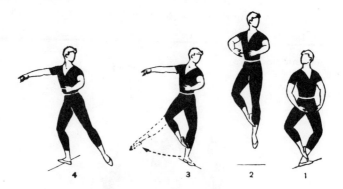

4   3   2   1

TEMPS LEVÉ TOMBÉ

Temps levé tombé is different from the one previously described only in the end, which is a transfer into Second or Fourth Position, as it is in performing the sissonne tombée. The arms, head and body perform in the same manner.

The rules for the temps levé tombé require that, in flight, one leg remain in the sur le cou-de-pied position and the other remain vertical. The finish of the jump by the pushing leg in demi-plié finds the other leg stretched from sur le cou-de-pied position and ready to receive the transfer of the body as pas tombé. The movement is light and with no lagging behind in tempo of placement of the legs. (See illustration #135.)

The general rules for the temps levé simple and tombé are kept as previously described with the turnout and softness in the demi-plié visible and in harmony with the movements of the head, arms and body.

The movement may also be studied as a medium jump: sissonne simple croisée forward, temps levé tombé croisé forward and petit pas assemblé backward. The same exercise may be done in Second from the other leg and repeated from the beginning and done, finally, in reverse.

The count is 2/4. The first three jumps are done to 1/4 of the measure with 1/4 for rest; the same tempo accompanies all the other jumps.

Later, the temps levé tombé may be studied joined with other jumps and ending in sur le cou-de-pied and gradually increasing or diminishing in height. In its turn, the temps levé tombé may be used as an approach to big jumps starting on one leg.

TEMPS LEVÉ IN POSES

Temps levé in poses requires a jump to 45 or 90 degrees. In the temps levé in first arabesque, for instance, the demi-plié and the flight must keep the form of the pose. (See illustration #136.)

The demi-plié for this movement is done with energy and force. The flight must be clear and light, and the finish of the jump a soft landing without a lowered leg from the 45 or 90 degrees. The arms are kept exactly and freely without extra strain. The body is pulled up with open and lowered shoulders. The back is kept strong and at the finish of the jump is not weakened at the waist. The head is kept straight, without extra strain and the eyes look forward.

On the whole, the temps levé is performed with sufficient lightness but not with too much bounce. The height of the jump and the degree of the advance are always clear and sure.

The form for study is as follows: grande sissonne ouverte into third arabesque; temps levé in the same pose; assemblé croisé backward. Then perform a sissonne ouverte into écarté backward; temps levé in the same pose; pas de bourrée with a change of leg into Fifth.

All the rules are strictly observed that pertain to the construction of the pose. All is repeated from the other leg and in reverse. The measure is 2/4; first three jumps in 1/4 each; 1/4 for a pause. The second jumps are also in 1/4; 2/4 for the pas de bourrée. Later, the number of temps levés must be increased and the poses must vary.

As an approach, this jump may be used: pas tombé, pas failli, pas coupé, pas chassé, etc. Additionally, in combinations this jump may end with an exit into

136   Temps levé in first arabesque

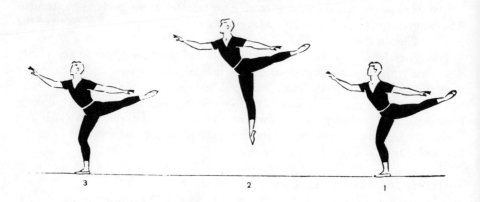

pas tombé with all the rules of its performance kept totally. A well-exercised temps levé in poses permits the study of more complicated jumps beginning or ending on one leg.

TEMPS LEVÉ WITH A CHANGE OF POSE

This form begins in one pose but ends in another. An instance would be the performance of a temps levé from a third arabesque during which the open leg is led through passé to effacé forward, which coincides with the finish of the jump. At the same time, the arm moves from First into Second. The body is vertical in flight, but with the opening of the leg forward it leans back a little. The head together with the movement of the arms turns toward the advanced shoulder. (See illustration #137.)

137   Temps levé from third arabesque into effacé

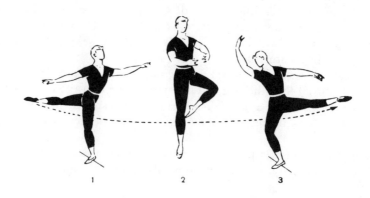

In this way, this jump may be combined with a variety of changes in the pose and with a great variety of movement of the arm, head and body. It is performed with the turnout throughout and with a supple demi-plié, a forceful stretch of the pushing leg and with an exact transfer of the open leg passing at the knee but not touching it. It must not be lowered from the knee position but, with the utmost stretch of the knee, instep and toes, must open to 90 degrees, unless the pose is an attitude, in which the knee is bent. The arms move freely, and clearly keep the lines of the movements as well as the starting and final pose. The body is always pulled up and keeps over the supporting leg; it changes its position at the change of legs. The shoulders must be free, open and lowered, the back collected and supple enough in the movements that lean or bend. The head, like the arms and body, moves freely and clearly throughout turns and inclinations and the eyes look in the same direction as the head.

The actions of the arms, legs, body and head must be united, clear and flexible throughout the duration of the flight. The image is light, strong, and the finish soft and stable. To study this movement this exercise may be used: grande sissonne ouverte in pose écartée forward, temps levé with a change of pose into croisé forward and pas de bourrée with a change of legs. Repeat from the other leg and repeat again and in reverse. The measure is 2/4; two jumps for each 1/4; pas de bourrée in one measure.

Then, the study of the temps levé in other poses, and also more complicated and varied combinations with jumps, may begin.

Notice that this jump may be done in combination with small poses or finish in pas tombé. But the study must not omit big poses, since this strengthens the technique.

There is one more temps levé with a change of legs: the open leg is transferred from pose to pose through grand rond de jambe. This transfer may be done en dehors or en dedans in 1/4 or 1/2 of a circle. All the rules are kept and have been previously described. The movement of the leg along a horizontal line must be done lightly and turned out, not lowered at the thigh or with a weak knee, unstretched instep or toes. The arms, head and body must act in one rhythm with the change of legs showing no extra strain or flabbiness.

This form may be studied at first with a change of pose along Second and Fourth, then from Fourth into Fourth through Second.

A beginning exercise for this form may be as follows: sissonne ouverte with the opening of the leg in croisé forward; temps levé écarté forward; pas assemblé backward; rest. Sissonne ouverte with the leg opening to effacé forward; temps levé écarté backward; pas de bourrée with a change of legs en dehors into Fifth Position. The exercise is done from the other leg and in reverse. The measure is 2/4. All jumps are done to a 1/4 count; 1/4 for rest; 2/4 for pas de bourrée.

PAS BALLONNÉ (BOUNCED)

The pas ballonné is done with an opening of the leg followed by a bending of the same leg into sur le cou-de-pied.

The pas ballonné is divided into a large or small form.

138   Petit pas ballonné

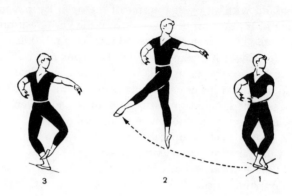

3   2   1

PETIT PAS BALLONNÉ

This movement begins in Fifth Position, épaulement croisé. The forward leg together with the flight and in a gliding movement is thrown croisé forward to 45 degrees, finishing in a demi-plié bending into sur le cou-de-pied. The arms, at the beginning demi-plié move from Preparatory into First; in flight, the arm corresponding to the opening leg is moved into Second. The body is pulled up and rises vertically, keeping the épaulement. The head turns toward the advanced shoulder. (See illustration #138.)

This petit pas ballonné may be performed in all other small poses. The rules for execution require an energetic starting demi-plié with a forcefully pushed jump and a stretched knee, instep and toes. The working leg moves with a light, gliding throw and is also stretched at the knee, instep and toes. At the crest of the jump, both legs must be completely stretched at the same time and fixed in this position. At the landing of the jump, the leg that did the push is pulled up to the toe of the open leg bringing the body to a new point of support. The final demi-plié is done lightly and elastically. The leg fixed in sur le cou-de-pied must not go behind the supporting leg or remain unattached to it. The turnout, the exact direction of the throw and a flow of movement are necessary.

The arms during the jump move freely into the suitable positions and remain until the final demi-plié. The head assumes the position suited to the given pose. On the whole, the jump is done with energy, with an advance to the opened leg, and with a clearly fixed flight and a stable ending. (See illustration #138.)

The pas ballonné must be studied first at the barre in Second Position without an advance; the forward leg does pas ballonné into Second ending the jump in sur le cou-de-pied forward; followed by a petit pas assemblé into backward. The exercise is repeated four times forward and four times backward. The measure is 2/4; 1/4 for the pas ballonné; 1/4 rest in demi-plié; 1/4 pas assemblé; 1/4 rest, etc.

Later, it may be done in the center of the floor *doubling* the pas ballonné in tempo and omitting the first pause. The three jumps will then be done consecutively and in a flow, with the help of a demi-plié that springs like a trampoline thrust. The second pas ballonné begins from the sur le cou-de-pied position.

The head and body remain en face and the arms stay in Preparatory Position.

Then pas ballonné with the advance and in small poses may be studied. It may be combined with petit pas jeté and pas coupé.

GRAND PAS BALLONNÉ

The grand pas ballonné is done as a big jump and a big pose. The previous description applies except that the opening leg is fixed at 90 degrees, raised from the position at the calf and returned to the calf position. The arms, body and head actively and strictly remain fixed in flight common to the performance of big poses.

The study must start in Fifth but then the approaches may be from Fourth, as from a pas tombé, pas failli, pas glissade or pas chassé.

The most frequently used poses of the pas ballonné are in croisé, effacé and écarté forward. The poses with the opening of the leg to the back are used onstage but are rarely performed. The student should, however, practice the technique of reversed advance in a big jump.

The study of grand pas ballonné may start after the small form has been well learned in combinations.

ROND DE JAMBE EN L'AIR SAUTÉ

Rond de jambe en l'air sauté is performed as follows: at the crest of the jump, the leg which has opened to the side at 45 degrees describes one or two (double) ronds de jambe en l'air. The arms are fixed in Second and the body and head are straight if the jump is en face. If the jump is done écarté, the body and head assume the épaulement positions. (See illustration #139.)

---

139 Rond de jambe en l'air sauté

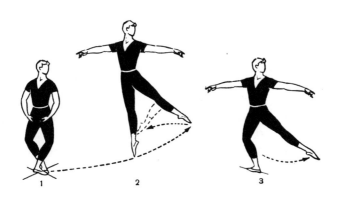

1   2   3

The jump may begin not only from the open leg, but also from Fifth Position with a gliding movement into Second together with a demi-plié on the supporting leg. The rest of the execution of this step is the same as previously described.

If the combination in which the movement is incorporated includes a pas jeté, or any other jump in which the final position is a sur le cou-de-pied, the leg may open directly into the rond de jambe in Second. Or the movement may exit into pas tombé in Second.

Regardless of the preparation given for the jump, the push from the supporting leg must be done with force and energy and stretched at the knee, instep and toes. Just as energetically and simultaneously with the push, the opening leg must "take up" the flight. At the crest of the jump the open leg must clearly and cleanly bend to the calf position for the rond de jambe and open at the demi-plié softly and with suppleness at 45 degrees to the side. The opening to 45 degrees must be with a stretched knee, instep and toes.

On the whole, the movement of pushing from the floor must be vertical without a reflex in the form of a lean in any portion of the body. The rond de jambe en l'air must be light without a lowering or raising of the thigh.

The double rond de jambe en l'air is performed just as clearly but must reach the highest possible level. The arms, head and body act freely and without strain.

The study should begin from the open position of the leg after a sissonne ouverte; then from Fifth; and finally from sur le cou-de-pied.

The first exercise may be as follows: sissonne ouverte on Second to 45 degrees on the front leg of Fifth Position; perform one rond de jambe en l'air sauté; petit pas assemblé; rest. Repeat the exercise four times and then repeat reversed.

Then the movement may be studied in a more complicated combination: double rond de jambe from Fifth Position with a pas assemblé after each jump.

When this form has been well learned, the jump may be studied from pas failli with an exit into pas tombé along Second. The arms, head and body are in écarté.

This rond de jambe may also be studied along a diagonal line after a pas tombé and followed directly by a pas failli. This combination is repeated four times from one leg and then from the other in diagonal. There too, one must strive for lightness, clarity and softness in the jump which is tied without separation to the pas failli and the pas tombé.

Later, the double rond de jambe may be introduced into combinations in big and complicated jumps.

CABRIOLE (CAPER)

The cabriole is a temps levé complicated by a beating of the stretched legs. (See illustration #140.) This movement is done in all poses at 45 degrees or 90 degrees with one or two beats in a big or small jump.

The cabriole may begin from an open position of the leg from Fifth or from sur le cou-de-pied; from approaches such as the pas coupé, pas chassé, pas failli or pas glissade. The cabriole may end with an open leg or with a leg closed into Fifth (fermé) and with pas tombé in Fourth. Regardless of the beginning or the ending, the cabriole must always be turned out and performed with stretched legs with clear beats at the calves, especially in a double cabriole. Both legs must energetically yet lightly touch in flight in the Fifth Position. The leg that pushes from the floor rushes to meet, for the beat, the raised leg, which has slightly lowered and which rises again for the final pose, maintaining that level in the final demi-plié.

The leg that pushes does so in a trampoline-like manner and accepts the weight of the body at the final demi-plié with softness. It may, however, be required to straighten immediately for the next jump.

During the beat, the knees, insteps and toes must be fully stretched so the movement may be light and resilient.

The double cabriole beat requires a beat at 70 degrees or it will seem small and constrained, which is incompatible with the technique of this virtuoso jump. At the same time, a beat that is too wide and harsh is also undesirable, as it may become gross in the performing style, and like a trick.

The arms must help in the liftoff. They must freely and clearly fix the design of the performing pose. The body must be kept collected with a held back and open shoulders.

The head, like the body, must not make any strained movement as a reflex to the efforts of the legs. Each cabriole must be done with clarity and resilience with a flow of action through the arms, head and body.

---

140   Cabriole ending in first arabesque

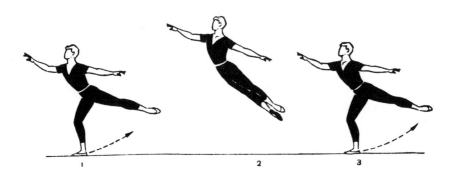

Totally inadmissible are inexact poses, flabby beats, rough and unstable endings for the jump.

The study begins at the barre with sissonne ouverte to the back at 45 degrees; petite cabriole, pas de bourrée with a change of legs into Fifth Position. Then again from the other leg, and again from the beginning. The measure is 2/4 with 1/4 for both jumps and the pas de bourrée in one whole measure.

Later, the study moves to the center floor in the pose of the third arabesque and in reverse.

Small cabrioles may be done in other poses, twice in succession on the same leg using a different beginning or ending such as fermé or tombé. Small cabrioles along Second should be practiced last.

The study of the cabriole should be undertaken only after the difficulties of the jump on one leg (temps levé) have been mastered. And when big jumps such as the grande sissonne ouverte, grand pas jeté, etc., have been mastered. The approaches should be simple at first and later complicated.

GRANDE CABRIOLE

The study of grande cabriole should be undertaken at first in effacé forward and backward, then in croisé and finally in écarté. At first the movement should finish with an open leg, then it should be practiced closing the leg in Fifth (fermé), then with a change into pas tombé.

The double cabriole is studied in the graduating class after the pupils have mastered the sum of technique for jumps.

The study is progressive, with a constant striving for lightness and softness of performance.

There is one more ultimate grande cabriole which is complicated by the addition of soubresaut—the collection of the legs at the moment they join in the air (collé—glued). The crest of jump is fixed in a horizontal position, after which the pushing leg, parting from the open leg, changes into a final demi-plié and the body takes the pose of the beginning of the flight.

This cabriole is done only in poses along Fourth with the aid of a powerful approach, maximum flight and a fast joining of the legs. Otherwise the soubresaut in the air will not be sufficient. An overly long soubresaut would lead to a harsh and sharp ending since the descending leg has no time to move with suppleness into the final demi-plié.

The study of grande cabriole may start as follows: in Fifth Position, épaulement croisé, sissonne tombée effacée forward and temps levé with a throw of the free leg through First forward in croisé, which means into a pose along Fourth. At the crest of the movement, the cabriole is done with the soubresaut in Fifth and a change into the final demi-plié. Then a temps levé tombé forward follows and a small pas assemblé back into Fifth ends the combination. All is repeated four times, then on the other leg and then in reverse.

The same exercise is useful for cabriole in effacé, changing the approach and the ending. Further along, the approaches may be pas failli, pas glissade, but only in the performance of the cabriole forward. The cabriole backward is studied with a turn (fouetté), since it is more compatible for this exercise.

The actions of the arms, head and body are the same as the cabriole without the soubresaut. The study of this form should be last and after the double cabriole. If the pupil has mastered the timing of a double beat, he is better able to deal with more technique for the single beat. If the study is in a different order, the pupil must develop the habit of only one beat, which will interfere with the free movement of the legs in double cabriole.

BATTERIE (BEATEN STEPS)

Beats are fast, clear hits of both legs by each other, which complicate jumps. They impart to the jump a filigree and virtuoso shine. The beats are done with turned-out and fully stretched legs, insteps and toes. The crossing of the legs is at the thighs, with the actual beating of the legs made with the calves in a resilient movement. The legs rebound from one another along a shortened Second equal to about the width of a foot.

Both legs participate actively in the performance of beats. It is inadmissible for one leg to remain passive while the other beats, since it would bring into the jump an element of flabbiness and unevenness.

Batterie require a higher jump, the more beats there are in the movement. If only one beat is performed in a high jump, it looks dragged out and without sparkle. Beats must be characterized by clarity, a compactness and gloss in performance. Too large a beat is unacceptable because it expresses unjustified trickery and gross technique.

It must be understood that each jump complicated by battu (beats) must be done according to all the rules: softness, elasticity, lightness, stability and with unstrained effort of the arms, body and muscles of the face.

Beats may only be performed with stretched legs, which complicates those jumps in which the legs are not bent in flight.

The steps complicated by beats are temps sauté, changement de pied and sissonne simple. These are called entrechats.

The steps complicated by beats in which one leg is open before or after the jump are given the word battu as their description: échappé battu, assemblé battu, jeté battu, sissonne ouverte battue, etc.

The steps complicated by beats which open along Fourth are given the word brisé as their description.

In this manner all jumps with beats are divided into three groups: entrechats, pas battus and brisés.

ENTRECHATS

The word entrechat is followed by a number: entrechat quatre; entrechat cinq; entrechat six; entrechat sept; entrechat huit. These are divided into even and odd. The number which follows the word does not indicate the beats required, but the number of separations and rejoinings.

Even-numbered beats are completed in the jump. Odd-numbered beats finish with one leg in sur le cou-de-pied forward or backward. The unit of measure is reflected in the odd number added after the word entrechat. For instance: the entrechat quatre ending in one leg in sur le cou-de-pied is called entrechat cinq. The entrechat six ending sur le cou-de-pied is called entrechat sept.

In this group of beats there is another beat called the royale. It has no number at the end of its name but the study of batterie begins with this beat.

ROYALE

The royale is a complication of the petit changement de pied. The legs open at the crest of the jump from Fifth Position very slightly, return to the starting position and open slightly again, finishing in an exchange of legs. In this way, the change of legs in the entrechat is a single beat and occurs at the finish of the jump.

If one counts separations and joinings of the legs and indications of exchanges, then the royale has as many as the entrechat quatre. But the configuration of the movement is different from the entrechat quatre. (The first beat is in the same position as the starting position.)

The study of the royale should begin facing the barre; with one stop; then without stopping and keeping to all the rules of performance of jumps and beats. When the royale is studied in the center of the floor, the arms are kept in Preparatory and one must see that they do not reflect the effort of the legs.

The royale may be performed not only in 1/4 of a measure, but in 1/8 as well. All the performance rules for the petit changement de pied apply to the execution of the royale.

ENTRECHAT TROIS

The entrechat trois is based upon the sissonne simple and is done in the pattern of the royale but ends on one leg with the other in sur le cou-de-pied. Convention has named this movement, which is a variety of entrechat cinq, since it has two separations and two joinings with the addition of a sur le cou-de-pied ending. But such is the immovability of tradition and the teaching of terminology, that its name, entrechat trois, prevails.

In the performance of the entrechat trois, all the rules for the execution of the sur le cou-de-pied must be followed so that the finished movement does not have a foot that is in back of the standing leg or separate from it. It must contain, like all jumps, the turnout, elasticity and a soft landing in demi-plié. The arms, head and body perform as in a sissonne simple.

The study must begin facing the barre with the following exercise: entrechat trois with the sur le cou-de-pied movement ending back; then the leg opens to the back with the toes on the floor and closes again into Fifth Position back. Repeat the entire exercise four times and repeat on the other leg. The measure is 2/4; 1/4 for the entrechat trois; 1/4 for the opening of the leg back; 1/4 for the closing into Fifth back; 1/4 demi-plié.

Later, the movement is studied in the center of the floor incorporating the change of épaulement. The arms are kept in Preparatory Position. Still later, the entrechat trois may be done in small poses combined with other jumps.

141   Exchange of legs in entrechats

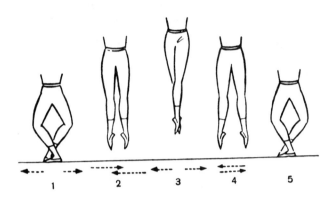

1   2   3   4   5

ENTRECHAT QUATRE

The entrechat quatre is a petit temps sauté in Fifth with the addition of one beat. The legs at the crest of the jump assume the position opposite to the starting position and return again to it. In this way, the change of legs in the entrechat is done twice: first, in flight; second, just before the finish of the jump. The rules are the same as for the royale and should be studied facing the barre. Later, in the center of the floor, it must follow the rules for petit temps sauté and for beats as well. (See illustration #141.)

ENTRECHAT CINQ

The entrechat cinq is based upon the sissonne simple and is executed like the entrechat quatre with the finish of the jump in sur le cou-de-pied. The sur le cou-de-pied position is counted as an additional unit. In the performance of this battu, the rules for beats must be preserved, as well as the rules for jumps and the sur le cou-de-pied position. The movement of the arms, head and body is the same as for sissonne simple. The study must begin facing the barre as the other entrechats, but then it should be followed by an opening of the legs to Second and a closing in Fifth front. The measure is the same, as is the rhythmic apportionment.

ENTRECHAT SIX

The entrechat six is a grand changement de pied complicated by two beats and three changes of legs, of which two occur in the jump and the third just before its ending. Naturally, the joinings and the separations of the legs in this entrechat must be even, more rushed and more compact. The technique is the same.

The study of the entrechat six may begin on the floor but only after the force of the jump and small beats have been well mastered. First, study the entrechat six with stops to the usual number—four to eight jumps. Then study it without stops from three to sixteen jumps. The arms must be kept in Preparatory Position. Then in Second and, finally, the arms may change from one position into another. After the entrechat six is well learned en place, it may be studied with an advance— de volée (flying)—while still observing all the rules of performance.

The new teacher must know that the practice of entrechat six with the waving of arms in Second does not answer the purpose. It may ease the flight, but it does not prepare the pupil for large complicated beats in which the arms must be fixed in varied designs with changes from one position to another. On stage, one sees this kind of waving around, but in school work, independence and plasticity in the use of the arms are more necessary than the trampoline-like image in flight. Therefore, the study must acquire freedom and exactness in the action of the arms before one may incorporate the exceptions.

ENTRECHAT SEPT

The entrechat sept is similar to the entrechat six except it ends in sur le cou-de-pied (like all odd-numbered beats), and this adds a unit of measure. It is done in the highest possible jump, following all its rules for the quality of the jump, beat and small pose ending as used in the entrechat trois and entrechat cinq.

The study of the entrechat sept begins only after the study of entrechat six has been mastered in the following exercise: the measure is 2/4; to the first 1/4, entrechat sept ending in sur le cou-de-pied back; 1/4 small assemblé croisé to the back; 1/4 straighten from the demi-plié; 1/4 the next jump, etc. Repeat four times and four times in reverse. Later, perform the movement without stopping and incorporate it into combinations of big jumps.

It must be observed that the exact position of sur le cou-de-pied in this movement is learned with difficulty and its position must be given special attention.

ENTRECHAT HUIT

The entrechat huit is a double entrechat quatre. It requires maximum height and extremely fast changes of the leg. Three changes are in the air and the last one just before the finish of the jump. Since this movement demands a very great technical preparedness, this movement is studied only by the graduating classes that strive for virtuoso performance.

As a starting exercise, perform three petit changement de pied and the entrechat huit followed by a rest. This exercise should be repeated four times. Later, the rests may be eliminated. Still later, the movement may be introduced in combinations of big jumps.

PAS BATTUS (BEATEN STEPS)

As we explained earlier, all jumps that begin or end with an open leg that are complicated with a beat are given the word battu as a description. If the battu consists of one beat, nothing is added to the name.

All battus are divided into simple and double or complicated battus. If the battu consists of two beats, then the description "big beats" is added to the name of the step. For instance, grand pas assemblé or sissonne ouverte may be performed with *big beats*. Conciseness, impetuosity, clarity and exact performance of the beats and the jump are necessary as in the entrechats.

The pas battus (beaten steps) are described in the same groupings as other jumps but without the actions of the head, arms and body as described earlier.

PAS ÉCHAPPÉ BATTU

The petit pas échappé battu consists of two jumps, each complicated by one beat. The first is done with a change of legs in the air opening into Second; the second jump is done from Second repeating the flight and the change of legs at the closing into Fifth back. In this way, the pas échappé battu may be performed immediately from the other leg.

It is studied at first only as a jump along Second into Fifth (the second portion of the movement). Then it is studied from Fifth Position into Second, which is more difficult, and then with the beats in both jumps performed consecutively.

Because beats are first studied with the help of the pas échappé, it is necessary that each portion of the pas échappé be learned very well. It may begin by facing the barre, then on the center floor without use of the épaulement or use of the arms, a turn of the head or body. The aim should be for a flow, for exactness and freedom of action.

Later, the beat on the second jump may end on one leg in sur le cou-de-pied front or back. Then the following jump is learned without beats.

GRAND PAS ÉCHAPPÉ BATTU

The grand pas échappé battu is done with double beats in a maximum jump beginning in Fifth with the right leg forward. The first beat is done like the entrechat quatre with the legs opening in Second; the second jump begins in Second and, like the entrechat six, beats first with the right leg backward. This permits the movement to continue on the leg. The double beat is studied progressively like an ordinary petit pas échappé, but in the center floor instead of at the barre, and after the entrechat six has been mastered.

The arms, head and body are included from the beginning of the study. The lightness, softness of the jump, the dynamics and force for beats is required as in the petit pas échappé. The finish of the second beat in sur le cou-de-pied is a possibility. The movement may also be done several times in a series with an advance along a diagonal line—de volée. In the second act of *La Fille Mal Gardée,* the leading male character, Colin, performs this movement as the second coda.

The advance in the diagonal is kept even on both jumps and performed energetically with ballon in the flight and with meticulous beats.

PETITE SISSONNE OUVERTE BATTUE

This step has one beat, which, as a rule, is done with a change of legs in the air and ends in any small pose. As an exception, the opening of the leg along Fourth may be done as the royale, with the beat in the starting Fifth Position and a change of épaulement both in flight.

The beat in the petite sissonne ouverte battue is done according to all the rules, but at the moment of flight, the legs fall behind a bit from the movement of the whole body trajecting itself into the advance. The beat is then not done with perpendicularly hanging legs since to do otherwise would lead to difficulty in repositioning the body for the correct sissonne pose and would lead to a harsh demi-plié.

The study begins at the barre opening the leg along Second and is followed with a pas assemblé. Then the study may move to the center floor and the performance of the step with the beat ending in Fourth ouverte with no change in the épaulement and then with a change of épaulement.

Still later, this beat is studied with a final closing of the working leg into Fifth—fermée. In executing that form, the beat and the opening of the leg must be somewhat forced to gain time for a clear and rhythmic closing into Fifth. If the working leg opens late and is flabby, the entire movement becomes heavy. The arms, head and body, as in any sissonne, should show no sign of extra effort reflecting the difficulty of the beat.

GRANDE SISSONNE OUVERTE BATTUE

The grande sissonne ouverte battue has two beats done like the entrechat quatre and ends in a big pose. The rules are the same as for petite sissonne and the leg lags a bit behind the body on the takeoff of the jump. This beat is done at maximum height, clearly and quickly with energetic and even beats of the legs. Shortening the length of the jump makes "sticky" beats as well as a coarse final jump, both of which are inadmissible. Unacceptable as well are weak or overtense movements in the arms, neck and body and a lowered leg after its opening. This warning may seem exaggerated, but at the beginning of the study of this step these faults sometimes occur.

The study of the double beat is followed in the same progression as the simple form. The pas battu with a double beat is not done ending in fermé (closed) since that form does not make it possible to move quickly to a high point in the jump from a big pose into Fifth in a soft demi-plié or to prepare the next big jump with needed force.

PETIT PAS ASSEMBLÉ BATTU

The petit pas assemblé battu is done with one beat as the royale. At the crest of the jump, the legs repeat the starting position as the beat and exchanges the close into Fifth. The pas assemblé battu is only done along Second and strictly in one place. The turnout, elasticity and evenness of the beat, a soft ending, free arm, head and body movements are obligatory. And the pas assemblé itself must be faultless in every way.

Begin the study of pas assemblé battu facing the barre, with a pause after each jump, performing it four times forward and four times backward, or reversed. Then execute three jumps in a row, twice forward and backward and finally with eight jumps in a row forward and backward. Then the study is ready to move to the center floor.

The arms remain in Preparatory Position and later may be changed to the positions for small poses as described in the simple form of pas assemblé along Second.

GRAND PAS ASSEMBLÉ BATTU

The grand pas assemblé battu is done with a double beat like the entrechat six. In this step, the throw of the leg is made only to the Second and is somewhat lower in height than the grand pas assemblé without the beat. This difference permits the double beat to be cleaner and bigger. The force of the push from the floor, however, for height and advance, must not be shortened by this requirement. On the contrary, in shortening the throw of the leg, the sendoff must be strengthened to its utmost. Ballon in flight and softness in landing in demi-plié are required. All other rules of performance of the beats and the grand pas assemblé must be scrupulously kept, which means correct use of the head, body and arms as well.

This assemblé is studied at first with stops and forward since this beat is not done backward. It should be repeated four times on each leg, then without stops alternating each side. It may then be introduced into combinations.

PETIT PAS JETÉ BATTU

The petit pas jeté battu is done like a small assemblé battu except that it ends on one leg with the other in sur le cou-de-pied. It is important that the leg doing the push from the floor be exact in the sur le cou-de-pied position after the beat. The arms, head and body must be light, flexible and show no extra effort. The study begins facing the barre and then continues on the center floor.

JETÉ PASSÉ BATTU

The jeté passé battu is complicated by one beat of the legs and in its performing techinque resembles the cabriole rather than a pas battu, since the beat begins from Fourth instead of Second.

However, this trait brings to the jump a new color in the movement that is obvious only if the beat is large and clear along Fifth Position and does not become reduced into a Third Position.

The study of the jeté passé battu may begin at once on the floor joined with big sissonnes ouvertes forward and backward. Clear and free action of the arms, head and body are required, as well as lightness in the flight and a soft and stable finish. The jeté dessus en tournant or grand jeté entrelacé is also complicated by a beat but is described in the next section on jumps that turn.

PETIT BALLONNÉ BATTU

The petit ballonné battu is done with the opening of the leg only to the side and with one beat done like the entrechat quatre or royale ending in a sur le cou-de-pied.

As in all other jumps, the beat must be energetic, clear and quick without apparent effort in the arms, head, body or muscles of the face.

The study begins facing the barre without an advance. It continues onto the floor, en face, with the arms in Preparatory Position. Then the advance may be introduced into the movement and the use of the head, arms and body as previously described for ballonné.

It must be remembered that the sur le cou-de-pied position must be very clear at the end of the jump, which is a difficult element in this step. The landing in demi-plié must be soft at the end of the beat.

GRAND BALLONNÉ BATTU

Grand ballonné in the classes for males is not complicated by a beat since the flight is fixed at 90 degrees by the open leg, which is more necessary to the shape of the step than the one beat. Big jumps for male dancers harmonize better with a double beat—and there are many such steps—than with a single beat, and the grand pas ballonné is not done with a double beat. Therefore, it is better to prolong the pose in the air in the grand pas ballonné and to beat the small pas ballonné with a clear and fast movement.

TEMPS LEVÉ BATTU

The temps levé battu is a double beat in a big pose with the leg open along Fourth forward or backward, in effacé or croisé. This jump is much like the double cabriole except that it is done like the entrechat six with a change of legs during

the beats. For instance: using the pas failli as an approach, the free leg is energetically thrown through First into effacé; the other leg which has performed the
push from the floor immediately makes a beat at 70 degrees on the open leg,
then exchanges its place during the second beat and separates from the other leg
and rises a bit; this frees the leg that pushed from the floor to descend vertically
and catch the weight of the body in a demi-plié.

The arms, head and body fix the big pose in effacé forward and remain for
the duration of the jump.

The temps levé battu may be done in croisé forward or backward, in arabesque
from several approaches such as the sissonne tombée, the pas glissade, etc.

In the performance of this step, the beats must be executed in Fifth Position
and not be waving about in the air in First Position.

The movement is studied first forward, then backward and separately. This
step may also be performed as a fouetté with a turn from pose into pose, which
is described in the next section on jumps that turn.

BRISÉS

Brisés are performed in two ways: one ending in Fifth, and the other on one leg
dessus-dessous.

The brisé along Fifth is done like a small assemblé battu, but with that the
resemblance ends. The throw of the leg is done to 45 degrees, not directly side
but in effacé forward by the leg standing in back in the starting Fifth Position.
The step, if performed backward, begins with the throw of the leg that is forward
in the Fifth Position. The jump is not en place but in the direction of the throw,
and the beat starts along Fourth, not along Second. The beat is done like the
entrechat quatre, not like the royale. The closing of the legs at the finish is in
Fifth Position, from which the jump started and from which it starts again without
a change of legs.

The arms in the jump are open into a lowered Second but during the beat the
arm corresponding to the advanced leg moves into a lowered First. The body,
during the performance of the jump, leans in the direction of the jump—forward,
or backward—if the step is reversed. The head is turned in the direction of the
movement. This underscores the movement of the body and the character of this
beat.

(The brisé backward or reversed is termed brisé dessous and the brisé forward,
brisé dessus. The brisé, however, in other schools is opened to Second for the
beat instead of Fourth.)

In the execution of the brisé, all the rules of technique for jumps and beats
must be strictly kept. It is inadmissible to throw the leg too high or to perform
too short an advance, which must be even with the size of the step opening
forward to 45 degrees. A sharp, flabby or tense movement weakens the coordination. Inexact or flabby movements of the head or body interfere with the
flow and lightness. No difficulty in the execution must be seen.

The study of brisé begins in the center floor and moves along a diagonal forward or backward. Begin with brisé forward at first, then backward with stops after each jump. Perform each movement four times on each leg. Later, brisé forward and backward may be studied as one movement with stops and finally without stops.

BRISÉ DESSUS-DESSOUS (VOLÉ)

The brisé dessus-dessous is done like the petit jeté battu, but it has its own characteristics. It ends on one leg with the other in sur le cou-de-pied. (The Russian and French schools end the movement in this position. The Cecchetti system ends each brisé volé—flying—with the working foot passing through First Position to Fourth Position after the beat, instead of ending in the sur le cou-de-pied position.)

The form of the brisé dessus-dessous conforms to the rules of the brisé, ending in Fifth except for the foot's ending in sur le cou-de-pied. The arms, head and body follow the same pattern as the pas jeté battu (leaning in the direction of the thrown leg).

It must be remembered that the sur le cou-de-pied position must be exact. The step must be flowing, clear, light.

It should be studied at first with stops after each jump, in a series of several, and then joined with other steps that are beaten.

It is not necessary to practice dessus-dessous separately, since by this time the students have mastered the technique of jumps and beats in general.

The brisé dessus-dessous is sometimes done from eight to sixteen times in a row with an advance on a diagonal line. This is a very useful exercise, but the advance, in this case, must be done only on the brisé dessus without losing the character of the movement of the entire figure.

PART FIVE

TURNS
AND
TURNING

In classical dance, there are movements to which a turn is added as a new element. The essence of the movement is not changed by this new element; it remains the same with or without the turn.

There are, as well, movements that become a new form with the turn as an element. These turns are very fast, repeated consecutively, and are unfragmented, such as the various pirouettes, tours chaînés, tours en l'air, etc. These movements are studied separately as turns.

Turns and spins may be performed on the floor—à terre—or in the air—en l'air. They are also performed in two directions, en dehors or en dedans.

Turns and spins introduced into classical dance add virtuosity and an imaginative component. These movements must be learned in classwork not only for their technical value but also as another means of expressiveness.

TOURS PAR TERRE (ON THE FLOOR)

The elementary movements, with a tour or turn, develop the ability to orient to changes in space. This ability will have greater value if practiced systematically.

A description of the movements has been given earlier. At this point, only the special qualities are described pertaining to the technique of tours and to the methods of study.

BATTEMENT TENDU WITH TOURS

The battement tendu should be studied to the side from First or Fifth Position with a partial turn of 1/4 circle.

The turn is made by displacing the heel of the supporting leg at the moment the free leg begins its gliding movement into Second. (The heel movement is very slight and is on the floor at the moment the movement is fixed.) The leg in tendu is closed into the starting position without a turn and the movement is ready to be repeated.

If the turns are done toward the right on the supporting left leg, the direction is en dehors. The arms, head and body perform as in the simple form of battement tendu with a turn.

The supporting leg must remain turned out and make an exact 1/4 circle. The

277

heel must barely separate from the floor and the free leg must be guided by the toes toward that point on the floor or in space where it is going to finish.

The body is always pulled up over the supporting leg and the head and arms are kept free of showing extra effort. The turn must be made with the active participation of the entire body without obvious involvement. The body must turn in a compact manner, clearly and with stability.

The study should start from First with 1/8 of a circle at each turn. It is done eight times with each leg and in each direction. Then the study may be done with 1/4 turns. In this way, the exercise performed on each leg and in each direction (en dehors and en dedans) may be alternated with battements tendus without the turn. Then the movement may be performed from Fifth Position with 1/4 turn. All the rules for the correct execution of the battement tendu must be kept.

Each movement may incorporate a demi-plié before or after the turn in the starting position only after the pupil has mastered the turn.

Finally, it would be useful to practice the battement tendu jeté with the 1/8 and 1/4 turn. All the rules for turns remain unchanged with the only new element added of a throw of the leg to 30 degrees to a faster tempo.

It must be noted that all battements tendus with a turn along Fourth are not practiced independently. There are single turns to 1/4 of a circle beginning in Fifth croisé from which the leg opens to effacé forward with a change of épaulement. In this movement, the supporting leg has turned 1/4 en dehors at the same time the other leg moved forward into effacé.

This same movement may be done en dedans with the leg led to the back in effacé along Fourth. The leg led into effacé along Fourth forward or backward may close into Fifth with a 1/4 turn at the same time. This same closing of the leg with the turn may start in croisé and end in Fifth in effacé. All these possibilities offer a variety of construction for the study of battement tendu en tournant (turning).

In all these examples, the rules are undeviatingly observed, learned and practiced with the opening of the leg along Second, en dehors and en dedans.

GRAND BATTEMENT JETÉ WITH TOURS

The technique for 1/4 and 1/8 turns is the same except that the battement is now thrown along Second to 90 degrees. The 1/4 turn coincides with the throw and is made following the rules for grand battement. The arms, head and body keep their given position.

The study begins along First Position with 1/8 of a circle and a stop after each turn. Then the series of unbroken turns to 1/4 circles with stops may begin. The study continues along Fifth in the same pattern.

This form demands a great deal of strength, which means that the student must be persistent in eliminating inexactness and a mechanical performance. Each battement must be done freely and clearly with aplomb and ease.

As a single exercise, the grand battement jeté may be done with a turn along Fourth with a change of épaulement as in the battement tendu described earlier.

BATTEMENT DÉVELOPPÉ WITH TOURS

This movement with a turn is done with the displacement of the heel, not as a separate movement, but as a component of the exercises of adagio movements.

All the elements of battement développé are joined for the turn of 1/4 circle: the movement through sur le cou-de-pied to the knee; the straightening of the leg along Second or Fourth; the return to the starting Fifth Position. These turns may be done at each développé, but not consecutively. The movements are separated as a change of épaulement in order to open the leg into another post, or as a lowering of the leg into Fifth. The turn on the supporting leg in all instances is done at the same time as the movement of the free leg, except when lowering the leg into the starting Fifth Position. In that instance, the turn on the supporting leg is done when the leg *closes with a gliding movement along the toes into Fifth Position.*

The arms, head and body are free and move with the transfer into the développé or other poses.

The study of this movement may begin with a développé from Fifth into sur le cou-de-pied moving at once to the knee, then opening into Second and Fourth. The first study should be in a turn en dehors, then en dedans. The study may also include ending in demi-plié and, finally, be performed on demi-pointe. (The heel movement is the same in this most difficult movement and lowers softly, usually into a demi-plié, or may simply lower, abaisser.)

ROND DE JAMBE PAR TERRE WITH A TOUR

This movement coordinates the 1/4 turn with the movement of the leg from Fourth to the completed Fourth. The transfer of the leg through First remains without a turn.

This movement may be done en dehors and en dedans, repeating from each leg into every direction. The free leg must be light and glide with the toes along the floor. Its course must not be shortened along its arc. The arms, head and body perform as for the simple rond de jambe par terre. The body must be pulled up over the supporting leg and the arms and head must be fixed freely without slowing the turn of the body.

This study must be done in combination with a rond de jambe first en dehors, then en dedans, with all the rules strictly observed. The study may include ronds de jambes from demi-plié, for instance, after the second simple unturned rond de jambe par terre. The pupil should strive for lightness, exactness and stability in the turn of the entire body. The arms, head and body keep the rules of performance of rond de jambe par terre with demi-plié.

ROND DE JAMBE EN L'AIR WITH A TOUR

This movement follows the pattern of the par terre movement for 1/4 circle. The turn coincides with the bending of the open leg when it is at the calf of the supporting leg—that is, with the first part of the rond de jambe. The second part of the movement, the straightening of the leg into Second, has no turn. This movement may be done en dedans or en dehors repeating on each leg several times. All the rules for the simple form of rond de jambe en l'air should be observed. The supporting leg must turn with ease and in exact 1/4 circles. The working leg must be kept turned out at the thigh and it must remain immovable.

The study plan is the same as for simple rond de jambe en l'air. It may be joined with demi-plié after the second simple rond without a turn. The arms, head and body are kept according to the rules.

GRAND ROND DE JAMBE

This movement is done with the leg at 90 degrees, held horizontally from Fourth into Second and back; from Fourth front into Fourth back; or reversed (en dehors or en dedans).

The turn is done at the same time as the transfer of the open leg and goes in the same direction as the leg, en dehors or en dedans. In addition, if the open leg is transferred from Second into Fourth, the supporting leg makes only one 1/4 turn. If, however, the leg is transferred from Fourth into Fourth, the supporting leg makes two 1/4 circles.

The technique here for the supporting leg is the same as for the previous movement, which means lightness, suppleness and a flowing movement. The body flows with the movement into the large poses that begin or end this large movement.

This movement and the turn may be combined with demi-plié at the transfer of the leg from Second into Fourth and back. The transfer of the open leg may begin from a demi-plié and finish with the straightened supporting leg, or it may be the other way around.

The arms, head and body perform in harmony with the composition of the poses that usually accompany this movement.

The grand rond de jambe en tournant usually finds a place in complicated combinations of adagios or becomes a single instance. It is not an independent exercise such as the battement tendu with a turn.

The study must be progressive, beginning with 1/4 circle and then 1/2 circle. It should be included gradually in increasingly complicated adagios, with special attention given to a flowing performance of the turn and transfer of the open leg. The movements must coordinate exactly at the start and at the finish.

BATTEMENT SOUTENU

At the end of this movement the open leg is pulled up into Fifth Position into demi-pointe. This is the beginning moment of the turn done in a complete circle in the direction of en dehors or en dedans.

After the leg is pulled into Fifth Position en dedans, the turn is done en dedans. This means that the turn exchanges the legs during a complete turn ending in Fifth Position. The support during the change within the tour should be even on both legs. This, however, does not permit more than a half-circle turn. Therefore, before the turn begins, the open leg moving into Fifth Position must overcross on demi-pointe. This allows the turn on both legs to exceed the 1/2 circle. The finish finds the support on one leg, the other leg closing lightly and tightly with it and ending in Fifth. (The movement is an exchange of heels which permits a more exact Fifth Position to end the movement.)

When the movement is done with the opening of the leg along Second, the arms rise from Preparatory Position at the same time into a lowered Second. Then, actively helping the turn, they move into a lowered First and rise straight up to the Third Position. During the gathering of the legs together in Fifth, the body leans very slightly in the opposite direction from the turn as if stressing its start. At the movement of the turn, it straightens. The body and the legs must turn at the same time. The head, when the body leans, turns a bit and bends in the same direction. At the beginning of the turn it lags a bit, then overtakes the body in assuming the final position. The entire movement must flow, be smooth and have no sharp movement of the head.

If this movement is done along Fourth, the legs turn with the same method as above. The arms, regardless of the position during the preceding movement, must move into the lowered First and then into the given position.

The study of battement soutenu en tournant begins with the leg opening to 45 degrees along Second. It is studied first at the barre moving into a 1/2 circle. The study is without crossing the legs or the final particulars of the full turn. In the study, the turnout must be fully retained. The knees must be kept straight during the turn and the lowering to the heels from the demi-pointe after the turn must be even with both heels lowering at the same time. The body must be pulled up and kept shapely with the weight divided evenly on both legs. One arm at the turn moves into lowered First as the other lowers to the barre. The head turns at the same time with the body.

The study of the movement with the full circle may begin, but without the lean of the body and head. Then the study with the full turn in the center floor and with combinations may follow. The demi-plié may be introduced or it may be studied without the demi-plié. Combined with elementary movements at the barre and on the center floor, the movement in 1/2 circles, then in full circles, may be learned.

Obviously, this is a form of turn that differs from the others since it is done on demi-pointe on the structure of a relevé and is not just a displacement of the heel of the supporting leg. The rules pertaining to relevé, consequently, must be followed.

BATTEMENT FRAPPÉ

This movement is complicated by a turn of 1/4 circle at the moment of lowering from demi-pointe to the entire foot. At the same time, the working leg opens the toes to the floor. If the turn is made on the left leg in the same direction, it is an en dedans turn. If the turn is made in the opposite direction using the left leg for support, the turn is en dehors. This form is usually done with the third frappé ending in a small pose in demi-plié.

The turnout must be kept throughout and the working leg kept elastic but with a forceful and clear opening of the leg. If the finish of the exercise is in demi-plié, the supporting leg must bend no sooner than the working leg begins to stretch to the final pose.

The arms, head and body move as in simple battement frappé without the turn. On the whole, the turn must be clear and the finishing pose light, especially in a demi-plié ending.

It must be remembered that in demi-plié in small poses forward in effacé or croisé, the body leans toward the open leg. In performing the movement to the back, it leans in the same direction.

In the écarté, the body also actively and clearly harmonizes with the pose but without additional bending. The arms and head coordinate suitable to the bending of the body.

The study begins at the barre with 1/8 of a circle in this form: Two battements frappés are done to the side on demi-pointe; then one is executed with the descent into effacé forward. The same exercise is done in the opposite direction and to the back. The tempo is 2/4. All three frappés are done to 1/4 with a 1/4 stop.

Then the study may include a 1/4 circle: two battements frappés in effacé forward; one with the descent into écarté forward. The same is reversed; repeated once more from the beginning; and finally three frappés, to the side en face and on demi-pointe, end the exercise.

Later, the turns may be studied with demi-plié in the center of the floor.

It must be noted that variations of the battement frappé may be very different, but they must always be light, clear and quick. Speed which develops the feeling of free aplomb is preferred to a fussy haste. The speed for these turns must be practiced very gradually with a gradual increase in tempo.

Turns to 1/8, 1/4, 1/2 may be complicated with double frappés. The moment of the turn coincides with the rising onto demi-pointe with the other leg in sur le cou-de-pied position. The descent must coincide with the opening of the toes to the floor. The turns may be done with a frappé each time and end in a small pose. The rules applicable are for the small poses along Fourth in demi-plié.

The study of the double frappé begins at the barre with a 1/8 turn and follows the pattern of learning of the single battement frappé. Next it is studied in 1/4 circles: double frappé with the descent forward in effacé; repeat the same to the back; then once again to the effacé and to the side en face. Then practice the reverse side. The measure is 2/4 and all battements are done on the first 1/4 of the measure and every second 1/4 is a pause.

Now begin the descent forward into en face from the double frappé; descend forward into écarté, again into effacé; to the side en face and reverse sides. The measure is 2/4. All frappés are performed to each 1/4 of the measure.

Turns may be added with demi-plié and the exercises studied at the barre may be moved to the center floor.

Back again at the barre, the exercise is studied with a 1/2 turn at first without and then with the demi-plié: double frappé forward en face; then back with a half turn en dedans; again forward with a half turn en dehors and to the side en face. The exercise is done in reverse. The measure is 2/4 and all the turns are done to each first 1/4 of the measure and every second 1/4 is a pause.

During the half turn, transfer of the free arm must be done strictly following the rules of port de bras. On the center floor, these half turns are studied last, at first en face, then in small poses.

BATTEMENT FONDU

This movement is complicated by a turn of 1/8 or 1/4 circle at the moment of transfer of the supporting leg from demi-pointe and into demi-plié and with the close of the other leg into sur le cou-de-pied. The turn may be en dehors or en dedans. The legs must be supple and turned out and the entire movement must have a flow with a soft, light and clear finish in a small or large pose.

The study begins at the barre with a 1/8 turn; two battements fondus with the opening of the leg forward in effacé; two along Second; en face. Reverse. The measure is 3/4. To each measure there is a demi-plié and an opening of the leg. Then the turn is added in 1/4 of a circle: two battements fondus to effacé forward; two in écarté forward; two in effacé forward; two to the side en face. Then all is repeated in reverse.

When these movements are well learned, they may be practiced in the center.

There is another form of turn in the performance of the battement fondu which is done to 1/8 and 1/4 of a circle. At the same time as the opening of the working leg, the supporting leg rises to demi-pointe. In this movement, all the rules of relevé to demi-pointe are followed. A smooth turn, a flowing opening of the leg and a clear fixing of the pose should be preserved. This form may be studied after the pattern of the other exercises.

Both turns may be combined, but not in each battement fondu and not in each lesson.

The double battement fondu may also be complicated by the addition of a turn of a 1/2 circle to the first part of the movement. It is done at the moment of the first stretch of the leg from the demi-plié and change to sur le cou-de-pied. After the second demi-plié, the leg opens without a turn. The turn is kept turned out and supple and the bending and straightening from demi-plié is smooth with an even transfer to sur le cou-de-pied position. The second part of the double fondu is done according to the rules with the head, arms and body performing the same with or without the turn.

The study of the double fondu with the turn begins at the barre and with 1/2 circle: perform the double fondu with the half turn en dedans and opening the leg backward at the second demi-plié; then reverse opening the leg into Second; then the movement is done backward. Or another exercise might be: two double fondus with the leg opening into Fourth and two with the leg opening into Second. The half turns alternate in direction and the movement is repeated in reverse.

Both of these movements at the barre must be performed without épaulement, then in the small poses. The same order is brought to the center floor. The measure is 4/4. To the first 1/4, demi-plié; to the second, half turn; the next 1/4, demi-plié and open the leg; then straighten from demi-plié, etc. Later, each battement fondu with a turn may be made to one measure of 2/4.

It must be remembered that all battements fondus with or without the turn must be combined in equal measure. They must not be crammed with turns.

If any of the elementary movements mentioned here are not yet fully learned, they must not be studied with a turn.

FLIC–FLAC

This form of flic-flac is done in a full circle en dehors or en dedans. The turn starts in the first sur le cou-de-pied (flic) but is basically done with the transfer of the foot in its second position (flac), when the supporting leg rises to demi-pointe.

If the flic-flac is done en dehors, the open leg is transferred back of the supporting leg and the turn is done in the same direction. It may also be done the other way around.

The arms at the moment of the turn from Second give an energetic push to the body and transfer into a lowered First. The body is straight and pulled up. The head, at the start of the turn, lags a little, then, overtaking the body, assumes the starting position. Flic-flac must be done clearly and in tempo, keeping all the basic rules.

Flic-flac with the turn may end in a large pose with a stop on the whole foot or in demi-pointe or in demi-plié. In each case, the leg opens energetically through a développé.

The study starts with a smooth movement: battement fondu; then with a faster rond de jambe en l'air; battement frappé, etc. This movement may be introduced into adagios and be used as a transfer from one pose into another.

BATTEMENT DIVISÉ EN QUARTS (DIVIDED INTO QUARTERS)

In classical dance, there is a form of turn called the fouetté. This turn permits a move from one pose into another without transferring the open leg along a horizontal line through a rond de jambe en l'air, but by leaving it in a given direction and turning the body on a vertical axis in a 1/4 or 1/2 circle en dehors or en dedans. The open leg is kept in place with the leg stretched and unswerving. The toes of the open leg remain in the same place on the floor or in the air, as the body turns.

The technique is to permit the top of the thigh bone of the open and turned-out leg to rotate in the pelvic cavity as it does in the performance of the grand rond de jambe en l'air. These turns may be done from pose to pose with the leg at 22 degrees, 45 degrees or 90 degrees. The height of the working leg must be kept strictly on the same level during the course of the movement.

To master this technique, the battement divisé en quarts is a useful exercise. Its basis is the battement développé and relevé on demi-pointe. Beginning in Fifth Position, en face, battement développé is done forward in a demi-plié; at the same time a relevé to demi-pointe is made by the supporting leg and a fouetté turn of 1/4 circle en dedans. The position is now fixed as à la seconde (facing corner #7 or corner #3). The open leg then bends into the passé position (at the knee) as the standing leg remains on demi-pointe.

The arms during the développé are moved from Preparatory into First and during the turn open into Second. At the bending of the leg, they return to Preparatory Position. The body is pulled up at all times into a straight position, turning with the supporting leg. The head, at the moment the arms move from Preparatory Position, bends a very little forward and the eyes focus on the hands. During the fouetté the head returns to its erect position.

The exercise is repeated four times in 1/4 circles. The first développé begins from Fifth while the other three begin from the passé position at the knee. The fouetté ends lowering the open leg into Fifth Position in back and the entire exercise is done with the other leg. Backward or reverse, the exercise is done with the leg opening en dedans and the turn en dehors in 1/4 circles. Everything else is done according to the rules except for the position of the body when the leg opens backward. The body at that time leans a bit forward and at the fouetté returns to its erect position.

In the performance of the exercise, the student must rise high and with flexibility onto the demi-pointe and hold fast to the turnout at the hip, knee and foot. The center of gravity must be kept over the supporting leg and the body fixed in the pulled-up and collected position. The arms should move in a pliant manner, in one rhythm with the movement of the head and body. The entire exercise must be clear in a moderate tempo, not too fast or too slow in the turning. There should not be even the slightest weakening of the supporting leg, the body or the arms.

To reestablish the balance during this difficult movement, the student may make a very short push with the supporting movement to find a more stable perpendicular alignment, but shifting about with the whole body or falling off demi-pointe is not permitted.

The measure is in a 4/4 tempo with 1/4 for the développé; 1/4 for the turn; 1/4 for the fixing of the pose à la seconde; 1/4 for the bending of the leg to passé, etc. If the measure is 3/4, every portion of the movement is done to one full measure.

These turns may be studied only after the pupil has mastered the battement développé combined with relevé to demi-pointe and with the demi-plié in the center floor.

Before taking on the study of this exercise, which may be practiced first, it may be best to master the simplest form of this turn—doing the fouetté with the toes in the tendu position on the floor. It is studied with the help of the displaced heel of the supporting leg. The fouetté should be in a combination with battement tendu, then with the working leg in 45 degrees in a double battement tendu. The fouetté turn is done after the second demi-plié at the moment of the transfer of the supporting leg to demi-pointe.

Later, this form of turn may be studied in combination with battement tendu in a faster tempo with the transfer from one small pose into another pose.

POSES IN TURNS

TOUR LENT (SLOW TURN)

The name indicates that this turn is slow. The method involves a small displacement of the heel of the supporting leg at the moment when the large pose has been fixed. This turn is usually done in a full circle en dehors or en dedans. The displacement and movement of the heel must be even and supple, not too big or too small, and no more than four moves for a full circle. The turn must be smooth and free, strictly rhythmical and properly timed. It is understood that all the poses held during this turn are correctly aligned.

The movement of the head depends upon the pose. In arabesque, for instance, the head is immovable. In poses where the leg opens along Fourth croisé forward or back, the start of the turn coincides with the lag of the head movement until the effacé pose is assumed. The head then remains in its proper position for that pose during the turn. The same is true for the poses in écarté when the turn is done en dehors and the leg opens to corner #2 or #8 of the room or when the leg is opened to corner #4 or #6 and the turn is en dedans.

In performing the pose à la seconde, the head is kept back slightly as in the écarté turns. The arms, body and open leg as a rule are immovable. But, during these turns, additional elements may be introduced such as the demi-plié, which may be incorporated into the turn during its duration or which may begin or end the turn.

Various forms of port de bras may also be introduced, such as an arm in First Position in the first arabesque, which lowers toward the end of the turn and stretches out again at the end of the turn into its former position.

Another example: The turn may start in first arabesque and end in second arabesque. Both arms begin and finish the movement together. One arm from First goes into Second, the other from Second goes through Preparatory and moves into First. The head leans slightly forward and gradually turns to the advanced shoulder. The lean of the body is slightly increased; the shoulder with the arm opening into Second, is lowered a bit and led back. Such a change of arabesque during the turn may occur in any variation from second into third or fourth arabesque.

Another variation: The turn begins in attitude and ends in arabesque or the opposite. The turn may begin in écarté in the usual position and ends in a transfer of the arm from Second into Third as the other arm moves from Third through First into Second allongé, etc.

All turns may be done en dehors or en dedans but always with a smooth transfer of arm, head and body.

It is useful to join the tour lent with big pirouettes by increasing the speed of the end of the turn through a demi-plié preparation.

The study of tour lent may be sensible to start in pose à la seconde with a 1/2 circle tour en dehors. This half-circle turn must be divided into four equal parts, each with a short fixing of the position, so that the pupil may learn to work the supporting leg sufficiently and carefully correct the pose during the performance of the turn. The music should be in 3/4, a slow waltz. The first two measures are used for a relevé lent à la seconde; the following first 1/4 of the third measure is used for the displacement of the heel of the supporting leg; each second and third 1/4 of the same measure is used for a rest; repeat measures 4, 5 and 6 as measure 3; the seventh measure is used for a relevé to demi-pointe and the eighth is used for lowering the leg and the arms into the starting position. The next half of the exercise is done en dehors. All is repeated on the other leg to the same sixteen measures of 3/4. Then the half turn is studied en dedans.

The pose à la seconde is learned with the full turn. If it is well learned, stable and correct in performance, the student may then study the turn in the first arabesque; in poses with the leg raised forward, in attitudes and second and third arabesque, in écarté poses and fourth arabesque. The music is slow, in the form of an adagio, 3/4, 4/4 or 6/8.

Each turn is usually done to two measures. As each is learned separately, it may be introduced into the adagio portion of the class where the final study is the joining with demi-plié, and various transfers of arms which change the construction of the poses. (Tour lent is called tour de promenade in the French School.)

FOUETTÉ TURNS (WHIPPED)

In the elementary exercise, battement divisé en quarts, we mentioned the fouetté turns. At this point, we will describe several aspects of this means of turning from one pose into another.

The turns are slow or fast, en dehors and en dedans. The slow turns are made with the displacement of the supporting leg as in tour lent and the fast ones by means of relevé on demi-pointe.

The opening of the leg into the starting pose before performing the fouetté may be done by different means: battement développé, battement lent, grand battement jeté, pas glissé, pas tombé, etc. The turn itself is performed with a stretched open leg, or bend, to the passé position at the knee, or a combination of the two.

The supporting leg may remain straight or begin or finish the turn with a demi-plié. The arms, body and head during the turn may perform in different ways, but always according to the rules of port de bras.

The peculiarity of the fouetté turn is that with an open leg forward it may only turn en dedans. With the leg open to the back, it may only turn en dehors. With the leg open to the Second Position, it may turn either way.

These turns may be made in 1/4 or full circles. They serve as a means of joining a variety of poses.

Here are some examples and basic forms of the fouetté established in our teaching practice:

From the à la seconde pose, a slow turn is made en dedans in 1/4 of a circle, ending in a second arabesque. The supporting left leg does a displacement of the foot at the same time it straightens from the demi-plié. The open right leg remains outstretched and is kept firmly in the position. The body turns in profile and the right arm goes through Preparatory into First as the left is led backward into second arabesque position and the head takes its usual pose. (See illustration #142.)

This turn is made smoothly with a flow and no delays or sharp twists. The starting pose must change into the final pose with assurance and clarity.

Another example: From third arabesque, a slow turn is made en dehors of 3/4 of a circle ending in croisé forward. The supporting leg makes three displacements of the heel, the last ending in demi-plié.

The open right leg has made a smooth move through Second. The body is pulled up and the arms are kept moving evenly into the final pose. The right arm has opened into Second and the left into Third. The head, together with the arms, has turned the advanced shoulder. (See illustration #143.)

This turn from pose into pose must be done with fluidity, without fixing the leg in one special point, and by moving with the body during the 3/4 turn.

From the effacé pose forward the turn may be made with a relevé en dedans of 1/4 circle ending in attitude effacée. The supporting leg does the relevé from a demi-plié onto demi-pointe with a push. (See illustration #144.)

This movement is done with a flow, and with an energetic rhythm. At the moment of the culmination of the relevé to demi-pointe, the body is pulled up and lifted upward.

Still another example: From a third arabesque a turn is made in relevé en dehors in a full circle ending in écarté to corner #6 or #4 (if reversed). The supporting leg makes the relevé to demi-pointe with a turning push. The open leg bends into the passé position smoothly and straightens into the Second at the finish. The body is kept straight and at the end of the turn leans slightly away from the open leg. The arms join in a lowered First during the turn and, at the end, one arm rises into Third as the other opens into Second. The head leans slightly toward the arm in lowered First and at the opening of the arms turns to the advanced shoulder.

142 Tour lent with fouetté of ¼ turn from à la seconde to second arabesque

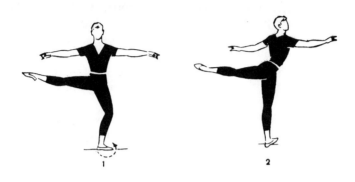

143 Tour lent with fouetté of ¾ turn from third arabesque ending in croisé devant

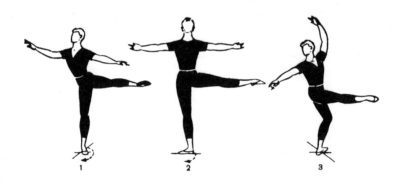

144 Fouetté from effacé devant with ½ turn to attitude effacée

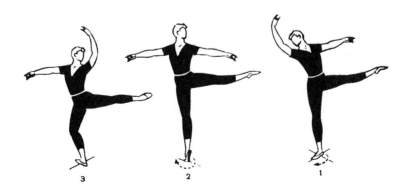

All of these examples follow the strict elementary rules of movement for the arms, legs, head and body. The center of gravity must be fixed correctly over the supporting leg. The shoulders and thighs must be kept strictly level and the open leg must not be lowered during the turn through Second, whether bent or outstretched. The passé position is from a firmly held thigh which simply bends at the knee to passé position. The starting and final pose must be performed with a clear design and a definite rush of expression.

All these examples must be done in reverse and alternating the bend and open leg positions. Altogether, there must be a variety of joinings and poses in the study of these turns.

Next, the study of the grand fouetté reveals a turn which has its own firmly established form and clearly expresses the lashing out of the open leg.

GRAND FOUETTÉ (WHIPPED TURN)

The grand fouetté is begun with a grand battement jeté followed by a turn of a full circle en dedans or en dehors.

If it is to be performed en dedans, the open leg rushes with a wide and energetic movement into Second en dedans passing through First forward, or backward if the turn is en dehors. Therefore, the name grand fouetté is justified in the form and character of the movement.

---

145   Grand fouetté en dedans

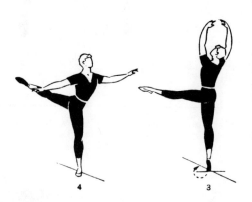

The grand fouetté en dedans begins from à la seconde and ends in third arabesque. The starting pose may be done in various ways. The most comfortable one compatible in tempo is the grand battement jeté. It is done from demi-plié into a high demi-pointe. This throw may start from Fifth or from sur le cou-de-pied.

The supporting leg descending from demi-pointe must turn en dedans for about

1/4 of a circle in order to become turned out in relation to the leg which performed the throw (the heel leads this additional adjustment). The first descent to the supporting heel must be done in demi-plié in a short, elastic and uninterrupted sendoff. Then the second relevé to demi-pointe with the turn of 3/4 of a circle ends in a demi-plié.

The open leg during the throw rushes energetically but lightly to the upper corners of the room (#4 or #6), gliding the entire foot along the floor as it passes through First Position.

In Fourth, the leg must be retained at the same point in space, turn along its longitudinal axis and rise slightly at the final demi-plié. The arms during the throw of the leg to Second are also thrown into Second, palms down. At the moment of the throw through First into Fourth, the arms move in the same tempo through Preparatory from First into Third.

This position is a passing pose along Fourth forward through the upper back. At the final turn, the arms open into third arabesque. The body, during the turn, is straight and pulled up. At the end of the turn, it leans somewhat forward into the third arabesque pose.

Grand fouetté must be done clearly, in one tempo with a clear design and a free turn. (See illustration #145.)

The grand fouetté en dedans may be done in somewhat different detail: 1. The starting pose is écarté diagonal in #2 or #8; 2. The final pose of third arabesque

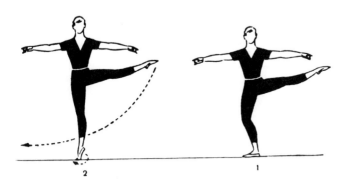

is replaced by attitude croisée; 3. The throw of the leg through First into Fourth is done without a demi-plié; 4. The degree of the turn may be increased by 1/4 circle, ending the movement in first arabesque or attitude effacée. These changes must not be studied until the basic form is thoroughly learned and can be done without serious mistakes.

The grand fouetté en dehors also begins in the à la seconde position, but ends in croisé forward. The turn of the supporting leg and the entire body move en dehors with the same throw of the leg through First into Fourth, but aimed at the lower corners (#2 or #4).

The arms at the first opening of the leg in Second are thrown into Second. Through Preparatory Position, they rise to First and into Third and finally open into pose croisée forward. The body is straight at the moment of the throw through First backward; then leans a bit forward; straightens out as the arms rise to Third, and assumes the position for the final pose.

All changes in the details of grand fouetté en dedans are permissible as previously described.

The study of fouetté turns may be started only after the battement divisé en quarts has been well learned. With the use of this remarkable exercise the basis is laid without which it would be impossible to master the technique of performing all fouetté turns, especially the larger forms.

TURNS RENVERSÉ (THROWN BACK)

The renversé is a turn in which the body is thrown backward. It is performed in two forms: renversé en attitude and renversé en écarté.

RENVERSÉ EN ATTITUDE

The starting position for this form is attitude croisée backward. The supporting leg does a demi-plié followed by an energetic relevé to demi-pointe, with a turning sendoff en dehors. Then a pas de bourrée is done during the turn with a change of legs. The movement ends in Fifth Position in demi-plié. The body, during the first demi-plié, bends forward to 45 degrees and at the relevé is straightened forcefully into the starting position and onward to a backward bend. At the first stepover of the pas de bourrée, the body continues in the backbend, but at the

146 Renversé en attitude

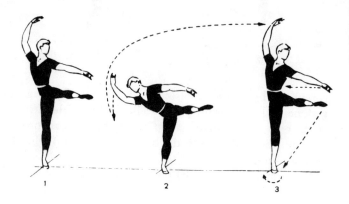

second stepover it straightens and at the final demi-plié is quite straight. The arms, when the body bends forward, remain in their position. At the relevé, one arm moves through First and Second to Third, as the other remains fixed in Second. At the stepover of the pas de bourrée, the arm in Second moves into First. At the second stepover, both arms move to First; and in demi-plié in Fifth Position at the end pose, both are in Preparatory Position.

The head at the first demi-plié turns en face and, together with the body, bends forward. At the relevé, it turns to the starting position and at the first stepover of the pas de bourrée it remains in profile. At the second stepover, it begins to turn into the final position, which it assumes at the second demi-plié. (See illustration #146.)

The head at the first demi-plié turns en face and, together with the body, bends forward. At the relevé, it turns to the starting position and at the first stepover of the pas de bourrée it remains in profile. At the second stepover, it begins to turn into the final position, which it assumes at the second demi-plié. (See illustration #146.)

The renversé en attitude must begin in a sweeping movement coinciding with the relevé at the start of the turn. The body actively continues the turn. The throw of the body backward, however, is controlled and constrained, yet supple.

The arms, head and body take an active part in the turn, increasing the flow of its performance.

All the elementary rules of movement for the head, body, arms and legs must be strictly observed.

In performing the renversé en attitude, other movements of the arms are permissible: 1. At the forward bend of the body, the arms join in First, and at the turn, the arm corresponding to the lifted leg rises through Second into Third. The other moves into Second. The rest of the movement is the same as the previously given version. 2. During the bend backward, the arms join in First, then the arm opposite the open leg moves into Third and the other arm into Second.

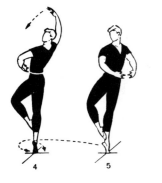
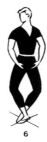

At the turn, the arm in Third moves into Second and lowers with the other arm into Preparatory Position.

This movement may begin with an attitude effacée. Then the relevé to demi-pointe is done with a turn of 1/4 circle en dehors.

En dedans, this renversé is done from attitude croisée or attitude effacée. The body here leans forward and then is thrown back. The arms and head move in the previously described pattern. The relevé starts with a turning push en dedans. The pas de bourrée is done with a reversed change-stepover.

This movement is also done as a fouetté. The croisé position is fixed forward as the body and head lean forward on the demi-plié and the arms join in First. The relevé is done to demi-pointe and the body straightens forcefully and turns en dedans. At the same time, the supporting leg makes a 1/4 circle; the open leg keeps the same point in space in the fouetté movement as the body turns. The arms and head take the pose écartée. After the turn, the open leg along Second performs the first stepover in front of the supporting leg together with the turn to 1/4 circle and the throw backward. The arm in Second goes into First and the other stays in Third. The head remains in the preceding position. The second stepover finds the body straight and the arms in First. The head starts the turn and the movement continues as previously described and ends in the Fifth Position.

The study of this complicated movement must begin with only a slight throw backward by the body. The movement gradually increases to the required size and force. The starting pose should be in Fifth and then may be changed to the pas tombé as an approach to this movement. Then the pas tombé may be used as an approach from croisé front or from pas tombé, attitude croisée back. From demi-plié where the change ends, the relevé to demi-pointe and all the other elements of renversé may be prolonged.

After learning the movement from this method, the student may study its variations and the fouetté version.

147　Renversé écarté

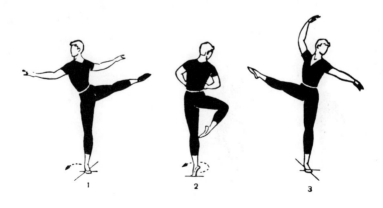

RENVERSÉ EN ÉCARTÉ

The renversé en écarté is done in a full circle beginning in fourth arabesque and ends in pose écartée into the upper corners (#4 or #6).

The turn is en dedans on high demi-pointe without a demi-plié. The open leg bends at the knee in the passé position, and the movement ends in a supple release of the supporting foot to the floor.

At the same time as the release, the free leg has opened to the écarté position. The body, at the start of the turn, bends forcefully toward the knee of the passé and forcefully straightens without losing the tempo, then throws the leg lightly into the écarté, where it remains fixed. The arms at the turn make an energetic move into a lowered First and, just as energetically at the end of the turn, rise into Third. The head, at the lean toward the knee, inclines in the same direction. Then, as the body is thrown back, the head lags a bit, clearly overtakes the body, and assumes its final position. (See illustration #147.) (Previous renversés began with a coupé or pas failli, with a grand rond de jambe opening devant to attitude ending in pas de bourrée en tournant with similar leanings.

This renversé is done with vitality, a flexible turn of the body, decided movements of the arms and a clear turn of the head. The final pose in écarté must be firm. The movement is not done in reverse and it is studied in the last two levels of the school.

STEPS DONE IN A TURN

PAS DÉGAGÉ

This turn is done as a fouetté at the end of a change from one leg onto the other leg. It is performed along Second into Fourth in 1/4 circle and from Fourth into Fourth in a 1/2 circle. The supporting leg straightens from demi-plié and turns with one displacement of the heel.

If the turn is done away from the supporting leg it is an en dehors turn. If it is done toward the supporting leg, it is en dedans.★

The free leg, at the moment of the turn, must straighten from demi-plié and the toes must be kept pointed on the floor.

The body, head and arms before and after the turn are fixed in a small pose. At the moment of the turn, they change smoothly into the next pose. The rules of pas dégagé are observed.

★ (One of the simple ways to determine the direction of a turn in any movement is to observe the direction of the heel of the supporting foot in demi-pointe or on the floor. If the heel of the supporting foot on the floor or in demi-pointe moves forward, the turn is en dedans—toward the body. If the movement of the heel of the supporting foot on the floor or in demi-pointe, or even in demi-plié, is backward, the turn is en dehors—away from the body.)

The movement must be studied in the center floor incorporated into adagio combinations as an element of transfer from one pose into another. At first, the turn of 1/4 with the transfer from Second into Fourth and back is studied. Then, from Fourth to Fourth is studied in 1/2 circle.

PAS GLISSÉ

The turn is done from Fifth in 1/4 circle at the moment of the relevé when both legs rise to demi-pointe. It begins in croisé, and ends in effacé with a light, gliding slide into Fourth forward, back or to écarté. The head, body and arms take the pose given. The relevé with the turn has a gliding exit, and a final demi-plié with the movements of the head, body and arms flowing softly and clearly.

This study may be begun by means of this exercise: pas glissé with a turn to effacé forward; repeat the same step without the turn; end on demi-pointe; the following demi-plié makes an exchange of legs to Fifth through a battement tendu écarté to the back corner (#4 or #6). The exercise is ready to be repeated on the other leg. Repeat the exercise once more and perform in reverse. Later, the exercise may be studied in the same pattern but in écarté instead of effacé. The arms, body and head assume the position for small poses. The pose is fixed during the turn and remains fixed during the glide.

PAS TOMBÉ

This turn is made as a fouetté at the moment of the fall onto the open leg. It is done in 1/4 and 1/2 circles toward the open leg—en dehors—or away from the open leg—en dedans.

The starting pose may be écarté and the finish, first arabesque. This turn equals 1/4 of a circle en dehors. As a 1/2 circle turn, the starting pose may be third arabesque into attitude effacée. The performance of the tombé and the turn must be simultaneous and smooth. The starting and final pose must be fixed clearly and with élan. As a whole, the pas tombé must flow with all the rules observed as it is without the turn.

The study is first done 1/4 or 1/2 circles in small poses, then progresses to large poses. It is best studied within adagio combinations as a method of changing from one pose into another.

The pas tombé may be done in place through Fifth Position in 1/4 turn en dehors and en dedans. In this case, the turn occurs at the moment of the change from one leg to another and is on the leg from which the movement started. This movement is usually done as a change of épaulement for a movement which follows. It is studied with battement fondu and other elementary exercises at the barre and on the floor.

PAS DE BOURRÉE

The forms previously described may be done with a turn (en tournant). The arms, body and head perform as in the simple pas de bourrée without the turn. With the turn, the turnout must be especially maintained as well as the suppleness of the stepover onto a high demi-pointe and the exact position of the sur le cou-de-pied. There must be a clarity in the turn.

The pas de bourrée with a change of legs begins with a turn in 1/2 circle. It is done during the two stepovers on demi-pointe in this way: beginning in the Fifth Position, right leg forward, épaulement croisé; demi-plié on the right leg as the left rises to sur le cou-de-pied in back; at the first stepover of the left leg onto demi-pointe a 1/2 turn is done to the left en dedans; the second stepover is done on the right leg and then the left turns en dehors. But the direction of the first half turn gives the name to the circle. It must be noted that both stepovers require that the free leg be in an exact sur le cou-de-pied forward and that the second stepover is a decreased Second, shortened to a minimum for greater stability and clarity in the turn. The final demi-plié is done in épaulement croisé.

The arms and body follow the previously described pattern for simple pas de bourrée. The head is held back a bit at the first half turn, and at the second half turn it returns to the starting position ending toward the advanced shoulder. (The French School calls this a pas de bourrée enveloppé en tournant.)

The pas de bourrée en dehors begins in Fifth Position as well. With the right leg forward, épaulement croisé, the demi-plié is done on the left leg with the first stepover and half turn on the right leg, turning to the left, en dehors. The second half turn is on the left leg to the left. In both stepovers, the free leg moves to sur le cou-de-pied backward. The arms, head and body follow the pattern for the first form for pas de bourrée en dedans. (The French term for this step is pas de bourrée détourné.)

This movement may begin from any pose. In that case, the open leg when the knee is straightened from the first demi-plié moves directly into the sur le cou-de-pied position. The rest of the movement is unchanged. If the demi-plié is done with the open leg and the first stepover onto demi-pointe is done with an advance to the side along Fourth or Second, it must be a broad or wide pas dégagé. Both turns are performed as described. The movement must be studied first separately, then added into combinations.

PAS DE BOURRÉE WITH NO CHANGE OF LEGS

This turn is done as a change of épaulement of 1/4 at the first stepover. This form may be repeated four times in a series in the same direction (or a diagonal) in a 1/2 circle. The first and third turns will be en dehors and the second and fourth turns, en dedans.

The direction of the first turn gives the step its name, but it may be done en dehors and en dedans.

The arms, head and body perform as previously described, but the study must start at first with a change of épaulement, 1/4, 1/2, then one circle for each pas de bourrée with no change of legs.

PAS DE BOURRÉE DESSUS-DESSOUS

This pas de bourrée is done with two full turns: dessus in en dedans, and dessous in en dehors. The technique for these turns is the same as for the pas de bourrée with a change of legs. The arms, head and body follow the prescribed pattern.

This movement must flow and be clear. Each demi-plié, each stepover onto demi-pointe and half turn must seem to be flowing from one movement into the other. The head at the first and third half turn must be somewhat lingering, but at the second and fourth, it returns a bit earlier.

Since both turns are uninterrupted, the stepover onto demi-pointe along a shortened Second is here reduced even more to a minimum or even eliminated altogether if the movement is performed at a quick tempo.

Both turns must be stable, *without* a lean away from the vertical axis. In the performance of the pas de bourrée with a change of legs, one turn allows a certain displacement from the beginning position. But not here.

The study of this form must begin only after the pas de bourrée with a change of legs has been well learned. Both forms must be used equally.

PAS BALANCÉ

The pas balancé is done with a turn of 1/4 at the time of the transfer to Second in demi-plié. The arms, head, body and shoulders take the position for second arabesque, which means they turn en dedans. The legs are kept turned out and flexible. If the balancé is repeated in another direction, the same rules apply. The turn and bend of the body must be supple but not overdone in male performers.

The study of balancé with the turn begins only after the pupil has mastered its basic elements.

There is another form of pas balancé which is performed four times in a row in a full circle. Each balancé is done in 1/4 circle without the turn of the body to second arabesque. The turn occurs not on the demi-plié in Second as in the first description, but at the moment of the stepover to demi-pointe. The entire movement is in the overall pattern of a square with the turn of exactly 1/4 at the corners of the square. The movement must flow, be exact and light. The study begins after the turns in 1/4 in elementary form have been mastered.

TURNING OR SPINNING MOVEMENTS ON THE FLOOR

The technique of turning in classical dance requires the ability of the dancer to orient himself in space, to transfer his center of gravity correctly to the supporting leg, to hold a vertical axis of the body with stability and to maintain the form of the given movement as well as to maintain the rhythm and dynamics of the turns.

The basis for correct and stable multiple turns requires well-practiced movements of the arms, leg, body and head as well as well-developed muscular strength, endurance, resoluteness and concentration.

The study of small and large pirouettes (multiple turns) begins with the elementary placement of the body at the barre and in the center floor in adagio and allegro portions of the class.

Large and stable pirouettes done in a fast tempo but on a low demi-pointe, with angular arms, distorted movements of the body or head, do not reflect the beautiful nature of this movement for the male dancer. In the art of classical dance, turning must always be harmonious in form, stable in technique, dashing in tempo and inspired in character.

SMALL TOURS (LES PIROUETTES)

These are divided into petite and grande forms. Pirouettes in which the free leg remains in sur le cou-de-pied position while the supporting leg turns are called petites pirouettes.

Pirouettes in which the free leg remains at 90 degrees are called grandes pirouettes. Both forms have their variations and may be done with the help of various approaches and in different directions, en dehors and en dedans.

The technique consists of three components: 1. the turning push; 2. the turn itself; 3. the ending. The forms and rules for pirouettes are given in this progression.

PETITES PIROUETTES

These turns are done from different approaches. Each has its own form and performing traits. But the pirouette itself, at the moment of the turning of the body, fixes the one and only performing method.

The beginning and ending of the petite pirouette is varied in form and in the degree of difficulty. All these factors must be given attention in the study of the small pirouette and must be practiced in equal measure.

PIROUETTE FROM SECOND POSITION

This pirouette en dehors begins in Fifth Position en face: demi-plié and rise to demi-pointe in relevé en face to begin the movement; the leg in Fifth forward stretches out to 45 degrees to the side while the supporting leg remains in a high demi-pointe. Then a demi-plié in Second on both legs prepares the turn. The turn begins as a transfer from the demi-plié in Second into one pirouette en dehors on a high demi-pointe. There is a turning push and a transfer of the free leg to sur le cou-de-pied forward. The turn occurs on the leg that was fixed in demi-pointe in Second while the other leg opened and, since the turn is opposite to it, it is en dehors. At the end of the turn the supporting leg descends into a demi-plié and the other leg lowers from sur le cou-de-pied *at the same time* into Fifth Position back. The movement is finished in épaulement croisé.

During the relevé to demi-pointe in Fifth, the arms move from Preparatory Position to First. As the leg goes to 45 degrees to the side, they open into Second. As the leg transfers into demi-plié along Second, the arm corresponding to the direction of the turn transfers into First. The other arm remains in Second. When the turning push is performed, the arms energetically join in a rounded and lowered First with a little sendoff into the en dehors direction. This helps the movement of the legs. At the final demi-plié, the arms open into a lowered Second.

The body is straight throughout the turn and its preparation. The three demi-pliés must be done evenly on both legs, but at the turning push the working leg moves over onto the supporting leg and with a small sendoff spins into the en dehors direction with the help of the arms. The head at the start and end of the movement, and also during the relevé on demi-pointe in Fifth, is fixed en face.

---

148   Preparation and small pirouette from Second Position

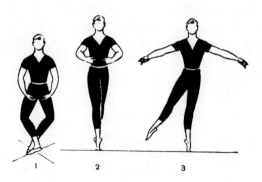

At the start of the pirouette, it is held back a bit, but turning sooner than the body, it returns to the starting position. In this way, the head seems to perform a turning push itself, first with a delay, then a movement faster than the body. (Spotting, which is the term given to the rapid movement of the head and gives the impression that the face is always forward, prevents the dancer from becoming dizzy. It requires a focus of the eyes on a fixed place slightly above eye level.) (See illustration #148.)

The rhythm is 2/4 to the measure. The demi-plié is before the measure; relevé in Fifth is 1/4; the opening of the leg to Second is 1/4; fixing the position is 1/4; demi-plié in Second is 1/4; the pirouette is 1/4; *the fixing of the stop on demi-pointe is 2/4;* the final demi-plié in Fifth is 1/4 in the position from which the movement may be repeated to the other side.

PIROUETTE EN DEDANS

The pirouette en dedans begins in Fifth Position en face. The demi-plié is done and the relevé to both legs in high demi-pointe is en face as well. The leg in back in Fifth stretches out and opens to the side to 45 degrees as the supporting leg remains in a high demi-pointe. Then a demi-pointe in Second is done on both legs and the transfer into one pirouette en dedans on a high demi-pointe begins. It is done by a turning push and a transfer of the open leg into sur le cou-de-pied forward. The turning may be done on the supporting leg in Second at 45 degrees and the direction is the same or toward it, en dedans. The supporting leg then does a demi-plié as the other leg descends into Fifth forward keeping the épaulement croisé. The arms at the relevé in Fifth to demi-pointe rise from Preparatory Position into First and, at the moment of the leading of the leg to 45 degrees, open into Second. At the moment of the transfer into demi-plié in Second, the arm that corresponds to the turn's direction moves into First. The other remains in Second. At the moment of the turning push, the arms ener-

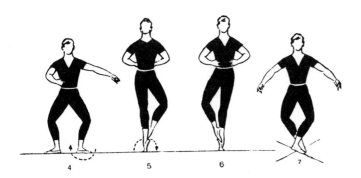

getically join in First in a rounded and lowered position and sendoff in the direction of en dedans, thus helping the legs.

At the final demi-plié, they open into a lowered Second. The body is straight throughout. In all three demi-pliés, the body rests on both legs. At the turning push, the center of gravity is moved totally onto the supporting leg and, with a small sendoff, spins in the direction en dedans helping the legs and arms. The head moves as previously described.

At the start and end, and at the relevé to demi-pointe in Fifth, the position is en face. At the beginning of the pirouette, the head delays a bit, then, turning faster than the body, returns to the starting position sooner than the body. The head does not coordinate with the legs, arms or body but is independently a force in the formation of the turn. The tempo is the same as in the en dehors pirouette.

PIROUETTE FROM FOURTH POSITION

The pirouette from Fourth Position starts in Fifth, épaulement croisé. It begins with a demi-plié followed by a relevé on the back leg to a high demi-pointe with a turn to effacé. The other leg, at the same time, rises in sur le cou-de-pied forward.

Then a demi-plié is done on the supporting leg at the same time the other leg transfers into Fourth back croisé. *The knee of the back leg is stretched* and the entire foot is on the floor.

Then both legs deepen into a demi-plié from which the pirouette en dehors is made on the forward leg (to the right).

The pirouette is made by means of a turning push by both legs as the one leg transfers to a high demi-pointe and the other moves to sur le cou-de-pied forward. At the end of the pirouette, the supporting leg again transfers into demi-plié and the other leg transfers into a croisé in Fourth back with the knee stretched out. The entire foot in back is on the floor.

To close the movement, the supporting leg straightens from demi-plié, and the leg standing in back keeping the toes on the floor closes into Fifth Position, épaulement croisé.

The arms at the first relevé to demi-pointe move from Preparatory Position into First. At the movement of the leg into Fourth in back, they open into third arabesque. At the movement of the leg back and during the pirouette they energetically, and in a rounded form, join in a lowered First with a little sendoff en dehors.

At the end of the pirouette, the arms open into a lowered Second and, at the close of the legs into Fifth, they smoothly lower into Preparatory Position. The body is held straight throughout the preparation and turn. During all three demi-pliés, it rests evenly on both legs. When the leg is stretched in back along Fourth Position and during the pirouette, the weight is totally on the supporting leg. During the turning push with the slight sendoff, the body coordinates with the en dehors movements of the arms and legs.

The head at the start of the movement is turned toward the advanced shoulder. During the following movement including the pirouette, the face and look are turned in the same direction as at the start. Only at the end of the pirouette does the head turn en face.

During the push, the head delays and increases in speed to catch up, returning to the starting position faster than the body. At the final closing with the arms in Preparatory Position, the head turns to the other advanced shoulder.

The measure is 2/4. The first demi-plié is before the measure; 1/4 for the first relevé in demi-pointe; 1/4 to hold the position; 1/4 for the transfer into third arabesque; 1/4 for the deepened demi-plié on both legs along Fourth; 1/4 for the pirouette; *1/4 to fix the stop on demi-pointe;* 1/4 for the second transfer of the leg into Fourth back; 1/4 for the final closing of the leg into Fifth. The movements may be repeated to the other side.

PIROUETTE EN DEDANS

Beginning in Fifth Position, épaulement croisé, a demi-plié is done. Then a relevé on the supporting leg which is in back on high demi-pointe with a turn into effacé as the other leg moves at the same time to sur le cou-de-pied in front. The supporting leg does a demi-plié at the same time the other leg is moved into Fourth back in croisé. The leg in back is stretched at the knee and the entire foot is on the floor. Then a pirouette en dedans on the forward leg is done from a turning push from both legs. The pirouette is on a high demi-pointe of the supporting leg as the other remains fixed in sur le cou-de-pied front. At the end of the pirouette, the supporting leg lowers into demi-plié and the other leg, at the same time, goes into Fifth Position front and joins in the demi-plié.

The arms at the first relevé onto demi-pointe rise from Preparatory Position into First. At the moment the leg moves into Fourth back, the arm opposite to the direction of the turn opens into Second as the other arm stays in First. When the turning push is made, the arms energetically, and in a rounded image, join in a lowered First, helping the leg with the momentum of the turn. The body is straight at all times. At the first and last demi-plié in Fifth, it rests evenly on both legs. On the demi-plié with the leg open to Fourth, it rests totally on the supporting leg.

At the moment of the turning push, the body, with a small sendoff, pushes in the same direction, thus helping the arms and leg. The head, at the start, is turned to the shoulder. During the movement of the leg back into Fourth, it turns en face with a very slight bend toward the arm opening into Second.

At the moment the leg opens into 45 degrees, the head straightens, delays a bit at the start of the pirouette, then turns faster than the body and returns to the starting position. (Notice the working leg in the en dedans turn opens to 45 degrees side before moving into sur le cou-de-pied front. The supporting leg remains in demi-plié until the foot is placed in sur le cou-de-pied.)

The measure is 2/4: demi-plié is done before the measure; 1/4 is for the relevé on demi-pointe; 1/4 pause; 1/4 for the transfer of the leg into Fourth in back; 1/4 pause; 1/4 for the pirouette; 1/4 to fix the pirouette ending on demi-pointe; 1/4 to make the final demi-plié into Fifth; 1/4 for the battement tendu to the side with a change to Fifth back into demi-plié, from where the entire movement may be repeated to the other side.

PIROUETTE FROM FIFTH POSITION

PIROUETTE EN DEHORS

The pirouette en dehors begins in Fifth Position, épaulement croisé and demi-plié. A relevé to demi-pointe with a turn en face follows. The next demi-plié in Fifth is followed by a relevé on the back supporting leg on a high demi-pointe as the other leg rises into sur le cou-de-pied in front as *both legs* coordinate in the turning push en dehors—the opposite side to the supporting leg—for one pirouette. Finally, the supporting leg goes into a demi-plié as the other descends at the same time into Fifth in back. The épaulement croisé is kept at the final pose.

The arms, at the first relevé in Fifth, rise from Preparatory Position into First. At the second demi-plié, the arm opposite to the direction of the turn opens into Second and the other stays in First. At the moment of the turning push, they join in a lowered First and, with a small sendoff en dehors, support the action of the legs. They keep the same position during the pirouette. Together at the final demi-plié, they open into a lowered Second and at the straightening descend into Preparatory Position.

The body is straight at all times. At the first and last demi-plié and in demi-pointe in Fifth, it rests evenly on both legs. During the pirouette, it moves the weight onto the supporting leg. At the turning push, the body with a slight sendoff moves in the same direction, helping the arms and legs. The head, at the start, is turned toward the shoulder and is there at the end. During the relevé onto demi-pointe into Fifth, it turns en face. At the start of the pirouette, it is delayed a little, but returns before the body to the starting position, and in this way seems to turn independently.

The measure is 2/4; demi-plié before the measure; 1/4 relevé onto the demi-pointe in Fifth; 1/4 demi-plié before the pirouette; 1/4 pirouette; 1/4 final demi-plié; from which the movement may begin to the other side.

PIROUETTE EN DEDANS

The pirouette en dedans begins in Fifth Position épaulement croisé. There is a demi-plié followed by a relevé to demi-pointe with a turn en face. Then there is a demi-plié in Fifth and the leg *in front* rises to a high demi-pointe as the other leg moves to sur le cou-de-pied in front. The pirouette is done by means of a turning push by both legs en dedans, in the direction of the supporting leg on which the one pirouette is made. Then the supporting leg is released into a demi-plié while the other lowers into Fifth front fixing the épaulement croisé.

The arms in the first relevé in Fifth Position rise from Preparatory Position into First. At the second demi-plié, the arm corresponding to the direction of the turn opens into Second and the other stays in First. At the turning push, they join in a lowered First with a slight sendoff en dedans helping the leg in the momentum of the turn. During the pirouette, they remain in the same position. Together with the final demi-plié they open into a lowered Second and, at the end of the demi-plié, descend into Preparatory. The body is kept straight. At the first and last demi-plié it rests evenly on both legs. During the pirouette it rests totally on the supporting leg. With the push, it is sent off in the same direction, helping the arms and legs.

The head at the start of the turn is toward the shoulder. At the relevé onto demi-pointe in Fifth, it turns en face. At the start of the pirouette, it delays somewhat and then speeds up and returns to the starting position before the body. The musical division is the same as the other example—en dehors from Fifth.

ADVICE ON TEACHING PIROUETTES

These are the general rules for the turning push, the pirouette and the steps which follow:

In all small pirouettes, in whatever starting position in demi-plié that permits a convenient position to take a turning push, the transfer of the weight to the supporting leg with proper force and consideration is involved. Both legs must maintain the turnout and the weight must be firm on both legs, especially the heels of the feet.

The pushing turn is done from both legs. The support at that moment, in an elastic and turned-out movement to relevé onto a high demi-pointe, moves the foot into a vertical position. With the vertical axis as its base, the turn should be harmonious, light and stable. If the turn is on a medium high or low demi-pointe, the turn becomes squat.

The other leg departs from the floor into sur le cou-de-pied just as actively, with good pressure on the entire foot, neither too strong nor too weak, in order not to disrupt the balance. It is very important that at this moment the pelvis, as well as every part of the body and every move, be timed correctly and that the alignment of the body be entirely over the supporting leg.

The arms, at the moment of the turning push, are sent with commensurate strength for one pirouette, no more, no less. During the pirouette, the arms actively take part in the movement of the entire body by holding the rounded position with aplomb. They must not be pressed to the body or led too far from it, as that would make an unstable movement and distort the lowered First Position. During the push and in the pirouette, they must act resolutely, clearly and exactly. After the pirouette, the arms must open boldly but softly, with more restraint underscoring the stable character of the pirouette and the final demi-plié.

During the pirouette, the knee, ankle and instep must be well pulled up and the toes tightly and elastically pressed to the floor.

The knee of the free leg is led back turned out and the foot stretches and fixes the sur le cou-de-pied exactly. At the end of the pirouette, the supporting leg moves into demi-plié with pliability and *no earlier than the touch of the heel to the floor*. The other leg, at the same time and with the same suppleness, is put into Fifth or Fourth, *from the toes through the whole foot*. The transfer to demi-plié after a pirouette must be soft and not flabby.

The body at all times is pulled up and collected. During the turning push, it must not turn in the opposite direction, as this would destroy the harmony of the starting position and the technique of the transfer to the supporting leg. It is very important that the shoulders and the thighs, in all phases of the performance of pirouettes, remain on one plane and with the center of gravity on the supporting leg. The body and the supporting leg, during the pirouette, must be one pivot, one center which supports a stable turn of the whole body. Therefore, the open and lowered shoulders and a strongly held upper back and waist are necessary.

The head, as described before, is delayed and then sped up. The active and independent participation of the head allows the student to look directly, and almost without interruption, at one spot in space without dissipating his attention. Additionally, the head must move along the same vertical axis as the body and the supporting leg, without tensing or relaxing the muscles of the neck. The head, during the pirouette, must move freely and lightly but with sufficient clarity.

All movements of the legs, arms, body and head must be coordinated, especially during the turning push when the slightest weakening of the unity of the movement will have a very negative effect on the stability of the performance of the pirouette and its ending.

When the pupil has learned the movement well on demi-pointe and the varied promenades (walks), the preparatory study of exercises for pirouettes may begin. They are done exactly in the pattern of the pirouettes from Second, Fourth and Fifth and in the same musical divisions. This will allow the pupil to better master the starting methods, from which the pirouette will be performed. The transfer and the fixing of the body weight on a high demi-pointe are part of the practice prior to the performance of a pirouette.

The practice of these exercises instills the sense of the vertical line as well as the pulled-up body that is necessary for the performance of the pirouette. It is necessary, as well, to master the many stops in which the pirouette will end.

As the movements are learned, the study of the pirouette may begin from Second, Fourth and Fifth at first; en dehors, then en dedans.

The pirouette must be done with restraint to allow the pupil to understand well and to feel all the stages of the turn of the body on the vertical axis. Once this is properly understood and sensed, the approach to pirouettes may be increased. For instance, the pirouette from Second en dehors may be done in this way: measure, 2/4; demi-plié before the measure; 1/4 relevé on demi-pointe in Fifth; 1/4 opening the leg side to 45 degrees; 1/4 demi-plié in Second; 1/4 pirouette; 1/4 stop on demi-pointe; 2/4 for the straightening from demi-plié; 1/4 for the demi-plié to begin another exercise from the other leg.

Later, the study may be sped additionally: demi-plié before the measure; 1/4 for relevé to demi-pointe; 1/8 for the opening of the leg to 45 degrees; 1/8 for the demi-plié in Second; 1/4 pirouette; 1/4 for the final demi-plié in Fifth.

When the study of two pirouettes begins, the approach is even shorter: demi-plié before the measure; 1/4 for the rise to high demi-pointe as the other opens to the side to 45 degrees at the same time; 1/4 for the demi-plié in Second; 2/8 for two pirouettes; 1/4 for the ending in demi-plié in Fifth. When three or more pirouettes are studied, the entire approach to demi-plié in Second may be made before the measure, and may even be in the form of a small jump—pas échappé—into Second. The same applies to the pirouette en dedans.

The pirouette from Fifth en dehors and en dedans may also have shorter approaches. For instance: demi-plié before the measure; 1/4 for relevé to demi-pointe; 1/8 to free the leg back into Fourth; 1/8 to deepen the demi-plié; 1/4 for the pirouette; 1/4 for the final demi-plié in Fifth. This approach is suitable for two or three pirouettes.

Later, the approach may decrease to: demi-plié before the measure; 1/4 for relevé to demi-pointe; 1/8 leg to Fourth; 1/8 for a deepened demi-plié; 1/4 pirouette; 1/4 final demi-plié in Fifth. This is suitable for two or three pirouettes.

Still later, the approach may be: demi-plié, relevé and transfer of the free leg into Fourth in back before the measure; pirouettes to one or two measures of 2/4 together with the final demi-plié. Pirouettes from Fourth and from Second may be done from pas échappé as previously described.

Even shorter is the approach for a pirouette from Fifth with the relevé to demi-pointe in Fifth omitted entirely, and the pirouette itself done before the measure to one or two measures of 1/4 together with the final demi-plié into Fifth.

All three forms of pirouette may be made from a small jump ending in Fifth, like the changement de pied, the petit assemblé, etc. Both jump and pirouette are joined in one tempo. The more pirouettes that are made, the more forceful and resolute is the turning push needed. The body must be pulled up even more, but not constrained. Multiple turns require economical and deliberate effort to allow a stable performance of the given number of pirouettes. The force of the turning push must always be commensurate with the number of turns, the tempo and character of the pirouettes. For instance, in the performance of three to five pirouettes or even more, the corresponding arm to the direction of the turn must energetically move from First into Second at the moment of the turning push (to provide centrifugal force) and the one arm must join the other arm at once. (Vaganova, the first Soviet pedagogue, suggests the use of the arm for centrifugal force to precede the turning push by a hair's breadth.)

The body is also more active and the head at each turn clearly and rhythmically does its turn.

Small pirouettes on stage may be done fast or slow, coolly or temperamentally, with a dynamic increase or decrease, thus becoming the means of a vivid and expressive presentation of an emotional condition of the artist-dancer. But for all this, one must have a turning push of sufficient force. This must be worked out and practiced during the school lessons. Of course, it is learned only through years of work with the gradual increase in the complexity of the approaches. But if the pupil does not develop resolve and comprehension of the components of the pirouette, he will not be stable or varied in the character of this movement.

Students who are not yet in mastery of the technique of turns must not be allowed to spin out more pirouettes than given, and must not turn in a tempo not yet fitting to their level of accomplishment. Untimely actions lead to the break in the balance between the unsureness of their forces and their desire to escape the difficulties of developing a correct and beautiful turn. This unbalance leads to their accepting for themselves deep-seated mistakes.

The increase in the number of pirouettes from year to year must be gradual and progressive with individual approaches to each pupil. It is possible for a pupil to be carried away by the number of turns at the expense of quality. It is better to learn a small number in a faultless form and truly classic style.

At times, pupils try to reestablish balance by contortions of the upper part of the body so it will pull out more turns. The reestablishment of balance is possible only in one way: by a light and hardly noticeable glide from high demi-pointe on an elastic and stretched supporting leg to find the proper point of support. If the pupil's body is properly aligned, this glide will eventually not be necessary. (A hop is to be discouraged as soon as it appears.)

In the higher and graduating classes, where the pupils make a great number of turns from one approach, the ability to squeeze out turns on the highest demi-pointe must be practiced. Gradually, the working leg must be raised from sur le cou-de-pied position to the knee or passé position. The smooth movement of the arms one about the other, still preserving the roundness of the First Position, should be practiced as well.

The body must be pulled up to its limit, as well as the diaphragm, with the deepest intake of air and the shoulders kept lowered and open.

The turns of the head should increase to the limit and there should be an active, general pulling up and collectedness to the figure.

In the performance of a great number of turns, the body cannot sag. The dancer must resolutely and harmoniously seem to grow along the vertical axis but not with contorted facial muscles. The face must be free, ready to present the inner striving of the role being performed.

The conscientiousness and will of the pupil must at all times be constantly ready to remove the possible loss of balance. The slightest inattention in this respect leads to technical and artistic dissolution.

Stable and emotional endings of pirouettes, especially after numerous turns, reveal the mastery of great artists. The proper ending of a pirouette must be performed in one tempo, with the stopping of the turning energy immediate but soft, with no special gestures to the spectator, and with very stable actions of the arms, body, leg and head.

The stability of the ending depends on not only the accuracy of the performance of the pirouette, but also the commensurate force of the turning push. If the force is too strong, the ending may be unstable in technique and casual in character. Therefore, in preparing for the pirouette, one must foresee the duration of its development from the push to the final stop. Calculating the quantity, tempo and character of the pirouette includes keeping in mind the ending which will not be stable or persuasive if not determined before the start of the turn.

The turning push, actually the turn and pause, is one whole and is the basis on which the technique of pirouettes is kept and practiced.

When the described pirouettes are well learned with the given endings, the student may go on to different forms: at the end of a pirouette en dehors, the free leg may move from sur le cou-de-pied back into Fourth in pose croisée; stretching out the knee and lightly touching the floor with the toes; the supporting leg remains stretched at the knee; arms open into lowered Second, the body is straight but with a very slight lean to the right or left; the head repeats this leaning, turning to the advanced shoulder; arms and look are in the same direction.

This ending for a pirouette en dehors is traditional and obligatory in classwork as the image of the male performer, and it is performed with strictness. The ending may also be done in any of the smaller poses with an opening of the free leg to 45 degrees or 90 degrees with the toes to the floor with demi-plié or without. The supporting leg always remains elastic and turned out firmly on the whole foot, with the heel tightly resting on the floor. The arms, body and head assume their position with aplomb and in the same tempo.

If balance is lost, it may be reestablished in all these endings by a light, hardly noticeable gliding of the supporting foot into a more stable support.

Here are some complicated approaches to small pirouettes.

PIROUETTE FROM GRAND PLIÉ

This approach to a pirouette is done from a grand plié in First, Fourth or Fifth Position. It differs from the previously described because *the heels of both feet are raised* during the grand plié before the pirouette. It is a new method of applying the turning push.

The approach must be made without the heels touching the floor. The demi-pointe position, already fixed at the lowest point of the grand plié, must be raised at the same time the knee straightens on the supporting leg. The pirouette must start not from the lowest point of grand plié, but emerging halfway from it, otherwise the supporting leg will stretch out too late and the other leg will go into sur le cou-de-pied too soon, which gives the performance a grotesque appearance.

During the performance of the grand plié, the arm opposite to the direction of the turn is moved from Second into First as the other stays in First. At the moment of the turning push, the arms are rounded and join in a lowered First and stay in pirouette from demi-plié. These pirouettes usually end in a big pose with the leg opening through a développé to Second or Fourth.

The study must start in First, Fifth or Fourth, first en dehors, and, later, en dedans. Both are in exercises of adagio. The musical division is a measure of 6/8: 1 measure for grand plié; 3/8 for pirouette; 3/8 for the stop in big pose. Later, this pirouette may be done with two or more turns to a full measure of 6/8 or 4/4. All the rules of grand plié, pirouette and final poses are kept strictly, as well as the turnout, the flow, softness and aplomb of the movement.

PIROUETTE FROM PETIT TEMPS RELEVÉ

The petit temps relevé has already been described in the chapter on elementary movements of classical dance. Now it is used as an approach to small pirouettes beginning on one leg. Therefore it will be described here only as the tie to a small pirouette and the technique of its performance will continue to be as previously described.

In performing the petit temps relevé before a small pirouette, the starting demi-plié on the supporting leg must be prolonged until the total opening of the free leg to the side at 45 degrees. Then, without delay, it bends energetically at the knee and moves into sur le cou-de-pied. At this moment, the position is fixed in back; or if the movement is en dedans, then the position is fixed in front. The arms, together with the turning push, join in First. The body and head are straight *without* a lean away from the vertical axis, as may have been demanded by the pose. The face and look are fixed in the starting position of each pirouette.

The pirouette ends in a small pose in a very exact design. This pirouette with one turn is studied at the barre and on the floor, or joined with battement fondu to 45 degrees, with battement frappé, petit rond de jambe en l'air. Later, it may be done with two or more turns.

Still later, this pirouette may be strengthened by moving the open leg into the starting point from which the small pirouette starts: battement fondu forward to demi-pointe at 45 degrees; from there the open leg is moved in a rond de jambe into Second and, with a passing demi-plié on the supporting leg and no delay, a pirouette en dehors is executed. Or, the leg may open in the back and move into Second, from where a pirouette en dedans is executed. All this may be done in reverse, moving the leg from Second into Fourth and doing the pirouette from there. The movement of the leg before the pirouette goes along with the direction of the turn and allows an active taking of the turn. The descent from demi-pointe in demi-plié must be light and supple, permitting the leg to go no further than Second or Fourth. The arm, head and body perform as previously described. This form must be studied first at the barre, then studied in the center of the floor.

There is another form of small pirouette from a large pose which, as a rule, ends in a large pose. In that case, the turning push is done without a preceding demi-plié and rises to a high demi-pointe with an outstretched leg together with the bending of the knee of the open leg to the passé position, as in the performance of the small pirouette from a small pose. The arms, head and body act as previously described. This method is considerably more difficult and only a small number of pirouettes is possible because the force of the turning push is less than with the use of a demi-plié.

Here is an example of this approach to a small pirouette: from a large pose croisée forward, the open leg at 90 degrees performs an energetic bend with a turning sendoff of the entire body, rises to a high demi-pointe and does a small pirouette en dedans. The arms are rounded and a forceful lowered First is co-ordinated into the movement. The head and body, during the turn, are straight, and at the end of the pirouette, together with the arms and opening leg, assume the position of écarté.

This example does not exhaust the possibilities of performing small pirouettes from pose to pose by this method, which is especially useful in teaching adagios.

The study of this approach at the barre and on the floor must be done only with one turn. When two or more are performed, the thigh of the working leg closing at the knee must always be turned out and high. When it is well learned, it may be strengthened with a demi-plié which, in this case, must be a more active deepening at the moment of the turning push.

APPROACHES TO PIROUETTES

PIROUETTE FROM PAS TOMBÉ

The approach of pas tombé to a small pirouette is made by means of a fall into demi-plié on the open leg from a pose, into Second or Fourth—not standing on one leg as in previous approaches. At the moment of the fall, the free leg rises to 45 degrees and immediately, and together with the turning push on the supporting leg, moves into a heightened sur le cou-de-pied in front or in back. In this way, the pas tombé and pirouette are done uninterruptedly through a trampoline-like demi-plié. All the rest of the movement is as described previously for small pirouettes, including the stop.

The performance of the pas tombé along Second or Fourth must not be shortened. It requires an exact transfer of the center of gravity to the supporting leg. Losing the tempo or rushing the tempo at the moment of the tombé is counterproductive. The force of the body falling into the demi-plié must be used at the right time to give impetus to the turning push.

The arms perform in the same tempo as the legs, body and head in executing a stable and clear turn. The placement and transfer of gravity must be assured and technically exact.

The study of this approach begins in the center, first en face, with the leg opening along Second for the turning push, then along Fourth. When it has been well learned with one pirouette the study should increase to two pirouettes en dehors and two en dedans. The ending may be in Fifth in demi-plié or in a small or a large pose.

Then the pas tombé may begin with a small pose with the leg at 45 degrees with suitably arranged arms, body and head. From this pose several turns may be made en dehors. The exercise may then be performed en dedans, ending after the pirouette in a pose at 45 degrees or 90 degrees. All the rules must be strictly observed for the given poses.

PIROUETTE FROM PAS DÉGAGÉ

The pirouette from pas dégagé is done in the form of a step along Second or Fourth, ending by rising on high demi-pointe and turning on that demi-pointe in either direction.

The movement begins from demi-plié on the supporting leg as the other assumes a front or back sur le cou-de-pied. The supporting leg makes a turning push with a transfer of the body onto the opening leg from sur le cou-de-pied to a height under 45 degrees. The freed leg under 45 degrees moves immediately to a heightened sur le cou-de-pied front or back. The arms, head and body assume the procedure for a small pirouette ending in Fifth in a large or small pose. The movements end with the transfer into demi-plié onto the free leg while the supporting leg moves into sur le cou-de-pied, a position for the repeat of the pirouette.

All this must be performed with suppleness but not in too wide a span. The step should be active and calculated so that the center of gravity moves with stability from one foot to the other. Otherwise, the turn will not be possible.

This pirouette is studied at first en dedans with a rise to demi-pointe along Fourth forward, then to the side along Second and, finally, along Fourth backward, ending in Fifth Position.

Then, in the same progression, the study is the same for the exercise, with an en dehors direction for the turn.

When the approach with one pirouette has been mastered, it may be studied with two or more turns ending in Fifth, as described, or in poses. In stage practice, this form is used usually in the en dedans direction because it is easier and more comfortable. But the en dehors form is used as well. In class, however, both directions should be studied equally, as they develop technique and stability in the ability to turn in general.

PIROUETTE FROM PAS COUPÉ

The pirouette from pas coupé is begun with a demi-plié on the supporting leg with the other leg open to 45 degrees. From this position, the stretched-out leg moves energetically forward to Fifth and rises flexibly to a high demi-pointe as if replacing the supporting foot. At that same moment, the supporting leg pushes off en dehors and transfers into a heightened sur le cou-de-pied back.

If the pirouette is en dedans, the open leg goes into Fifth back and the other goes into sur le cou-de-pied front.

The arms at the turning push go from Second into a lowered First. The body and head perform as described for the small pirouette. The ending may be in Fifth, in a large or small pose or a demi-plié on the free leg with a simultaneous throw of the supporting leg to the side at 45 degrees, from where the approach may be repeated.

All components of the movement must flow, be supple and with an exact estimate of the turning push in the en dehors or en dedans direction, including the number of turns and the ending of the movement.

The study of the approach from pas coupé begins at the barre and on the floor with one turn in either direction, ending in Fifth. Then two turns are incorporated and endings in small or large poses.

PIROUETTE FOUETTÉ AT 45 DEGREES

The pirouette with fouetté at 45 degrees is a small turn consisting of uninterrupted repetitions of one or two turns from a passing demi-plié of the supporting leg and a throw of the free leg to the side at 45 degrees.

This pirouette, like the others, is done on a high demi-pointe on the same supporting leg and in one direction. The opening and closing of the free leg is in the form of the petit rond de jambe en l'air through the passing demi-plié. In the starting moment of the turn, the free leg is moved to a raised sur le cou-de-pied in back and, if the pirouette is en dehors, the leg moves quickly around the calf of the standing leg to sur le cou-de-pied front. After the leg opens again to 45 degrees with the supporting leg in demi-plié, the movement is ready to be repeated.

If the movement is done en dedans, the pattern of the free leg is reversed. This helps the turning, as it coincides with its direction and gives it a clear and rounded design.

These pirouettes are usually performed by female dancers on pointe in a series of sixteen to thirty-two separate turns. The name fouetté at 45 degrees is correct because the opening of the leg to 45 degrees at every turn appears to be a rond de jambe but is *an opening to Second*. The student should perform this movement only on demi-pointe and in smaller numbers in succession. (This fouetté is more popularly known as the fouetté rond de jambe en tournant, which opens in demi-plié at hip level in croisé devant before whipping to the Second and closing at the knee in front of the supporting leg on pointe for the turn. It is the Cecchetti form. The Russian form opens to the side as described, at 45 or 90 degrees in demi-plié, then closes at the knee in front of the supporting leg on pointe for the turn. Both versions are performed by females.)

The first pirouette starts in Fifth or Fourth Position. The subsequent turns follow the rules for small pirouettes. The execution of the demi-plié and the joining of the petit rond de jambe en l'air movement must flow and be a supple yet firm lowering of the heel to the floor without moving from one place. The petit rond de jambe en l'air must be clear, pliable, and maintained at the thigh to the level of 45 degrees throughout.

It is very important to estimate the force needed for the turning push in order not to have it too big or too weak for one or two turns and in order to end each time exactly en face. It is also important during the demi-plié to correct the balance for the transfer to high demi-pointe with an elastic push from the floor into a collected and pulled-up body in a vertical position.

The arms at each opening of the leg are thrown energetically from a lowered First into Second and, at each turning push, just as energetically join into the same position. The body and head act clearly, retaining the vertical position of the entire body. On the whole, the fouetté at 45 degrees must be done with a dash and in one rhythm, but not too fast or in a mechanical manner. The student must strive for the end of each turn and the transfer into demi-plié to be the next turning push and sendoff.

These fouettés in the male classes are done many times, not as a separate exercise, but as part of a combination with a battement fondu, for instance.

At first, the fouetté at 45 degrees is studied en dehors with one turn and repeated no more than two or four times in succession. Then it is studied with two turns in the same number and, finally, gradually increases in difficulty in combined teaching examples. It must be noted that small pirouettes from pas dégagé or pas coupé in the male classes are not practiced in a series along a diagonal or in a circle, but only in combinations. They are performed two or three in a series. The same is true of the small pirouettes studied in the female classes from Fifth into Fifth which are practiced as sixteen in a series.

These small pirouettes, previously described, acquire a special technical and expressive importance when performed on pointe by female dancers and are therefore widely used in the profession. Male dancers have their own difficult, virtuoso turning movements for stage work. They are: a transfer from small pirouettes into turns in the air; grand pirouettes along Second in a series of sixteen to thirty-two; double saut de basque with pas tombé performed along a diagonal line; revoltade, etc. The small pirouettes from pas dégagé, pas coupé and turns from Fifth to Fifth are not part of the following explanation.

The factors for consideration in the performance of these turns are: a turning push of the proper size; a firmly placed supporting heel on the floor; a good spring from the demi-plié; a correct sendoff with the center of gravity on the supporting pointe; clear action of the arms; exact action of the free leg; precise action of the head and body; stable performance of each successive pirouette, especially the final or closing pirouette.

Important, too, is to observe that the force of the turn does not weaken at the end of each pirouette, but that each new pirouette is given fresh impetus and energy.

Finally, at the repetition of each pirouette, the transfer to the supporting leg must be short and resolute with a clear accent on the first quarter of the 2/4 musical measure.

The exercise must begin in a slow tempo with a gradual increase, including pirouettes, into more complicated combinations. Then the study with double turns, or two turns in a series using each approach, may begin. Or the turns may be joined in a short series.

The following descriptions of small pirouettes in various forms with various approaches require their own special technique and are widely used in teaching and in stage work.

PIROUETTE EN TIRE-BOUCHON

The peculiarity of this pirouette is that during the turn the working leg does not assume the usual sur le cou-de-pied position but moves to the knee. (See illustration #149.)

This method fortifies the pirouette's momentum, strengthens and elevates the entire figure of the performer and adds variety to the step's form.

This pirouette may be performed en dehors and en dedans, with the working leg at the knee in front or back of the knee of the supporting leg. It is performed according to the rules or to the directions given by the choreographer.

The transfer of the leg to the knee position (or passé position), regardless of how the pirouette was begun, must be sufficiently clear and energetic. It must be calculated without too strong a sendoff for the spin so as not to permit the student to fall from the supporting leg. The knee position must be kept elastic

149   Pirouette en tire-bouchon in the knee position

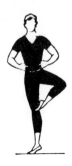

and stable, with a strongly pulled-up thigh and well-stretched foot of the sup-porting leg, so that the toes of the working leg at the level of the knee of the supporting leg are fixed. The position is high on demi-pointe.

If the pirouette en tire-bouchon ends in Fifth, the working leg must be lowered slowly, exactly along the calf of the supporting leg, as if doing a spiral or, more exactly, like a corkscrew (after which the step is named). The turnout must be preserved and all the rules for the finish in demi-plié.

When the pirouette en tire-bouchon ends in a big pose, the leg at the knee opens with flexibility to 90 degrees in a given direction following the rules of battement développé. On the whole, this pirouette must be done with sufficient dynamics and in strict cooperation with the classic, not the "grotesque" style. The study of tire-bouchon must begin with one turn and from the Fifth Position into the Fifth Position, and then from Fifth Position into Fourth Position and finally from complex approaches and with various endings.

All the rules of execution for small pirouettes must be undeviatingly preserved, especially the harmony of the figure in pulling up with clarity and stability in the spin itself.

If the small pirouettes are well learned, this pirouette will present no special difficulties.

HALF PIROUETTES

HALF PIROUETTE FROM PAS COUPÉ

The half pirouette may be done from several approaches as a single half turn or it may be repeated several times. The technique in performing these half pirouettes is more complicated and unique, thus demanding no less practice than a small pirouette.

When the study of the small pirouette in the center has been mastered along

Second, Fourth and Fifth, the study of the half pirouette may begin at the barre, en dehors and en dedans with a transfer to the supporting leg through pas coupé. These half pirouettes may be on a low or high demi-pointe with the preceding opening of the free leg in Second with toes on the floor in a tendu position. From there, the leg quickly closes into Fifth in front and, without delay, performs a half pirouette en dehors on a low demi-pointe. The free leg moves through sur le cou-de-pied in front and opens to the side, toes on the floor.

The free arm opens to Second before starting the movement. The other is resting on the barre. At the closing of the leg into Fifth, the free arm moves along a horizontal line toward the barre and descends upon it. The other arm at the same time opens through First into Second. The body is straight and is transferred exactly onto the supporting leg. The head at the start and end of the movement is turned toward the open arm. When this half pirouette is made en dedans, the leg that is moved from tendu closes into Fifth back of the supporting leg. The supporting leg transfers to a sur le cou-de-pied position back and opens to the side, toes on the floor. The free arm moves directly to the barre and the other remains in Second.

In high demi-pointe, the turn is done in the same way but the preceding and final opening of the leg are at 45 degrees. Pirouettes on a low demi-pointe should be combined with battements tendus and on a high demi-pointe, with all the exercises in which the openings are to the side at 45 degrees.

HALF PIROUETTE FROM PAS TOMBÉ

This half pirouette is done from a sur le cou-de-pied or from a leg open to the side at 45 degrees. From these positions on demi-pointe, the free leg lowers forward into Fifth in demi-plié (tombé) as the other rises into sur le cou-de-pied back. Then, without delay, the supporting leg does a relevé onto high demi-pointe with a half pirouette en dehors. The free leg moves into sur le cou-de-pied in front. The open arm at the start of the movement and at its end is kept in Second. The other is kept on the barre. During the tombé, the open arm goes into a lowered First, and at the pirouette rises and descends onto the barre. The other, at the same time, opens through First and into Second. The body is totally straight and exactly over the supporting leg. The head at the start and end of the movement turns toward the open arm.

If this half turn is done en dedans, the open leg moves in Fifth in back as the tombé, and the other rises to sur le cou-de-pied in back. Everything else is unchanged.

These half pirouettes may join with petit battement sur le cou-de-pied or with exercises in which the free leg opens to 45 degrees. The half pirouette is practiced from pas coupé and pas tombé and worked into the barre with the object of integrating them into more complicated combinations.

They also enter arbitrarily into certain complex forms of uninterrupted turning such as the pas emboîté or tours chaînés. These movements do not rightly belong to a chapter on en tournant movements. But because of the character, tempo and multiple performance of these turns, they clearly belong, despite their peculiarities, in a chapter on turns.

PAS EMBOÎTÉ

The pas emboîté is done with minimal advancement and no demi-plié. It starts in Fifth Position en face. The approach is a pas dégagé with an advance to the side beginning with a demi-plié on the back leg. The other leg goes into sur le cou-de-pied in front and opens to 45 degrees. Then, with a broad rise on high demi-pointe and a half pirouette, the leg moves from that pose to demi-pointe as the other moves to the sur le cou-de-pied front. The half turn en dedans ends with the student's back to the mirror or #1 of the room. Then, without delay, another pas emboîté, rising onto high demi-pointe with a minimal advance to the side, follows. The free leg goes into sur le cou-de-pied position not from a demi-plié, but from a high demi-pointe. The half pirouette is now en dehors, ending facing the mirror. Then a series of pas emboîtés en dedans with minimal advance and en dehors with half pirouettes follows.

This movement must be repeated no less than four to eight times in a series on a straight line from #7 to #3 or along a diagonal. If it is performed in reverse, then the first pirouette is en dehors and en dedans with the sur le cou-de-pied always in back.

It must be noted that when the pas emboîté is done in a quick tempo, a small degree of advance to the side in the direction of Second harmonizes more with a regular rather than a conditional (higher) sur le cou-de-pied position.

At the first demi-plié, the arm corresponding to the direction of the turn is in First. The other is in Second. During the opening of the leg to 45 degrees and the first rise on high demi-pointe, the arm from First moves into Second, and the other from Second moves into First. At the second rise and emboîté, the arms move into the same positions. In this way, the arms move first along with the pirouette, then in the opposite direction. The body, before each half pirouette and after it, passes en face in relation to the mirror. If the emboîté is done on a diagonal, the body is in épaulement. The head, before the first half pirouette, turns in the direction of the advance. During the first half pirouette it keeps the position and at the second half pirouette, turns somewhat faster than the body in the same direction.

When the movement is done in reverse, the arms and body act in the same way. The head, before the first half pirouette, is turned in the direction of the forthcoming advancement, and at the first half pirouette, it turns faster than the body in the same direction. At the second half pirouette, it retains this pose, etc.

The study of this movement should be in a sequence of four times to the right, four times to the left. The measure is 2/4; first pas dégagé before the measure; 1/4 for each half pirouette; 1/4 for the stop on demi-pointe. After the fourth half pirouette 1/4 is used to close the free leg in Fifth in demi-plié; 1/4 to transfer the supporting leg into sur le cou-de-pied in order to begin the movement once again to the other side. Then the half pirouette may be studied in reverse.

Then the number of half pirouettes should increase to six with no stops on pointe for 2/4 counts.

Finally, the study of emboîté to 1/8 of a measure introduces into the exercise a small jump. The arms move more energetically into a lowered First and remain until the last pirouette when they again resume the starting or any other given position. (This form of pas emboîté belongs to both the Soviet and the Cecchetti schools. The French School calls it petit jeté, preferring to reserve the term emboîté for the sur les pointes or demi-pointe version.)

These pas emboîtés require a clear and light rising onto high demi-pointe and a free and exact transfer sur le cou-de-pied, a shortened but not constrained transfer from one leg to the other, a harmonious coordination of the body, arms and head with a sufficient turning sendoff. There should be a rhythmic accent on each half pirouette.

PAS JETÉ WITH ADVANCEMENT

This movement is in the form of a petit pas jeté with a small jump, but is done without the jump, but with a small advancement. It begins from demi-plié on the supporting leg with the other in sur le cou-de-pied front. From that position it opens to the side to Second at 45 degrees. Then without delay, and together with a turning sendoff, advance and rise onto high demi-pointe through pas dégagé. The free leg goes into sur le cou-de-pied in back. From there, a half pirouette en dedans, ending in demi-plié on the supporting leg, completes the movement. Then the same movement is done, ending with a half pirouette en dehors. The freed leg is led into sur le cou-de-pied in front, etc.

This form of jeté is done no less than four times, starting with the leg in front in Fifth, with sur le cou-de-pied or an open leg to 45 degrees.

The peculiarity of this movement is that the first rise onto a high demi-pointe is en dedans and the second, en dehors, but the turning goes on all the time, in the same floor direction. It is explained by the fact that the half pirouettes change supporting legs in relation to the direction of the spinning.

Before the half pirouette, the arm corresponding to the direction of the advance is in First and the other in Second. During the opening of the leg to the side, the arm moves from First into Second. At the moment of the transfer of the open leg, the arm corresponding to the direction of the half turn moves into First from Second. At the second demi-plié from the back, everything is done the same way. The body on each demi-plié is kept front. If the pas jeté is done on a diagonal, the position is in épaulement. The head at the start of the movement is turned in the direction of the advance; at the first half pirouette en dedans, it stays in that position; at the first half pirouette en dehors, it returns a little faster than the body to the starting position. The movement may be reversed—starting the first half pirouette en dehors, with the opening of the leg from the back of Fifth Position or in a sur le cou-de-pied.

The study must be done four times to the right and four times to the left. The measure is 2/4; opening the leg before the measure; 1/4 for the half pirouette en dedans; 1/4 for the demi-plié and movement to sur le cou-de-pied, etc. Each fourth half pirouette ends in a transfer of the free leg into Fifth in back in demi-plié. Then the movement is ready to be performed on the other side.

Each part of the movement must be well learned and practiced. Each half pirouette and each opening to 45 degrees is a broad and resolute advance to the side into Second. There should be a harmonious turning push and the rise onto a high demi-pointe, a supple move. A supple lowering onto the heel of the demi-plié will provide a good support. The sur le cou-de-pied must be in an exact—elevated or conditional—position (higher than at the ankle) and the body must be straight and pulled up. The movement of the head must be clear as well as the movements of the arms. The turnout must be maintained, the shoulders lowered and the transfer of all the positions given a dashing finish.

Next, the study of these half pirouettes may be studied at 1/4 each to a 2/4 measure, and be included in combinations.

TOURS CHAÎNÉS (CHAINED)

Tours chaînés is a movement that dashes along in a chain of uninterrupted turns along a straight line, a diagonal or in a circle.

They are executed on a high demi-pointe with a pulled-up body and legs joined along First Position, in a half-turned-out position. Each turn in the tours chaînés is divided into two equal half pirouettes which are not evident to the observer because they are very fast and flow into a seamless whole.

The transfer from half pirouette into another half pirouette is done with a minimal advance measured only by the separation of the toes and *without separating the legs to the side in Second or Fourth Position.*

Some dancers in performing tours chaînés do not retain the First Position but place the foot where it is most comfortable for them. But for the attainment of the most virtuoso tempo, for an exact design, compactness, flow and stability, it is necessary not to perform this movement in a haphazard way, but to instill a definite method for the movement of the legs and to begin from there the study of tours chaînés.

These turns cannot be performed on a low demi-pointe, on half-bent knees, joined toes and separated heels. The legs in this movement must be exact and only in case of a mishap may the leg be separated to regain the stability of the body or the rhythm of the turning. And that should only be for a moment in one or two half pirouettes.

The turns start from a sendoff begun by a pas dégagé or a pas tombé along Fourth to the front.

In a start from pas dégagé, the tours begin on a high demi-pointe and begin en dedans, then en dehors, etc. In the start from pas tombé, the turns begin from the half pirouette in en dehors in this way: At the moment the supporting leg stretches out from demi-plié, it is placed in First on demi-pointe simultaneously with the turn of the body, making the first half pirouette en dehors. The stretching out itself must be done not immediately or sharply, but with a tasteful transfer onto high demi-pointe.

The turns may start as a rule in a fast tempo, increasing near the end, and are unexpectedly interrupted by a clear and stable stop in a small pose. The turning sendoff is taken energetically and resolutely, but with calculation, so as not to fall off the line of proper advance, and in order not to break the chain of half pirouettes. The amount of turning energy must be used economically to keep the evenness of the turns to 180 degrees and at an even distance between the feet with the legs in First. This adds to the greater flow and stability of the turns.

Of course, the increase in tempo must be compensated with a shortening of the distance between the toes, which will minimize the advance, but it will help to maintain the speed and stabilize the exit into the final pose. The exit must be very clear, without any falling from high demi-pointe, but should be, at the last two half pirouettes, a lowering from that position.

The final pose may be done into Fifth Position in back with a transfer of the free leg through the sur le cou-de-pied front. Or, the final pose may begin with a pas dégagé forward into a small pose in effacé derrière with a firm and turned-out leg put on the floor.

The arms at the start of the turning sendoff, together with the leg opening forward into Fourth, make a rush to the first arabesque position. They immediately round and join in a lowered First, remaining there until the last half pirouette, when they open into the given pose.

At each half pirouette en dedans, the arms, rounded and joined in First, help the turn by a barely noticeable impulse in the given direction. When the turns speed up at the end, the arms close in toward each other until the last pose. The arm corresponding to the direction of the turns is above the other when the tempo increases. At the last half pirouette, the arm in tempo opens into the given pose.

The body, during the first movement of the leg forward into pas dégagé or pas tombé, leans toward the movement. It then straightens out and stays erect until the end. It must not lag behind, nor lean too much in the direction of the advance, as this also would break the tempo and stability of the turns, forcing the legs away from an exact half-turned-out First, making them search for a more viable point of support. In the final pose, the body must act resolutely and with aplomb.

During the approach, the head turns in the direction of the forthcoming advance. The eyes look straight ahead in the same direction. At the first half pirouette, the head lags, but at the second half pirouette it turns swiftly and faster than the body into the starting position. At the end of the turns, the head takes the position suited to the given pose and lightly underscores the finale of the turning.

The ending may be into a first or second arabesque, a pose with the arms open in a lowered Second or Third, or one arm in First and the other in Second or Third. The body and head take the suitable position.

As an exception to the rule, turns may end in one of the big poses in demi-plié or on one knee, but they must always be done lightly with a resolve at the sendoff, a brilliantly technical but not showy effect.

Tours chaînés, like small pirouettes, are a very active stage expression. They tell much, bare much. Of course, there is a corresponding change in tempo, rhythm, character of the tours for this purpose. In other words, the exercise is turned into a dance gesture while keeping the basic rules of technique.

This is a fact the teacher must keep in mind after the method has been well learned. In incorporating these tours into combinations, the tempo, rhythm and character must change to develop virtuosity in turning and adaptability, so necessary on stage.

The study of these tours may start after small pirouettes on half pointe have been mastered, especially the emboîté which connects to the study of turns with a demi-plié.

The study must also be practiced in a slower tempo with the tours separated into parts. Start in Fifth Position, épaulement croisé; pas dégagé forward with a turn of 1/4 circle en dehors and four full turns along a diagonal. This equals eight half pirouettes, the last of which is done with a transfer of the free leg sur le cou-de-pied in front and fixed, and a lowering of it to the back in Fifth in demi-plié. This step is necessary because it teaches the student to end the tours without excessive force and exercises the stability of the transfer into Fifth or a final pose. In this exercise, every turn must start from a very small leading of the leg forward into Fourth in the direction of the advance. This is a temporary measure, but it allows a slower tempo for the feeling of rhythmic wholeness to develop in each turn. There is a detailed practice of the leg movements with this slower tempo.

Later, the study at a faster tempo, without mixing the movements and all the turns, flows with the legs joined in a half-turned-out position.

In teaching, turns from Third and Fifth give positive results, but I prefer to begin this virtuoso movement from the First Position, which is its basis.

The arms begin in Preparatory Position. During the demi-plié and transfer of the front leg into sur le cou-de-pied, the arm corresponding to the direction of the turn rises into First as the other rises into Second. At the pas dégagé, the arms are in the first arabesque position. Further on, at each full turn, they join in First in a rounded and lowered position. At the final demi-plié, they descend rounded and smoothly into Preparatory Position. At each arabesque, the arm pointing to First seems to indicate the direction of the advance as the other takes a turning sendoff. The arms join with no delay as a passing moment. The body, during the pas dégagé, leans toward the gliding leg, then is kept straight and pulled up. At the moment of the small leading of the leg and before each turn, the body gives a little in the same direction but with more constraint than at the beginning.

The head at pas dégagé is turned with the face toward the advance. During the turns, it delays somewhat, then, faster than the body, returns to the starting position as in small pirouettes. At the final demi-plié, the head turns toward the advanced shoulder, fixing the épaulement position.

The entire movement must be done without haste, clearly performing each half pirouette. The measure is 2/4 with pas dégagé before the measure; each half pirouette to 1/4 (8 in all); two measures to fix the sur le cou-de-pied after the fourth turn; 2/4 for the final demi-plié in Fifth; 1/4 for the transfer of the leg in front sur le cou-de-pied; 1/4 for the leg to open forward through pas dégagé and the whole movement is then ready to repeat from the other leg.

Then the tempo and number of chaînés may be somewhat increased by adding two more turns, ending in Fifth back with a passing, not a fixed, sur le cou-de-pied. Then the tempo may be increased for still more turns with the arms joined in a lowered First and the leg not separated before each turn. The ending is in Fifth, as in the other exercises. In this case the tempo must be slowed for each turn at 1/4. When all this has been mastered, the number of turns may be increased to eight, ending the last on pas dégagé through a passing demi-plié and into a small pose of first or second arabesque (par terre).

This exercise is done separately to each side, dividing the class into groups. When the first group of pupils ends the chaînés in a final pose of four measures, the other group begins.

Finally, the tours chaînés are introduced into adagio combinations and jumps with a diagonal of twelve to sixteen turns at a virtuoso tempo. The study may also include tours chaînés in a circle of thirty-two turns.

Tour chaîné from pas tombé must be done in the form of a turning push taken with more strength than the usual pas dégagé. The pas tombé is done from Fifth through a battement tendu jeté on demi-pointe; from sur le cou-de-pied; and even by means of a small sissonne tombée or a small jump.

The arms here do not take the first arabesque form, but remain in the same position at the start and very energetically move into a lowered First. The head and body follow the same pattern, but the tempo of the turns is increased to 1/8 for each turn.

In a circle, the tours must be studied in a medium tempo to be well learned and to maintain the proper outline of the circle. At the exit into the diagonal, the arms follow the usual pattern, and the body and head keep the former position, with the eyes toward the line of progress.

To master the technique of tours chaînés, it is useful to begin the movement at once after a small pirouette en dehors through a quickly passing small pas tombé. The finish may be aerial combined with jeté en tournant, saut de basque, etc.

Whatever the form, the design or combination in practicing tours chaînés must be worked out not only in its technique, but also in its musical and rhythmic requirements, in its clarity of performance, its constant flow and emotional interest. Otherwise, this virtuoso movement is cold and superficial.

GRANDES PIROUETTES

The grandes pirouettes are done in a big pose at 90 degrees, from various approaches on a high demi-pointe en dehors and en dedans. They are different from small pirouettes in tempo, which are slower, and in number, which are fewer. This does not require a simpler technique, but they have their own inherent difficulties, especially in maintaining a pliable line and musical rhythm.

The grande pirouette usually finishes in a pose fixed during the turn, but this pose may be altered at the end of each pirouette by means of an allongé, a grand rond de jambe en l'air, or a fouetté at 90 degrees.

In addition, the grande pirouette may be uninterruptedly repeated in any pose or changed into small pirouettes.

All approaches must be sure and clear without a shifting of the shoulders to the side opposite the forthcoming turn. The turning push itself is done with an exact sendoff of the center of gravity to the supporting leg with energetic and commensurate strength. The movement of the free leg, body, arms and head coordinate in a single tempo but not with too much sharpness or with drawn-out discord. The entire body lightly and harmoniously dashes into the performing pose with no extra effort or strain. The turning must be done in a brief and faultless form, but with feeling, a sense of dynamics, and not abstractly. During the turning, no change in the design of the pose is permitted in the lowering of the high demi-pointe, in the bending of the knee, in a flabby fixing of the open leg at the thigh, the body or the arms.

In performing the grande pirouette, the vertical axis must be kept throughout the body with an equal distribution of the body weight and the body itself must be pulled up and collected.

If the balance is broken, it can be restored as in the small pirouette, with a very slight displacement on high demi-pointe of the supporting leg, to find the correct point. But the balance must not be obvious in the body or arm movements.

The ending of the grande pirouette must be supple but firm with a heel on the floor in exact alignment in the pose along a diagonal or straight line. The foot, ankle, knee and thigh of the supporting leg must stop the entire body into a pulled-up and collected pose without a harsh movement. The ending of the turning must be a dancing gesture which continues the turning in its dashing manner or furthers the stage action or the teaching exercise.

Before beginning the study of grande pirouette, one must be well prepared with the ability to sustain a pose in high demi-pointe with correctness and stability, to stop in a big pose after performing small pirouettes, to perform slow turns in a big pose—tour lent, to do battements divisé en quarts and complicated transfers from one leg to another through various methods, to sustain big poses in jumps, and to perform preparatory movements and the elements that build big poses.

In addition, one must have endurance, strength, good concentration and musicality.

In short, the elements of grande pirouette must be well prepared in advance. True freedom in the performance of these pirouettes may be developed only in this way in order to bring the dancer priceless artistic help and to have the means of acting expressively.

The grande pirouette is described in the design of the pose and during the turning and along its approaches.

First, the approaches are given as performed from one onto two legs; then from one leg to the other; third, supported on one leg.

The basic rules of performance are described in the pirouette à la seconde. Further along, these will only be mentioned or omitted with an indication that they have been previously described.

---

150   Grande pirouette à la Seconde from Second Position

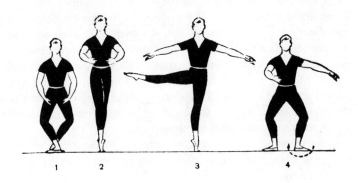

PIROUETTE À LA SECONDE

The starting position for this pirouette is en face, with the legs in Fifth Position. The first movement is a demi-plié and a relevé to a high demi-pointe in Fifth Position. The forward leg is then thrown into Second to 90 degrees in a grand battement jeté. From this position, a demi-plié on both legs in Second follows, and a turning push with a pirouette en dehors on high demi-pointe in the pose à la seconde at 90 degrees. With this position, the leg is fixed. It is the same leg which opened from Fifth Position front.

The grande pirouette ends by lowering the supporting leg from the high demi-pointe onto the entire foot and with the fixing of a pose. The arms at the relevé onto demi-pointe in Fifth move from Preparatory to First. As the leg is thrown to 90 degrees, it opens into Second; at demi-plié in Second, the arm corresponding to the direction of the turn moves into First as the other stays in Second. At the turning push, the arm from First is sent into Second; at the pirouette, both arms take a Second or Third Position. The head turns as in small pirouettes. (See illustration #150.)

When this pirouette is done en dedans, the leg in back in the Fifth Position is thrown to the side to 90 degrees, and the rest of the movement is as the above description except for the direction of the turn.

In doing the approach to this pirouette, all elementary rules must be kept in the relevé onto demi-pointe and demi-plié.

The leg, thrown into Second, must be done lightly and no higher than 90 degrees. This movement must be very clearly fixed, since it is the position which must be maintained throughout the turn. When it descends into the Second Position on the floor, the knees must be stretched and the toes flexible but stretched. The supporting leg at this moment moves with suppleness from high demi-pointe

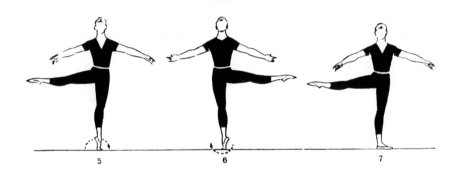

onto the entire foot and, with no delay, accompanies the other leg in a somewhat deepened demi-plié with a slightly widened Second.

Keeping these rules permits greater stability and a more forceful transfer of the body into the turning pose. At the turning push, the supporting leg energetically and *without a displacement of the heel*, goes into a high and elastic demi-pointe. The knee and thigh remain in a fixed position. The free leg, during the turning push, is sent no less energetically, but as it was in the transfer, it is no higher than 90 degrees. The free leg must not be thrown too forcefully or too high, as this would disrupt the balance. During the turning, the free as well as the supporting leg must keep the force, remain pulled up and stable throughout from preparation to ending, but not forced beyond reasonable stress or strain.

At the end of the pirouette, falling off the demi-pointe is inadmissible. The foot, and especially the heel, must be put down on the floor with firmness and flexibility. The knee must be pulled up and the thigh of the supporting leg must clearly and actively stop whatever turning momentum is left in the body. It is totally inadmissible for the supporting leg to weaken or the open leg to weaken. At the end of the pirouette, it must be firmly and strongly kept in Second Position with a well-pulled-up knee, instep and toes and turned out fully.

At the end of the pirouette, it is useful to check once more the harmoniousness and collected condition of the body by rising again onto high demi-pointe. End in this fixed pose smoothly and lower the free leg into Fifth, a passé or a given pose.

The ending may be in a deeper demi-plié that is flexible yet firmly fixed with pressure on the entire foot.

The arms in the approach must act clearly and surely, taking an active part in the turning sendoff. Together with the start of the pirouette, the arm in First is thrown energetically into Second; the other stays in place. On the whole, both arms are at the same time sent in the direction of the turn, keeping in Second freely and clearly.

If an arm is given the Third Position for the turn, both at the same time rise just as actively as in the other patterns. During the turn, they must be kept stable with neither too much strain, nor too much weakening. Successful turning in these grandes pirouettes demands the ability to manage the arms resolutely and freely.

At the end, the arms as well as the open and the supporting leg must be kept firm and exact.

If the arms are to be in Third during the pirouette, it is well to move the arms into Third from Second, or the other way around, during the additional rise of relevé to demi-pointe.

The body, during the approach, and at the end, must be collected, pulled up with open and freely lowered shoulders. In fighting the difficulties of the performance, the student may at times bend, lean back, strain and raise the shoulders, bend at the waist or loosen the diaphragm. These inaccuracies break the harmony of the figure and of the pose, as well as disrupt the technique.

Especially important is the correct placing of the center of gravity on the supporting leg and keeping it there to the end on high demi-pointe. The supporting leg and the body must all balance on a straight axis for the turning. If the center of gravity veers away from the axis, the balance of the body is disrupted and the turning becomes unstable. Therefore, the approach to the pirouette and the turning push must be done with an exact movement of the body onto the supporting leg. To keep the body firmly on the supporting leg, the side corresponding to the open leg must be "caught." (The hips must be kept equal and in one line, which means that the weight displaced by the open leg must be replaced in the hip by holding the working side level, firm and throughout the entire movement.) This helps the pupil to place the body onto the supporting leg and to keep it there until the end of the pirouette.

The head must be kept straight throughout the movement with no extra strain of the muscles of the neck or face. The eyes look forward quietly and surely.

During the turning, the head is kept on one vertical axis with the trunk and supporting leg.

On the whole, this pirouette must be done in an energetic tempo, especially for two to three turns, so that the dynamic of the turning is clear and persuasive but does not carry away the body at the stop, or disrupt its harmony, stability or suppleness.

The ability to calculate the force of the turning push for a specific number of pirouettes and for an exact and free stop must become the pupil's practiced habit.

The study of the à la seconde form, like the study of any other grande pirouette, must start at first from a preparatory exercise minus the turning and in a slow tempo: to a measure of 4/4; demi-plié in Fifth before the measure; 1/4 is used for a relevé onto demi-pointe in the same position; 1/4 to throw the leg 90 degrees to the side; 1/4 to fix this position; 1/4 for a demi-plié in Second; 1/4 for relevé on demi-pointe à la seconde—the moment of the turn in later practice; 2/4 to fix the pose on high demi-pointe; 1/4 to lower open leg into Fifth. The exercise is repeated to the other side.

The head, arms and body act as for the approach to the pirouette en dehors.

When this is mastered, the pirouette itself may be done en dehors or en dedans direction, with a stop on demi-pointe or a change into demi-plié.

An approach to the pirouette in a faster tempo is then studied. It is also done from demi-plié in Fifth, but the leg is thrown to 90 degrees by a gliding movement along the floor at the same time, with the straightening of the supporting leg from the demi-plié in Fifth Position. In this version, the throw of the leg is done before the measure followed by the turning push to 1/4 from Second and the pirouette itself.

This is followed by the study of two pirouettes, first with a stop on the whole foot, then on demi-pointe and on demi-plié.

Finally, there is the study of the stopping of the pirouette with a change of pose through a rond de jambe en l'air done at the moment of the descent from demi-pointe and in the same direction as the turn. If the pirouette was done en dehors, then the open leg is moved from à la seconde into third or fourth arabesque or attitude croisée derrière. If the turning was en dedans, the open leg goes into croisé forward. The change is finished on a stretched supporting leg or in demi-plié.

This change of poses is done in a flow, in the tempo of the turning or as a continuation of the pirouette which ends with an additional turn of the body into épaulement. All the rules for the grand rond de jambe en l'air apply exactly.

Later, the change of pose by means of a fouetté at 90 degrees is done as the supporting leg moves from demi-pointe onto the whole foot. The turn in fouetté is done in the direction of the turning. If the pirouette is en dehors, then the fouetté is done from à la seconde into effacé forward. If it is done en dedans, the fouetté is done into first or second arabesque or attitude effacée derrière. It ends on an outstretched leg or in demi-plié. The changing of poses must be done seamlessly and with a flow in the same tempo as the pirouette and as the continuation or addition to its end.

When the ending of grande pirouette is mastered, the study of a transfer into small pirouettes may begin.

When ending the grande pirouette en dehors or en dedans, the leg at 90 degrees must be lowered quickly and clearly to 45 degrees en face together with a short and flexible demi-plié of the supporting leg. In this way the turning push is prolonged in the same direction as the turn. Then, simultaneously and energetically with a relevé on high demi-pointe of the supporting leg, the open leg moves from 45 degrees to sur le cou-de-pied. The arms round and join from Second into lowered First. Then the movement is done as a small pirouette and may end in Fifth or Fourth, in a large or small pose.

In the performance of this movement the body must be collected and vertical. The coordination of the force for the turning sendoff and the number of turns, their character and tempo must be predetermined and calculated. In all the transfers there must be a melding of the changes, a clear and purposeful sendoff by the body into small pirouette. The study must be slowly practiced at first, with just one pirouette, then with two or three, etc.

PIROUETTE FROM FOURTH POSITION

In the pirouette from Fourth, the starting position in Fifth with épaulement croisé, the demi-plié and relevé to high demi-pointe turns to effacé at the same time the leg in front transfers to a sur le cou-de-pied front position. The supporting leg then goes into a demi-plié as the sur le cou-de-pied foot moves croisé to the back into Fourth. It stretches out at the knee, presses to the floor with the entire foot, and from there does a turning push en dedans with a transfer of the supporting leg to high demi-pointe. The other leg is thrown through a battement jeté, into à la seconde at 90 degrees.

The arms move from Preparatory during the relevé into First. At the transfer of the free leg into Fourth back, the arm opposite the direction of the turn opens into Second and the other stays in First. During the turning push, the arm moves from First into Second. During the pirouette, both arms are kept in Second or Third. The body is held straight and during the relevé it turns en dehors to 1/4 of a circle.

The head, at the demi-plié in Fifth, is turned to the advanced shoulder; at the relevé it stays the same, and at the moment of transfer of the free leg into Fourth back, the head turns en face and bends a bit toward the arm in Second. During the pirouette, the head is straight and follows the pattern for small pirouettes.

If from this approach the pirouette is done en dehors, the standing leg in Fourth back is thrown 90 degrees to the side by a fouetté. The entire body at this moment turns to 1/4 of a circle in the same direction as the thrown leg. At the turning push, the arm corresponding to the turn's direction is in First; the other is in Second in the form of third arabesque. The rest of the movement is the same.

The study begins with this exercise: In a 4/4 measure, a slow demi-plié is done in Fifth Position before the measure; 1/4 relevé to the demi-pointe; 1/4 fixes the position; 1/4 finds the free leg moving back into Fourth; 1/4 fixes this position;

1/4 throws the leg 90 degrees to the side; 2/4 fixes the pose à la seconde; 1/4 for the descent of the leg into Fifth in back. Then all is repeated from the other leg and again repeated.

The throw to 90 degrees must be well exercised, as well as the simultaneous transfer of the supporting leg to a high demi-pointe.

Following this pattern, the study of the pirouette en dehors and en dedans should begin at first with a stop on the entire foot, on the demi-pointe and in the transfer to demi-plié. In performance, the body must not turn ahead of time, nor should the head and arms turn or become disjointed from the thrown leg or the supporting leg.

Once it has been properly learned, the formula may be sped up with the leg going to sur le cou-de-pied before the measure, with 1/4 used for the turning push from Fourth.

When the approaches from Second and from Fourth are mastered, then the throw of the leg to 90 degrees side or its transfer to the raised sur le cou-de-pied—the transfer into Second or Fourth—may be replaced by a battement tendu, fondu or frappé. This is done on the floor and in combined exercises in the higher classes and not in the Fourth croisé, but in effacé.

PIROUETTE FROM PAS TOMBÉ

Unlike the approaches from Second and Fourth which perform the turning push on both legs, this form of pirouette performs the turning push from one leg.

The starting position is en face in Fifth. A battement développé or a battement relevé lent to the side to 90 degrees, with a relevé to a high demi-pointe, begins the form. Then, with no delay, a pas tombé to Second with an energetic lifting of the free leg to the side is done. A turning push en dehors or en dedans follows with a grande pirouette à la seconde to 90 degrees. The arms in pas tombé are in Preparatory Position to begin and during the push they may remain or rise energetically into Third. The body and head are straight.

The body's fall onto the open leg must be practiced well for exactness. It must be an uninterrupted and springy transfer into a turning push which must be assisted by the entire body, including the leg rising to 90 degrees with a light, harmonious and sufficient force.

The study at first should be for one pirouette and done somewhat slowly to a measure of 4/4; 2/4 for the battement développé in Second, 1/8 for the relevé to demi-pointe; 1/8 for pas tombé; 4/4 for the pirouette en dehors and a stop on demi-pointe; 1/4 for the lowering of the open leg into Fifth in back. Then, the same is repeated from the other leg. Practice with the pirouette en dedans follows, then practice in both directions and both sides with two pirouettes.

PIROUETTE FROM PAS DÉGAGÉ

In this form the turning push is done with the support on one leg. Beginning in Fifth Position en face, a battement développé to the side at 90 degrees is done with the supporting leg ending in the demi-plié. Then, the supporting leg starts a turning push as the open leg lowers in a broad movement onto a high demi-pointe. The free leg is thrown into à la seconde and remains there until the end of the pirouette.

The movements are continuous, energetic, and in one tempo so that the turning push, at the moment the working leg is on demi-pointe, is increased by the sendoff of the entire body into an en dehors or en dedans direction.

At the moment of moving onto high demi-pointe, the center of gravity must be put exactly over the supporting leg, with the body well pulled up and the arms fixed in Second or rising energetically into Third. The head remains straight.

The study begins with this exercise: The measure is 4/4 and slow; in 2/4 battement développé to Second ending in demi-plié; 1/4 for the beginning of the turning movement and the transfer to the open leg; 1/4 for the pirouette en dedans; 2/4 for the fixing of the stop on high demi-pointe; 1/4 for the lowering of the open leg into Fifth front; 1/4 for rest. Then all is done from the other leg and is repeated, then reversed with the pirouette en dehors. Then the study should include two pirouettes in both directions.

The pas dégagé approach to a grande pirouette à la seconde may also be done with the leg opening to 45 degrees followed by the same movements as in pas tombé.

PIROUETTE FROM THE À LA SECONDE POSITION

In an à la seconde position, from any suitable approach, a grande pirouette may be made in the following way: From the à la seconde position, the supporting leg does a relevé to high demi-pointe, then from a passing demi-plié with a turning push, en dehors or en dedans, makes an uninterrupted transfer into a grande pirouette, fixing the à la seconde position. While the relevé onto demi-pointe is made, the whole body prepares for the turn. When a vigorous descent into a demi-plié is made, it starts the sendoff of the entire body in the given direction. This increases to the maximum the force of the turning push. In this way, the supporting leg and the entire body in the descent to demi-plié is already turned about 1/8 of a circle and with the sendoff onto high demi-pointe provides an energetic turn. Care must be taken that in the 1/8 circle a strict Second Position is maintained.

This movement must have vitality and flow so that the supporting leg in demi-plié pushes away from the floor from the entire foot and transfers with flexibility to the high demi-pointe. There should be no slackening in the action of the open leg, the body, the arms or the head. On the contrary, the entire body must be collected and pulled up throughout the pirouette, which may end in a variety of ways.

The study begins with one pirouette en dehors: To a measure of 4/4; 2/4 is used for a battement développé to the side at 90 degrees; 1/4 for the relevé to demi-pointe from the demi-plié; 1/4 to fix this position; 1/4 to descend from the demi-pointe and make a turning push from the demi-plié; 2/4 for the pirouette en dehors and its ending; 1/4 to lower the leg into Fifth front. The exercise is then repeated from the other leg and both sides repeat the pirouette en dedans.

In the study using this approach to grande pirouette, especially with two turns, a turning push that is too strong should not be developed as it may easily push off the balance, interfere with free turning and with the stability of the ending. Free, exact and stable turning depends upon the harmonious performance of all the elements, especially the correct positioning of the center of gravity upon the supporting leg.

PIROUETTE IN GRAND ROND DE JAMBE EN L'AIR

This form of performing a grande pirouette à la seconde may be fortified and made more complex by the use of grand rond de jambe en l'air, which is done from Fourth into Second preceding the turning. In other words, the leg opening to 90 degrees in Fourth transfers vigorously into Second, as the supporting leg, through a passing demi-plié, makes a turning push and a pirouette on high demi-pointe. If the pirouette is to be made en dehors, the transfer of the leg and the push are done in the same direction. The same applies to en dedans. In this way the transfer of the open leg, with the active participation of the head, body, arms and supporting leg, makes a forceful spring into a grande pirouette.

The study begins in the following exercise: To a measure of 4/4 and beginning en face in Fifth Position; 2/4 is used for développé forward; 2/4 for the relevé onto high demi-pointe; 2/4 for the rond de jambe into Second and a turning push; 1/4 for a pirouette en dehors; 2/4 for a stop on high demi-pointe; 1/4 for the lowering of the open leg into Fifth.

The arms in développé move from Preparatory Position into First, and at the rond de jambe open strongly into Second and stay in that position until the end of the pirouette. During the lowering of the leg into Fifth, they return to Preparatory Position. The head and body follow the rules for these movements.

Here again, the movement must flow. Whatever the given pose for the start of this movement, the arms must take the most comfortable position for the turning push. For instance, for a pirouette en dedans, a convenient form would be the first or fourth arabesque. For a pirouette en dehors, a convenient form would be the second or third arabesque. For a pose with the leg at 90 degrees, transfer one arm corresponding to the direction of the turn, from Third to Second, or transfer both arms at once. The transfer must be light, harmonious, vigorous and in one tempo with the action of the legs. The body is pulled up and exactly over the supporting leg. The head takes its position rhythmically for the pirouette à la seconde. The supporting leg is firm but elastic, open and somewhat heightened, with stretched knee, instep and toes. The turnout is preserved without deviation.

PIROUETTE FROM GRAND TEMPS RELEVÉ

The method of performing the grand temps relevé and the grande pirouette à la seconde have already been discussed. Here we are concerned only with the turning push on one leg.

The usual grand temps relevé is a turned-out turning push to grande pirouette: Beginning in demi-plié on the supporting leg and straightening to high demi-pointe, the throw of the free leg moves along 90 degrees in an arc as the arms open from First into Second. All of this is done with the sendoff of the entire body en dehors or en dedans.

The grand temps relevé is done with a flow and a spring that is light and calculated to preserve the center of gravity over the supporting leg. The rhythm should be maintained and the plasticity of the movement of the supporting leg, especially the heel during the push, which must press firmly to the floor. The turnout must be maintained especially at the throw of the leg and the axis of the turn held with deliberation in a vertical line reaching upward.

All other rules of the performance of the movement apply.

This form is studied at first with the pirouette en dehors, then en dedans. Then it is studied with two pirouettes after the turning approaches from two legs to one have been mastered—that is, from Second and Fourth positions (previously described).

The exercise is in a measure of 4/4; grand temps relevé before the measure; 1/4 for the turning push; 2/4 for the pirouette en dehors and the stop; 1/4 to bend the open leg to the passé position at the knee. Then repeat the entire exercise from the other leg followed by performing the exercise en dedans on both sides.

PIROUETTES WITH UNINTERRUPTED REPETITION

The grande pirouette à la seconde without an additional movement of the open leg may continue uninterruptedly from two to thirty-two turns at a fast tempo.

The pirouettes begin from a demi-plié in Second. All the demi-pliés following are with the open leg remaining in à la seconde. The movement finishes with a transfer into small pirouettes which end in Fourth Position.

Because of the rushing transfer from one pirouette into another, the demi-plié is minimal. The foot of the supporting leg must act *firmly with the pushing accent up, not down to the floor*. The firm heel does not delay the rise to the next pirouette, but in fact helps the continuous turning in the same direction. The knee acts forcefully and flexibly as part of the supporting structure. The open leg, thigh and body, correctly and with coordination to the whole, maintain their position throughout. The head turns clearly in the small pirouettes and the body participates actively in the turning sendoff. The arms, too, participate even while moving in Second.

Totally forbidden in the study are: the loss of the structure as a vertical axis; displacing the foot from its point of support on the floor; lowering the open leg from 90 degrees or permitting it to veer from its position à la seconde; weakening the work of the thigh, ankle, instep or toes; permitting the body to slacken or stoop; raising the shoulders; using the arms with strain or indifference; turning the head arhythmically or moving the eyes without a steady focus; grimacing or straining the neck; incorrectly keeping the body en face at the moment of each turning push; breaking the rhythm of the turning, its vigorous tempo or classic style. A show of will and resolve is necessary, but without any acrobatic tricks or outside effects.

The study must be slowed in tempo and from four to eight turns with a passing demi-plié. This demi-plié will gradually be lessened as the tempo increases.

The exercise is in a measure of 2/4; with two measures for two battements fondus to the side at 90 degrees; two measures for four pirouettes en dehors. It is all done again in reverse, then on the other leg and repeated again.

Later, the study may be with eight pirouettes only, en dehors, speeding up after several classes. Then twelve pirouettes may be performed with a transfer into small pirouettes and finally sixteen.

Ultimately, the third turning push for two pirouettes without lowering from demi-pointe should begin. The tempo is at the utmost speed possible to the student.

There is still another form of grande pirouette en dehors à la seconde (grande pirouetette sautillée), which is very fast and in which the heel of the supporting leg is displaced in 1/2 circles. This is done flowingly without the rise to demi-pointe. It is as virtuosic as the one previously described. The actions of the arms, body, head and open leg are the same.

As a long series of pirouettes, it usually begins from small pirouettes en dehors with a transfer to à la seconde in a demi-plié en face in a deliberate movement, not a haphazard one. The series ends in small pirouettes which also begin en face from a demi-plié before the pull-in to the last turns. The head is comfortably involved in the movement and the arms at the final turns are rounded and energetically join in a lowered First. It is studied also in a slowed tempo with each displacement of the heel at 1/8 of a circle to a 2/4 tempo. This form is studied only after the other approaches have been properly mastered.

PIROUETTES IN ATTITUDE

PIROUETTE IN ATTITUDE FROM FOURTH POSITION

The pirouette in attitude from Fourth is easier to perform than from Second Position, which is the reason the description begins with this form.

Beginning in Fifth Position, épaulement croisé, a demi-plié and relevé onto high demi-pointe opens the movement with a turn to effacé. Simultaneously, there is a transfer of the forward leg into a heightened sur le cou-de-pied front. Then the supporting leg does a demi-plié as the other moves to croisé back into Fourth, and stretches out at the knee. The whole foot is placed on the floor. From this position, there is a turning push en dedans with a transfer of the supporting leg onto high demi-pointe and the other leg rises to the back to 90 degrees in the attitude position.

The arms during the demi-plié are in Preparatory Position. At the relevé, they rise into First and at the transfer of the free leg into Fourth back, the arm opposite to the direction of the turn opens into Second as the other stays in First. During the turning push, the arm in First is thrown into Second and the other, at the same time, moves into Third.

The body at the transfer into pirouette assumes the position for attitude. The head, during the demi-plié in Fourth, is turned toward the advanced shoulder; at the relevé it remains the same; at the transfer of the leg into Fourth in back, it turns en face and leans a bit toward the supporting leg. During the turn the head is fixed straight as for a small pirouette. If the pirouette is en dehors, then during the transfer of the leg into Fourth, the arms and head take the position for third arabesque. At the turning push, the arm rises energetically from First into Third as the other stays in Second. The head follows the previously given pattern.

During the turning push, the free leg is sent to 90 degrees with a turned-out, exact and pulled-back thigh, stretched instep and toes. The angle of the bend of the raised leg is about 120 degrees. The ending with an addition of a grand rond de jambe en l'air and a fouetté turn is not practiced here. However, this pirouette in attitude may end in arabesque with the arms, body and head following the rules of port de bras.

The attitude effacée may end in first or second arabesque and the attitude croisée, in third or fourth arabesque.

The transfer into a small pirouette is used here and, if done en dedans, the open leg at the same time straightens at the knee and lowers to 45 degrees, from where it is moved into a sur le cou-de-pied front during the turning push.

The arms at the passing demi-plié straighten—allongé—and at the start of the small pirouette, round and energetically join in a lowered First. The body is quite vertical. The head at this time keeps its position. At the turning push it turns en face, straightens out and acts as in small pirouette. The push itself must be done exactly through effacé, not in profile, so as not to interfere with the correct action of the head and the direction of the forward look.

If the transfer is done en dehors, the turning push, for the same reasons, must be done from croisé, not effacé or en face. To begin the study of this form, the exercise for pirouette à la seconde from Fourth may be used.

PIROUETTE IN ATTITUDE FROM SECOND

This movement begins en face in Fifth Position with a demi-plié and a relevé to high demi-pointe. The leg in front is then thrown sideways to 90 degrees. From here a demi-plié on both legs is done in Second Position and a turning push en dedans with a pirouette in attitude on high demi-pointe. If, before the pirouette, the throw is done on the right leg, then the same leg straightens from the demi-plié at the knee and rises into the performing pose.

The pirouette in attitude ends by lowering the supporting leg from demi-pointe onto the whole foot and fixing the pose in attitude effacée. The arms at the relevé to demi-pointe in Fifth rise from Preparatory into First. At the throw of the leg, they open into Second; on the demi-plié in Second, the arm corresponding to the direction of the turn moves into First; the other stays in Second. At the turning push, the arm from First is *thrown* to Second, and the other from Second moves to Third.

The body at first is straight and at the demi-plié in Second bends a very little toward the arm in Second; at the transfer to the pirouette, it leans toward the supporting leg and assumes the attitude position.

The head at first is straight, but on the demi-plié in Second, it turns with the body. During the turn it acts in the pattern for the small pirouette. If this approach is done en dehors, then the leg thrown to the side to 90 degrees is the leg that was in back in Fifth Position. The arms during the push rise directly and with energy into Third from First and the other stays in Second. The body takes the attitude position. The rest of the rules are the same.

It is important to remember that during the push the free leg must be sent to its position turned out, with a stretched instep and toes, and kept exactly in back and in a high position. The angle of the bend of the raised knee is 120 degrees.

An ending with the addition of a grand rond de jambe en l'air or a fouetté is not used here. There may be a transfer into a small pirouette as in the attitude from Fourth: The open leg at the same time straightens at the knee and lowers to 45 degrees, from where it is moved sur le cou-de-pied front during the turning push. This movement has no preparatory exercise.

PIROUETTE IN ATTITUDE FROM PAS TOMBÉ

Beginning in Fifth Position in épaulement croisé, this pirouette begins as a big pose effacée forward with a relevé on high demi-pointe. It is followed by a pas tombé forward into attitude effacée and a pirouette en dedans from a turning push.

During the pas tombé, the arms and head assume the suitable position until the end of the movement. The body gives a little over the supporting leg and the head turns as in a small pirouette. (Giving a little, in these movements, means placing the torso well over the supporting leg and even slightly forward over it. There should be no break in the connection of the line through the hip and thigh.)

This pirouette may also be done with a pirouette en dehors. In this case it begins from a pas tombé en croisé.

The study begins with one pirouette in a somewhat slower tempo, in the pattern of the pirouette à la seconde from pas tombé. Later, this approach may be made with the leg opening to 45 degrees in a battement, fondu, frappé, etc.

PIROUETTE IN ATTITUDE FROM PAS DÉGAGÉ

This movement begins in Fifth Position, épaulement croisé. From a big pose forward and effacée, with the supporting leg in demi-plié, the open leg moves together with the straightening supporting leg, in a broad movement to high demi-pointe. The freed leg, without delay and with energy, rises in back to 90 degrees into attitude effacée and remains until the end of the pirouette. The arms and head in pas dégagé keep their pose to the end, and the body favors the supporting leg slightly. The head turns as in a small pirouette.

Special attention should be paid to achieve a flowing push and a smooth transfer to the leg that makes the pose.

The study at first is with one pirouette, or the exercise for pirouette à la seconde from pas dégagé may be used.

PIROUETTE FROM A POSE

The pirouette from a pose follows the same rules as the pirouette from a pose in à la seconde. There must be a flow, energy and a spring from the passing demi-plié for a stable and harmonious turning.

The study, at first en dedans, should be from attitude croisée, so that the entire body and supporting leg, as it lowers into demi-plié from a high demi-pointe, is already turning in 1/4 of a circle.

The arms, head and body follow the usual pattern. If the pirouette ends in demi-plié, then the attitude is made more complex by the addition of allongé. In addition, during the push, the arms, head and body may change positions. For instance, both arms may be joined in Third; or in starting the movement en dehors, they may change positions suitable to the head and body.

The study is done after the exercise scheme of the pirouette à la seconde from a pose.

PIROUETTE FROM GRAND ROND DE JAMBE EN L'AIR

The approach to this pirouette may be complicated by means of a transfer of the open leg from Second or Fourth for the en dehors or en dedans pirouette. For instance, from the pose ecartée forward, the open leg is transferred into attitude croisée derrière by means of a grand rond de jambe en dehors. At the same time, the supporting leg from the entire foot on the floor or lowering from a high demi-pointe makes a passing, springy demi-plié for the turning push. The pirouette is en dehors. From a pose croisée forward, the open leg is led through Second en face into attitude croisée back. At the same time, the supporting leg performs as above into a pirouette en dehors.

The arms, head and body change positions during the transfer of the open leg. During the push, they assume and from there, they maintain the attitude position.

The transfers and the turn must flow and be energetic. For the study, the exercise for pirouette à la seconde should be used. This movement is later used in adagio movements in center floor.

PIROUETTES WITH UNINTERRUPTED TURNING

The rules for this form of turning in attitude are the same as the pattern for pirouette à la seconde, except that the turns are in attitude and repeated no more than four times.

If it is done eight to sixteen turns in a given series, it is performed by means of a demi-plié and a displacement of the heel in 1/2 a circle. In this case, the attitude allongée is fixed and the turning is usually en dehors.

The study is the same as for grande pirouette à la seconde, keeping all the rules, the flow, the clarity of design. Remember that this method usually begins and ends in small pirouettes and follows the rules for the grande pirouette à la seconde.

PIROUETTES IN ARABESQUE

PIROUETTE IN ARABESQUE FROM FOURTH POSITION

This pirouette from Fourth Position has the same approach as the pirouette in attitude from Fourth croisé derrière. The push is for an en dedans turn with a transfer of the supporting leg onto a high demi-pointe and the raising of the other leg to 90 degrees in an arabesque position. The arms at this moment, in allongé, are sent in the same direction as the turn. The body favors forward over the supporting leg, aiding the turn. The head turns toward the extended arm and is fixed in that position during the turning. On the whole, the arms, head and body, in one tempo, are sent into the first arabesque pose and kept there until the end of the pirouette.

If the pirouette is en dehors, the head, arms and body, during the push, assume the pose for third arabesque, which becomes the fixed pose for the pirouette.

The pirouette en dedans, as a rule, ends in first arabesque and the pirouette en dehors ends in third. But at the end of the pirouette in first arabesque there may be a change into second arabesque through a change of arms.

The third arabesque may be changed into fourth. The pirouette en dedans may start in fourth arabesque from Fourth croisé as well as from Fourth effacé. Finally, each pirouette in arabesque may end in an attitude. For instance: the first arabesque pirouette may end in attitude effacée; the third and fourth arabesque may end in attitude croisée. The rules must be kept.

New to these forms is the placement of the body as a counterweight to the stretched leg derrière and the immovable position of the head. These difficulties must be well practiced.

The transfer into small pirouettes is used here as in the pirouette from attitude. If the transfer is en dedans, the open leg lowers to 45 degrees and the turning push moves into a raised sur le cou-de-pied forward.

The arms join in a round, low First. The body, at the same time, straightens and the head turns en face and follows the pattern for small pirouettes. The push must be done only through the effacé position with a delay of the head en face so it may be included in the pirouette with freedom. If the transfer into small pirouette is done en dehors, the push must be from croisé keeping all the rules above.

The study may be without preparatory exercise after the scheme for the pirouette à la seconde from Fourth.

PIROUETTE IN ARABESQUE FROM SECOND POSITION

This pirouette is done in the same manner as the attitude from Second Position. In the en dedans direction, the transfer of the supporting leg onto high demi-pointe occurs during the push as the other leg moves to 90 degrees derrière. The arms are in allongé sent in the same direction. The body is at first straight during the demi-plié in Second, and leans a bit toward the arm in Second. During the transfer to the pirouette, it favors the supporting leg and assumes the first arabesque pose.

The head is at first straight, and at the demi-plié turns and leans in the same direction. At the pirouette, it is straight and fixed in the first arabesque position.

If this approach is en dehors, the arm corresponding to the direction of the turn will be in First and the other in Second. During the pirouette, the arms rush into third arabesque allongée as does the body and head. The position remains fixed until the end of the pirouette.

The study without a preparatory exercise follows the same scheme as the pirouette à la seconde.

PIROUETTE IN ARABESQUE FROM PAS TOMBÉ

This pirouette begins in Fifth Position, épaulement croisé. If it is performed from a big pose in effacé forward, the supporting leg does a relevé onto high demi-pointe and a pas tombé forward into first arabesque, followed by a push and a pirouette en dedans. The arms at the tombé are moved to First and rushed allongé into first arabesque. The body, at the same time, favors the supporting leg. The head turns toward the arm pointing forward and the pirouette ends in first arabesque.

This approach may precede a pirouette en dehors. In that case, the pas tombé is done croisé forward and the turning starts and ends in third arabesque. The arms, in this case, are not led through First, but rush directly into third arabesque. The same approach may later be done with the leg open to 45 degrees, as in battement fondu, etc.

PIROUETTE IN ARABESQUE FROM PAS DÉGAGÉ

This pirouette begins in Fifth in épaulement croisé. From a big pose in effacé forward, the supporting leg does a demi-plié, and in a broad movement the open leg goes onto a high demi-pointe.

The freed leg unbends energetically from the demi-plié and at once does a sendoff en dedans into 90 degrees. It remains there throughout the pirouette. The arms at the demi-plié are joined in a round movement in First. At the transfer of the leg through a dashing movement in allongé into an en dedans turn, the arms move into first arabesque. The body favors the supporting leg as it moves in the same direction and the head follows the arm, pointing forward. The end is in first arabesque.

The study is first practiced with one pirouette, as the scheme for pirouette à la seconde from pas dégagé.

PIROUETTE FROM A POSE

A pirouette from a pose already assumed follows the rules for the pose in à la seconde with a passing demi-plié that has a spring. This provides a stable and harmonious turn of the body.

The study of this pirouette begins in first arabesque in en dedans. When the supporting leg descends from the high demi-pointe, it and the body have already turned 1/4 of a circle. The arms, head and body assume the first arabesque pose for the en dedans turn. If the turn is en dehors, the position is third arabesque. It ends in the same arabesque as the turn. During the push, the arms, head and body may change position; for instance, from first arabesque into Second, etc.

It is studied in the same scheme as the pirouette in attitude.

PIROUETTE IN ARABESQUE FROM GRAND ROND DE JAMBE EN L'AIR

This pirouette is performed in the same manner as the pirouette in attitude and, like it, only moves in the en dehors direction. From pose effacée forward, the open leg energetically transfers through a grand rond de jambe en dehors, as the supporting leg, from the entire foot on the floor or from a high demi-pointe, passes through a springy demi-plié to a push en dehors.

The head and body, as well as the arms, coordinate their movements at the moment of the transfer of the open leg and during the push are already in the third arabesque. Here, as in all previous forms, there must be a flow and smoothness.

This study follows the same scheme as the pirouette à la seconde.

PIROUETTE WITH UNINTERRUPTED TURNING

The rules for this pirouette in arabesque follow the rules for the pirouette in à la seconde and the movement is repeated no more than four times.

If the pirouette is in the en dedans direction, it is fixed in first arabesque. If it is in en dehors direction, it is fixed in third arabesque.

If it is done eight to sixteen times or more, it is done through demi-plié at each turn with a displacement of the heel in 1/2 of a circle, as in the pirouette à la seconde. In this case, the position is fixed in first arabesque. If the pirouette is en dedans, the fixed position is first arabesque; if en dehors, the position is third arabesque.

The study follows the scheme for pirouette à la seconde with especial attention to the flow, stability and dash of the turning.

PIROUETTE INTO A POSE WITH THE LEG OPEN TO 90 DEGREES

All the approaches to this pirouette are done as in the cases discussed above except that during the push there is a transfer into a pose which is fixed during and after the pirouette.

PIROUETTE FROM SECOND POSITION

This pirouette is done from a demi-plié in Second with a push en dedans and a transfer of the supporting leg to high demi-pointe and a throw of the other leg to croisé forward to 90 degrees with a stretched-out position.

The arms move with the throw; the arm from First is sent into Third; the other arm moves from Second into First. The body at the move into the pirouette favors the supporting leg a little, and is kept straight. The head delays a bit, then turns as for a small pirouette, and the pirouette ends in croisé.

If the push is en dehors, then the free leg is thrown forward into effacé by means of a fouetté. The arm from first opens into Second and the other from Second rises into Third. The head and body follow their pattern. The pirouette ends in effacé forward.

Through a grand rond de jambe, the pirouette may also end in a third or fourth arabesque or an attitude croisée derrière or on a stretched leg or in demi-plié. The arms, head and body follow the rules of transfer from one pose into another.

The study follows the scheme of the pirouette à la seconde.

PIROUETTE FROM FOURTH

From a demi-plié in Fourth croisé, there is a push en dedans with a transfer of the supporting leg onto high demi-pointe and a throw of the other leg forward in an even 90-degree grand rond de jambe.

The arm in First rises into Third; the other may move into Second or close in First. The body remains strictly on the supporting leg in a vertical position. The head acts as in the small pirouette and, at the end, fixes in a pose croisée forward position.

If the push is en dehors, then the free leg is thrown in effacé through a fouetté, finishing the movement in back in regard to the mirror or corner #1.

The arm from First opens into Second; the other moves from Second into Third. The head and body act in the same pattern. The pirouette ends in effacé forward. It may also end through a grand rond de jambe in a third arabesque or in an attitude croisée in back, with or without a demi-plié. The arm from Second moves through Preparatory to First, as the other arm moves from Third into Second. If the leg is moved into attitude, the arm from Second goes into Third, and the other from Third descends into Second.

The study without a preparatory exercise follows the scheme for the pirouette à la seconde.

PIROUETTE FROM PAS TOMBÉ

From a big pose croisée or effacée derrière, or from any arabesque or attitude, a relevé onto high demi-pointe begins this approach. There follows a pas tombé back into croisé, or into effacé forward with a push en dedans or en dehors into a big pirouette in the same direction and into the same pose.

The arms, head and body from the tombé position take the pose in which the pirouette will be performed. When the pas tombé is done in effacé derrière and the pirouette is en dehors, then, as a rule, the fixed pose is effacé where it ends as well.

From this approach, if the pirouette is done en dedans, the pose is fixed in croisé. This rule is for the pirouette from pas tombé in croisé derrière.

The arms, in addition to the usual position, may take Third, and in the pirouette en dedans, one may go into First and the other into Third.

The pirouette en dehors may end through a grand rond de jambe into third or fourth arabesque or in an attitude croisée derrière. The arms, head and body act acccording to the rules of transfer from one pose into another. This study follows the scheme for pirouette à la seconde.

PIROUETTE FROM PAS DÉGAGÉ

This is a very difficult and complex pirouette. It has no convenient or firm point of support for the push, as in the pas tombé. Therefore it should not be omitted from class practice since it develops general stability.

As an example: From first arabesque, a demi-plié is done for a pirouette en dehors. In this case, the leg open to the back lowers in a wide movement and rises onto the high demi-pointe. The freed leg then straightens from demi-plié and without delay rises forward to 90 degrees and, with a straight leg, remains to the end of the pirouette.

The arm, during the push, moves from First actively into Second as the other, just as actively, rises from Second into Third and stays to the end.

The body at the pas dégagé, at the same time, energetically leans back toward the supporting leg. The head acts as for the small pirouette. The end is in effacé forward.

This approach may be done with a pirouette en dedans as from third arabesque or fourth arabesque or in attitude croisée with suitable actions in the head, arms and body.

The study should begin for one pirouette.

PIROUETTE FROM A POSE WITH THE LEG OPEN FORWARD

This pirouette is done in the same scheme as the pose in à la seconde with the exception that the demi-plié must be done with a flexible spring for the performance of the pirouette.

The study is at first in the en dehors direction from a pose croisée forward. As the supporting leg and the entire body descend from a high demi-pointe into demi-plié, it has already performed a 1/4 circle before assuming the effacé forward.

The arms, head and body during the pirouette en dehors are kept in the position for pose effacée, and during a pirouette en dedans, are kept in a pose croisée.

The pirouette ends in a pose fixed during the turning push. The arms and body may change their position during the push. For instance, they may join in Third if the pirouette is en dedans, or, if in Second, close into First.

The scheme for this study is the same as for the pirouette attitude.

PIROUETTE FROM GRAND ROND DE JAMBE EN L'AIR

This approach is like the one for the pirouette in arabesque or attitude, but en dedans. For instance, from the écarté pose derrière, the open leg is led energetically forward to croisé by means of grand rond de jambe en dedans. At the same time, the supporting leg from the entire foot moves to a high demi-pointe through a passing and springy demi-plié to make the turning push for a pirouette en dedans.

The head, arms and body act together with the opening leg and, during the push, clearly fix the position with the leg open in croisé forward. The study follows the scheme of the pirouette à la seconde, and the flow into the pirouette must be well practiced.

The plan for the study of the subject recommends one excellent exercise: quarter pirouettes. When the pupil shows insufficient aplomb, exactness and suppleness, then, instead of doing an abstract adagio, this exercise should be given. It reestablishes what was lost and improves what was poorly learned. Beginning in Fifth Position épaulement croisé, the Sixth port de bras is done with a pas tombé into Fourth instead of the final transfer forward of the Sixth port de bras. The turn will be en dedans so the arm corresponding to that direction moves with a round form, from Third through Second and Preparatory into First as the other stays in Second.

The body favors the forward leg and the head is en face but leaning a bit toward the arm in Second. Then there is performed a pirouette in attitude en dedans with a stop in effacé on the entire foot.

Then the supporting leg does a demi-plié and a relevé to high demi-pointe with a turn en dehors to 1/4 circle. The leg changes into a croisé position. The arm corresponding to the open leg during the turn in 1/2 of a circle, stays in Third and the other moves to Second. The body turns the 1/4 circle en dehors taking the pose for attitude croisée. The head turns toward the advanced shoulder. This pose, the attitude croisée, is then fixed on high demi-pointe.

From here the Sixth port de bras is again performed with the approach in Fourth forward from pas tombé followed by a pirouette en dedans into first arabesque with a stop in effacé.

This is all repeated a third time for the study of the pirouette en dedans and ends en face à la seconde. Finally, and at the fourth time, the open leg in à la seconde moves back into attitude croisée through a grand rond de jambe and a pirouette en dedans is done by means of a tire-bouchon (corkscrew): The leg in back in Fourth is bent to the knee of the supporting leg and gradually lowers along the shin into Fifth, a descending spiral like a corkscrew.

Then the entire exercise is done from the other leg and repeated. The tempo is a quiet 3/4. Two bars are used for a preparation in the form of the first part of a temps lié; four measures are used for the Sixth port de bras to pirouette en dedans; three measures for a grande pirouette in attitude and its end; one measure for demi-plié and relevé to demi-pointe with a turn to 1/4 circle in attitude croisée. From here all is repeated with a pirouette in first arabesque and a pirouette à la seconde. At the performance of the tire-bouchon, the leg descends into Fifth to the seventh measure. To the eighth, a preparation is done and all is repeated from the other leg. At first the study is with one pirouette for the tire-bouchon, then with two or three or more.

These tours, like all complex movements of classical dance, demand practice in combinations at every class for a free, detailed and exact performance.

It is useful to introduce these exercises at the barre from a big demi-plié from some pose with the leg open in Fourth, or from pas tombé. In such a case, the demi-plié into the à la seconde pose is not used because the barre would obstruct the movement. The demi-plié may be done for an en dehors or en dedans turn, but always for a movement with the open leg moving away from the barre and for the same reason.

First, these tours must be practiced on high demi-pointe, lightly pushing away the hand from the barre. Then, practiced from demi-pointe into demi-plié, and back as well, as with a springy pas tombé. In this last case, the arm, together with the body movement, must glide lightly in the same direction along the barre and lightly push away from it. At the moment of the ending, the other arm must lie exactly on the barre with a light push. Grasping the barre at the end or the beginning of the pirouette is inadmissible. During the demi-plié or placed on the barre, it takes the place of the free arm or goes from arabesque, for instance, into attitude and back.

In all these exercises, the proper placement of the center of gravity on the supporting leg must be carefully practiced. There must be a plasticity of movement through the whole body, especially in the arms, which leave the barre in observing all the rules of port de bras. There must be no evidence of strain.

TURNS AND TURNING IN AIR

Some jumps in classical dance may be done with a turn—en tournant—in a 1/4, 1/2, 3/4 or full circle in the air—en l'air.

For these turns, there is an added sendoff of the entire body en dehors or en dedans which must be of suitable force and start together with the jumping push of the legs. This action must be combined with the movement of the arms, body and head and, in some cases, with the throw of the free leg. Lacking all this leads to unstable endings of the jump, especially if the jump contains an advance.

These movements demand the most thorough study and practice, for the performance must be of maximum lightness and ease. Only then may they become part of the art of dance. A heavy, inexact or unstable performance of these jumps is not acceptable. These things may happen if they are not studied systematically, or if they are studied irregularly.

Different from turns and turnings par terre (on the floor), they have no point of support and therefore no point of reference for direction en dehors or en dedans. The leg which ends or begins the jump determines the direction.

For instance, in a sissonne en tournant, done *away from the leg on which it will end,* the jump will be considered en dehors. If a petit pas assemblé en tournant and turn are done *toward the pushing leg,* it is considered en dedans.

In a double tour en l'air ending in first arabesque at 90 degrees, the direction is en dehors because the turning is done away from the leg on which the jump ends.

If a tour en l'air is done from Fifth into Fifth, the turning, coinciding with the leg standing forward in Fifth, is considered en dehors. If it coincides with the leg in back, it is en dedans.

In tour en l'air, it is more convenient to spin toward the forward leg and because it coincides with the method of performing tours in small or big poses in Fourth back, from which it derives the en dehors direction.

The exception must be considered the temps sauté en tournant in First or Second. The direction of the turn, determined in respect to the supporting leg, is impossible because both feet before and after the jump are on the floor in one line and position. Therefore the direction here is "right" or "left." Moreover, this jump with a turn is learned only as a starting form and is later totally discarded in favor of more complicated forms.

Movements with turns are discussed in the same groupings as movements without turns as jumps. Tours en l'air are discussed separately.

JUMPS WITH TURNS

These jumps differ from other jumps because a new method of performance appears in them, a new means of dance expression allowing for more dynamic, colorful and virtuosic daring on the stage. All movements with tours do not exclude beats, but they are done only after mastering the turn separately and in combinations for study. Beats with turns demand thorough preparedness. Haste here is not permitted. The performance of jumps with beats and the cabriole are described at the end of this section.

TEMPS SAUTÉ WITH TURNS

This movement is performed only in First or Fifth Position. Second Position is excluded in these jumps with a turn, since it is performed more suitably from pas échappé.

PETIT TEMPS SAUTÉ

This jump is done in 1/4 circles from a very small sendoff. Both legs perform the sendoff at the moment of the push from the floor. The body must be collected and participate actively in taking the turning push. No turn in the air can be done if the body is inert during the turning push of the legs.

The arms are in Preparatory Position and the body is straight. The head turns with the body.

The study begins in First Position dividing the circle into four equal parts turning to the right. Then the left side is practiced. At first, there is a stop after each jump, and then it is done without interruption in four jumps, one circle. The push must be even in force and done according to the rules for the temps sauté without the turn.

The movement is then studied in Fifth Position, in 1/4 circles and then in 1/2 circles.

The arms, head and body follow the pattern as described above. The exercise may be in a measure of 2/4. To each 1/4 of the measure two temps sautés en dehors are performed in a 1/4 circle. Then in one measure, two temps sautés are performed in 1/2 circle, each followed by a battement tendu to the side with a change of Fifth Position. Then the exercise is repeated on the other leg. This is followed by repeating the exercises en dedans on both sides.

A more complicated exercise may be done in 2/4. To each 1/4 of the measure, two temps sautés en dehors are performed in a 1/2 circle, followed by three petits changements de pied each to 1/8 of the measure. Then it is repeated on the other side; repeated once again on both sides; then repeated on both sides en dedans.

The pupil must develop an exactness and a stability in orientation to the turns.

GRAND TEMPS SAUTÉ

This movement is performed with a high jump with a turn of 1/2 of a circle or a full circle. It is first practiced in First Position, then in Fifth Position. A premature turning of the body toward the turn or to the opposite side of the turn is not permitted. The sendoff must be from both legs evenly and together with the movement of the body.

The arms, head and body for the 1/2 circle turn follow the pattern as described for the petit temps sauté. In the performance of the full circle, additional movements of the arms and head are required which will have a considerable importance at a later time in the mastery of the technique of the tour en l'air.

At first, the full circle turn is done with the arms in Preparatory Position, but with the head moving as for a small pirouette. This helps to perform the turn with lightness and clarity.

When this has been mastered, the arm movements are introduced in First and Second positions as they are used in small pirouettes. At the movement of the push from the floor, the arms must join energetically in a lowered First Position and be kept in that position until the end of the jump.

This movement, performed with a turn en dehors or en dedans, is very useful and suitable. It prepares for the performance of other more complicated jumps which require the same position of the legs. For instance, the sissonne simple with a turn is performed with the legs in flight and, almost to the end of the movement, in Fifth Position. The pas chassé with a turn, as well as the grand assemblé with a turn, require the legs to be in the same Fifth Position during the turn.

The exercises for this movement are the same as for the petit temps sauté.

CHANGEMENT DE PIED WITH A TURN

This movement is performed with a small or large jump and a turn of 1/4 or 1/2 or a full circle.★ All the rules for temps sauté with a turn apply. The study begins with a stop after executing a 1/4 circle, and then is practiced without stops. All the rules for the movement without a turn must be strictly applied.

In a 2/4 measure, the starting position is épaulement croisé; four measures are used for four petits changements de pied en dehors in 1/4 circles with an elastic and deepened demi-plié. Then two measures are used for three petits changements de pied with a change of épaulement, followed by one grand temps sauté with an advance forward in croisé. One measure is for the jump; one measure for the stop. The exercise is then repeated on the other side; repeated once more from the beginning; reversed, repeated on each side en dedans in the same pattern.

Another exercise might be: Beginning in épaulement croisé to a 2/4 measure; three petits changements de pied en dehors in a circle in two measures; repeated twice fully, ending with a grand temps sauté with an advance forward in croisé. The exercise is repeated on the other side and the exercise on both sides, en dedans.

The arms in both exercises are in Preparatory Position except during the temps sauté, where they may be given different positions. The body must be straight

---

★ Tarasov's note: I believe that to call this changement de pied with a full circle turn a tour en l'air is incorrect, since the sissonne tombée and the sissonne ouverte each with a turn, retain their same names. However, when this turn is a double turn, the term tour en l'air is more correctly used, although it is performed with the same sissonne.

and the head at each first jump turned to the shoulder opposite the direction of the jump.

GRAND CHANGEMENT DE PIED

This movement is performed in a 1/4, 1/2 or full circle. The arms, head and body follow the pattern described above.

The study should begin with a 1/4 circle with a stop after each jump, then without the stop. The study should progress to include a 1/2 circle with a stop after each second jump with a suitably increasing sendoff with the entire body. Here also there must not be a premature turn of the body in the same or opposite direction to the direction of the turn. The body turns together with the legs during an even pushoff from the floor.

151   Grand changement de pied with a full circle turn

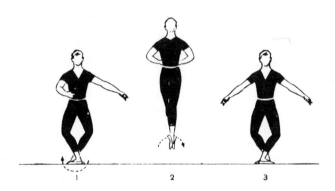

Then the study of the full turn, with the same rules and increased energy in the sendoff, should begin. The additional movement of the arms and head as used in the small pirouette should be included. In performing a turn en dehors, the arm corresponding to the leg that is front in Fifth Position rises to First Position. The other arm is in Second Position. During the turning push, the arms help the push by joining energetically in a lowered and rounded First Position and remain in that position to the end of the jump. (See illustration #151.)

When the turn is en dedans, the arm corresponding to the leg that is in back in Fifth Position rises to the First Position. The other arm moves to Second. In other aspects, the movement is performed in the same manner as the turn en dehors.

The study of the full turn should begin with the additional movement of the head alone, without the additional movement of the arms. The change of position of the legs in flight must be carefully observed.

The demi-plié must be elastic with firm placement of the heels pressed to the floor. The body should be pulled up, the shoulders open and lowered; the arms tensed a bit but kept strictly rounded; the head, free and clear in the turn; the look assured and focused directly forward. There must be no indication of strain in the muscles of the neck and face, caused by the difficulty of the turn.

Later, the movements of the arms may be added at the same time as the turning push but without too much strength, yet without flabbiness, in order to add to the force of the turn and to give it perfection.

The exercises described above serve as a preparation for more complicated forms of the full turn and the double tour en l'air. They exercise the basic elements well.

As an example of suitable exercises, in a 2/4 measure beginning en face and before the measure, a grand changement de pied with a full turn en dehors is performed; a stop in demi-plié for one measure follows; the three petits changements de pied en face to 1/8 of the measure each finishes the exercise. Repeat the exercise four times, then repeat from the other side and from each side en dedans.

Then, in a 2/4 measure beginning en face and before the measure, a grand changement de pied with a full turn en dehors is performed with the arm movements, followed by two petits changements de pied en face to 2/8, and in 1/4 an entrechat quatre. Repeat from the other side and from each side, en dedans.

Then, in a 2/4 measure beginning before the measure, a grand changement de pied with a turn en dehors is performed, followed by two entrechats quatres in 2/8, a sissonne tombée croisée forward in 1/4, and an assemblé to the back into Fifth Position in 1/4. Repeat from the other side, then from each side en dedans.

Further in the study, even more difficult approaches to the turn may be given, such as the petit pas échappé battu, the petit pas assemblé battu, etc.

Finally, the study of grand changement de pied with advances forward or backward (de volée) in turns of 1/2 circles en dehors or en dedans may begin. The arms and head, as well as the body, follow the pattern as the movement, without the turn. At first there should be a stop after each jump. Then, this movement may be included in combinations.

PAS ÉCHAPPÉ WITH A TURN

This movement consists of two jumps, each with a 1/4 or 1/2 circle turn. The turning push is from the legs as in other jumps and the sendoff follows the rules as described.

PETIT PAS ÉCHAPPÉ

In this movement, both jumps are with a 1/2 circle. The first jump from Fifth Position along Second Position is with a 1/4 circle; the second jump is from Second Position into Fifth Position with a 1/4 circle turn. The two jumps make a 1/2 circle and may be performed en dehors or en dedans. The arms, as a rule, are in Preparatory Position. The body is straight, and the head turns with the body.

This study begins immediately with the 1/4 turn in a 2/4 measure, from Fifth Position épaulement croisé. The first jump ends in Second with a turn of 1/4 circle en dehors. *Without delay* the second jump from Second Position into Fifth Position, without a turn, follows. The exercise is repeated four times, but at the end of the second jump into Fifth, the other leg is placed forward in order to begin the exercise on the other side. The exercise is then repeated en dedans on both sides.

As another example: The above exercise is performed as given except the second jump adds a 1/4 circle turn. Both exercises are, at first, performed in a slowed tempo to 1/4 of each measure. Then, with a minimal demi-plié, at a moderate tempo, with lightness and elasticity.

The petit pas échappé with a turn may be done in Fourth Position ending on one leg as it is performed without the turn. The movement is then added to combinations.

GRAND PAS ÉCHAPPÉ

Both jumps in this movment are done in a 1/2 circle en dehors or en dedans. The jump is high and there is a more active turn of the body to send off the movement.

The arms in the first jump rise from Preparatory Position through First into Second. At the second jump, they return to Preparatory Position. The body is straight and the head turns along with the body. In a measure of 2/4 beginning in épaulement croisé, the first jump is done ending in Second and the turn is en dehors in 1/2 circle; then the second jump from Second into Fifth is done without the turn. It is repeated twice, ending with a grand changement de pied with a turn en dehors of 1/2 circle with an advance forward in croisé. Then the exercise is performed on the other side. Both sides are done with the turn en dedans.

Another variation: Both jumps are performed with a turn of 1/2 circle en dehors, repeated twice, ending with a grand changement de pied with a full circle turn.

In combinations which include this movement, the second jump may end in a large pose in Fourth with a turn of 1/4 circle through a fouetté en dehors or en dedans. For instance, the ending may be a turn en dedans into first arabesque, second arabesque or attitude effacée derrière. Or from a turn en dehors, the ending may be in effacé with the leg open forward. All the rules for fouetté and the pose performed with an advance must be strictly kept for the second jump.

SISSONNE SIMPLE WITH A TURN

This movement, in its small form, is usually done with a medium jump and a turn of 1/4 or 1/2 or full circle, en dehors and en dedans.

Because this movement ends on one leg with the other in sur le cou-de-pied, it is rather difficult to perform and requires a graded study. The first study is en dehors in 1/4 circle with a stop after a jump. Then the study is without stops.

To a measure of 2/4, the movement begins in Fifth Position, épaulement croisé.

Before the measure, a sissonne simple with a sur le cou-de-pied forward and a turn en dehors of 1/4 circle are done; 1/4 is a stop; 1/4 for petit pas assemblé forward or effacé; 1/4 for another stop.

The arms during the first flight rise from Preparatory Position into First. At the end of the sissonne simple, the arm corresponding to the supporting leg stays in First Position as the other opens into Second Position. The body remains straight throughout the turn and the stop. The head turns with the body toward the advanced shoulder. At the pas assemblé the arms, head and body keep this position. This movement is followed by a sissonne simple (sur le cou-de-pied back) with a turn en dedans of 1/4 circle and a petit pas assemblé to the back. During the sissonnes, the arms do not lower into Preparatory Position and the head and body turn with the movement. The pattern to the music is the same as above.

Then the exercise is repeated again in the same direction, but at the end of a full circle the petit pas assemblé is not done to the back but to the side with a change of épaulement.

This prepares the exercise to be performed on the other side and other leg. It is then reversed with the same movements of the head, body and arms. In this exercise, the necesssary force for the turn should be practiced carefully for a stable ending and the proper fixing of the sur le cou-de-pied position.

This same exercise may be done without the stops. Then the study may include a 1/2 circle turn with stops after each jump, then with no stops.

The study may continue in the 2/4 measure, from Fifth in épaulement croisé with a sissonne simple before the measure, en dehors in 1/2 circle; 1/4 stop; repeat the tour of 1/2 circle to 1/4; along a diagonal a petit pas assemblé forward croisé is performed into Fifth; 1/4 for a stop.

The arms, head and body follow the pattern as in the previous exercise. Then it is all done in 1/2 circles en dedans. Both demi-turns are repeated without the stops. An ending may be sissonne tombée in croisé front, assemblé croisé back, and a changement de pied with a full turn en dehors.

The study of sissonne simple with a full turn may begin. In this case, the arms, during the demi-plié in Fifth, assume this position: The arm opposite the direction of the turn is in Second, the other is in First. Together with the turning push, they join in a lowered First or in Third. The body is held straight and the head is held as in a small pirouette.

The study of the full turn is done with an increased jump and a stop following the jump. This procedure corrects and stabilizes elements which will later enter into the double tour en l'air from one leg.

In the study of the full turn, the measure is 2/4 in Fifth Position and begins before the measure with a sissonne simple (sur le cou-de-pied forward) with a full turn en dehors in 1/4; 1/4 for a stop; 1/4 for pas glissade to the side with a change of leg; 1/4 for a stop. Then the turn is done to the other side, but the pas glissade is done forward in croisé. The exercise is repeated from the other leg; again from the beginning and then from both sides, en dedans. Later the exercise is done without stops and the movement is integrated into other combinations and with complicated jumps.

SISSONNE TOMBÉE WITH A TURN

This movement is done with a medium jump, with turns of 1/4, 1/2 or full circle, en dehors or en dedans. The arms, head and body act as in the sissonne simple with a turn. But during the tombé, they act as a sissonne without a turn depending upon the performed pose.

In this movement, the sendoff must be calculated for the entire body in the direction of the jump and the free leg. At the moment ending the jump, the free leg, through sur le cou-de-pied, does a pas tombé into Fourth or Second Position. If the sendoff is weak, then the pas tombé will end weakly, with insufficient advance. If the sendoff is too forceful, or too soft, the exit onto the opening leg will not be done with exactness in the given direction and will not be stable. Therefore this jump must be studied at first with a turn to 1/4 circle as a change of épaulement and as a first attempt at learning this method. It also prepares for the tours en l'air to come.

The beginning exercise is as follows: To a 2/4 measure from Fifth Position épaulement croisé and beginning before the measure in time to end on the first 1/4 note, a sissonne tombée effacée forward with a turn is done; on the second 1/4 a small assemblé forward into Fifth completes the movement. Then the exercise is repeated on the other side from the other leg. Then the exercise may be done in écarté along a diagonal to the back (en arrière) ending with an entrechat quatre. This is repeated to the other side and both sides are practiced with the turn en dedans.

Next, the turn may be increased to a 1/2 circle and then a full circle as in the described movement above. Beginning in Fifth Position, épaulement croisé, the sissonne tombée is done forward with a 1/2 turn en dehors followed by a small assemblé to the back. It is repeated to the other side. Then the sissonne tombée is performed to the side with a full circle turn en dehors followed by a small assemblé into Fifth Position forward. This exercise may be finished with two pas glissades from side to side with a change of legs in Fifth Position. Then it is repeated on the other leg and both sides with the turn en dedans. Each jump is made to 1/4 of the 2/4 measure.

Still another form of sissonne tombée with a turn is used incorporating a full circle turn en dehors or en dedans. During the jump, the legs change in Fifth Position. The rest is the same.

The movement should be done without stops, four times en dedans with an advance forward and four times en dehors with an advance to the back. The leg, in this exercise, is placed in sur le cou-de-pied only when the turn is to the side, and it remains there to the final demi-plié. The pas tombé is made by the free leg.

This form must be practiced well as it is used in complicated forms of the tour en l'air.

SISSONNE OUVERTE WITH A TURN

The turn in this movement may be 1/4, 1/2 or 3/4 and a full circle, en dehors or en dedans into a small pose, through a développé and jeté.

SISSONNE OUVERTE PAR (BY WAY OF) DÉVELOPPÉ

This movement is performed with the opening of the leg through the sur le cou-de-pied position in the small form, and through the passé or at-the-knee position in the large form. It is done with no advance in space.

PETITE SISSONNE OUVERTE PAR DÉVELOPPÉ

This jump is performed at medium height with a turn of 1/4 or 1/2 circle, ending in a small pose with the leg open to 45 degrees. The arms, head, and body, as in the sissonne ouverte without the turn, follow the same pattern. The sendoff and the turning push is done as in the preceding jump. The correct and stable ending of the jump in a small pose must be learned in small poses at first, with a 1/4 and later a 1/2 circle turn. For instance, in a 2/4 measure, beginning in Fifth Position, épaulement croisé, a sissonne ouverte is done with the turn en dehors in 1/4 circle ending in écarté to one of the back corners of the room; pas assemblé forward into Fifth Position ends the exercise. It should be repeated to the other side with a 1/4 circle, then performed with a 1/2 circle on each side. The ending is a royale for the 1/2 circle exercise. It is all repeated on the other leg and en dedans on both sides. Each movement is performed to 1/4 of the measure at a somewhat slowed tempo.

Another example: Beginning in Fifth Position, épaulement croisé; two sissonnes ouvertes, with a turn en dehors in 1/2 circle ending in écarté and assemblé into Fifth forward, begin the exercise. They are followed by a sissonne tombée to the side with a turn en dehors in a full circle, a pas assemblé backward into Fifth Position and a royale. The combination is then performed on the other leg. It is repeated from both sides with the turn en dedans. The tempo is a normal one for a medium jump.

Then the study of this jump, ending in a small pose in Fourth forward and backward, should begin with a 1/4 then a 1/2 circle turn.

GRANDE SISSONNE OUVERTE PAR DÉVELOPPÉ

This movement is done with a high jump and a turn of 1/2 or full circle, ending in a big pose with the leg opening to 90 degrees. The rules for the use of the head, arms and body in this movement are the same as for the movement without the turn. The sendoff and the turning push are more forceful than necessary for the smaller form. As a beginning exercise: To a measure of 2/4, and beginning in Fifth Position, épaulement croisé, two grandes sissonnes ouvertes, with a turn en dehors to a 1/2 circle into an écarté to the back corner of the room, are performed ending with an assemblé into Fifth Position forward. Then, a grande sissonne with a turn en dehors in a full circle ending in a pose à la seconde follows. This is followed by a pas de bourrée with a change of legs in a full turn in the same direction and, finally, a glissade to the side in the direction of the turn ends the exercise in Fifth Position. The exercise is ready to be repeated to the other side and on both sides with the turn en dedans.

Another example: Beginning in Fifth Position, épaulement croisé, a grande sissonne ouverte with a turn en dehors to 1/2 circle into a pose with the leg opened in a forward position followed by an assemblé forward is performed. The same sissonne with a turn en dedans into third arabesque follows. Then a grande sissonne with a full circle turn en dehors into attitude croisée back—through the passé position—is followed by a pas assemblé to the back and three small entrechats quatre, which end the exercise. Each jump in both examples is done to 1/4 of the measure and the entrechats quatre to 1/8 counts. The rules for the grande sissonne ouverte with a turn are the same as the rules for the small form, petite sissonne ouverte.

In the full circle jumps, the arms act as for a large jump. Before the jump, the arm opposite the direction of the turn is in Second and the other arm is in First. At the moment of the pushoff and the turning push they join energetically in a round and lowered First Position where they stay during the turn. They open together into a given pose at the end of the turn.

SISSONNE OUVERTE PAR JETÉ

This movement opens directly from the Fifth Position after the push from the floor. This jump is always done with an advance to the side of the leg on which the jump ends.

PETITE SISSONNE OUVERTE PAR JETÉ

This movement is done in a 1/4 and 1/2 circle in all small poses from a medium jump. The push from the legs and the turning sendoff of the body, and the advance, are calculated during the flight to a new point of support, as in the sissonne tombée. In the sissonne tombée, the advance is done with the transfer to the opening leg. In this movement, the transfer is from the leg that remains open at 45 degrees.

The arms, head and body follow the pattern for the movement without the turn. The study follows the pattern for the petite sissonne ouverte par développé.

It must be remembered that the advance in this jump is in proportion to the leg at 45 degrees which, at the moment of the final demi-plié, must not be lowered.

GRANDE SISSONNE OUVERTE PAR JETÉ

This movement is done from a high jump with a turn of 1/2 to 3/4 of a circle ending in a big pose with the leg opening to 90 degrees.

The arms, head and body follow the pattern for the movement without a turn.

The push from the legs must be more energetic, especially for a 3/4 of a circle turn. An example for an exercise: To a 2/4 measure, beginning in Fifth Position, right leg forward, épaulement croisé; sissonne ouverte is performed with an advance backward into the opposite corner, and with a turn left of 1/2 circle, en dedans. The jump ends on the left leg in attitude back, followed by a pas assemblé derrière into Fifth Position. All is then repeated but with the advance into the starting corner and with a turn to the right of 1/2 circle. Then sissonne tombée forward in effacé is followed with a turn en dehors of a full circle, and a jeté passé into third arabesque and a pas assemblé derrière into Fifth Position.

The movement is repeated from the other leg and en dedans.

Each jump is 1/4 measure and is somewhat slowed.

Another example: Sissonne ouverte is performed with an advance into the upper left corner of the room with a left turn of 1/2 circle, en dehors. The jump ends with the right leg in écarté derrière, followed by pas assemblé derrière into Fifth Position. Then all is repeated, but with an advance toward the lower and opposite corner of the room and with a turn to the right, en dedans. This is followed by a sissonne tombée to écarté forward and a royale with an advance forward. The combination is repeated to the other side and reversed.

In both exercises, the arms, head and body follow the rules for performing jumps and the conditions for the turn.

The sissonne with a turn of 3/4 of a circle is done only in Fourth with the leg opening forward or backward. The turn is done as follows: Beginning in Fifth Position, right leg forward, épaulement croisé, sissonne ouverte with an advance into the lower right in respect to the observer; a turn to the left of 3/4 of a circle is done in a jump that ends on the left leg; the right leg is thrown energetically back and the entire body, turning en dedans, ends in a third arabesque or an attitude croisée.

This same turn may be done en dehors. Sissonne from Fifth with the right leg forward is performed backward into the left corner with a turn to the left of 3/4. The jump ends on the right leg as the other is energetically thrown forward and the entire body, turning en dehors, takes a pose with the open leg in croisé forward.

In the performance of this jump, the displacement of the foot during the push from Fifth in the direction of the turn is not admissible, nor is the premature turn of the body in the same direction.

The beginning demi-plié must be done with a sendoff of the entire body into the direction of the place where the jump will end. And all the rules for this movement without the turn apply.

Another example: In two measures of 2/4, Fifth Position, épaulement croisé, and before the measure, a sissonne ouverte is performed into third arabesque with a turn en dedans of 1/2 of a circle; 1/4 is used for a stop in demi-plié for the landing; 1/4 for a pas assemblé derrière; 1/4 is used for a stop to straighten the legs from the demi-plié. The exercise is then repeated from the other leg and twice more.

Then the exercise is repeated en dehors, then without the stops and with turns:

From Fifth Position, épaulement croisé, sissonne ouverte is done with an advance back into the upper corner of the room with a turn to the left of 1/2 circle en dedans; the jump ends on the right leg in attitude effacée derrière. Then a pas assemblé to the back into Fifth Position is performed. This is followed by sissonne ouverte with an advance into the left upper corner and a right turn of 1/2 circle, en dehors. This jump ends on the left leg into écarté forward followed by a pas assemblé into Fifth devant (front). This is followed by a sissonne ouverte with an advance into the lower right corner with a turn to the left of 3/4, en dedans. This jump ends on the left leg in third arabesque from where a cabriole in third arabesque is performed, followed by a pas chassé croisé forward, and a pas assemblé derrière completes the combination. This exercise is repeated on the other leg and reversed on both legs.

In this form of sissonne, there are two elements bound together which must be clearly understood and mastered. They are the direction of the turn and the turn itself, which do not always come together and are not always easy to perform. If the pupil has mastered all the exercises and combinations in the study of the performance of the sissonne—and these are very difficult, especially in reverse—he can then orient himself in space. He will then have received an excellent basis for the further development of a virtuoso technique in jumps with a turn, and for spins.

PAS ASSEMBLÉ WITH TURNS

This movement is done with a 1/4, 1/2, full or double circle turn.

PETIT PAS ASSEMBLÉ

The first example is with a turn of 1/4 of a circle, but it is difficult because this requires a simultaneous throw of the one leg to the side at 45 degrees and its return to Fifth Position.

The study at first is in a slowed tempo of 2/4 for the measure and begins in Fifth Position, épaulement croisé. A petit assemblé to the side with the back leg in Fifth Position is performed. In flight, the entire body turns en face. The end of the movement has the open leg descending forward into Fifth Position and the body ending in épaulement croisé (opposite from the beginning), completing a 1/4 turn en dedans.

Then this same assemblé is performed from the other leg with a turn in en dehors of 1/4 circle. This is continued twice more, completing a full circle, and ends with a pas glissade along Second to the side of the forward leg, with a change into Fifth Position. The exercise is then ready to be performed on the other leg and then reversed on both sides.

Each jump is done to 1/4 of the measure with a stop in demi-plié on the second 1/4. The pas glissade is done to the last 1/4 of the last measure. Later, the exercise is done without stops and is joined with other, more difficult jumps, such as a petite sissonne en tournant, etc.

It is studied with the arms in Preparatory Position, then follows the rules for small poses, as does the head movement. All the rules for petit assemblé minus the turn are kept, especially exact Fifth Position, elasticity in the demi-plié, and the correct throw of the leg in Second Position. It requires lightness and stability.

GRAND PAS ASSEMBLÉ

This movement is done with a 1/2 circle turn, a full or double turn, and is performed only en dedans.

The approach is usually from a pas chassé in Second and turns in the same direction. At the moment of the pas assemblé, both legs join in Fifth Position simultaneously with the turn of the body in a 1/2 circle en dedans. The jump is done with the usual advance and ends with the open leg closing in Fifth Position front. The arms, during the assemblé, rise energetically from Preparatory to Second and into First, and into their usual position. The body is straight and the head turns toward the advanced shoulder.

The grand pas assemblé with a full circle turn must be done with a high jump, but the smallest advance, which allows the body to remain collected and stable at the end of the jump. The arms for a full circle turn move energetically into Third Position and remain fixed in that position until the final demi-plié. The body is straight and pulled up during the pas assemblé. The head turns toward the direction of the throw of the leg and at the end of the jump is toward the advanced shoulder. It is performed the same as for the double turn.

In doing a double turn, it is necessary to send off the body with a strong accent upward and a minimum advance after the throw of the leg. The body must be pulled up and collected. The arms and head take the same position as for the lesser turns but move with more vigor.

As an exercise: Beginning in a lower corner of the room, in Fifth Position, épaulement croisé, a preparation for a small pose in second arabesque on demi-pointe is performed. This is followed by a pas chassé along Second along a diagonal (step onto the leg that is forward in the chassé) and grand assemblé with a 1/2 circle turn. The jump ends in Fifth Position facing upstage with the head, arms, and body in écarté (to corner #4 or #6). This is followed by a sissonne tombée with a turn en dehors of 1/4 circle with an exit into third arabesque. The ending is a jeté passé into second arabesque and the entire exercise is ready to be repeated to the other side and repeated twice more. The tempo may be a 3/4 with a preparation of two measures before the execution of the combination. The exercise is done without stops in a somewhat slowed tempo.

The grand assemblé with a full or double turn may be studied in the same pattern. This will require that the assemblé end in épaulement croisé and without a 1/4 turn for the sissonne tombée.

The first example may be constructed differently but the assemblé with a turn must always be done from pas chassé along Second. No free run is permitted, since this disturbs the teaching methods of classical dance.

In performing a full and, even more, a double turn, the center of gravity must be placed exactly onto the pushing leg with a simultaneous throw of the other leg no higher than 45 degrees in flight. The legs must be quickly and tightly joined in Fifth Position and kept in that position into a soft ending of the jump.

In addition, the entire body during the turn must be completely perpendicular. Leaning away from the axis by the legs or body is inadmissible. The body must be harmonious in the movement, pulled up with open and lowered shoulders. The arms, during the turn, must also be kept perpendicular but maintain plasticity. The head, as well as the arms and the body, must not lose the tempo of the movement. *The look or focus must be exact and, in proper time, transferred to the starting and finishing point in the air.* This is especially important in the double turn to maintain aplomb.

The performance of these turns, especially the double turns, must be light and in strict dance form, with no special accents. Its study should start only after the tours en l'air in Fifth and Fourth positions have been mastered.

PETIT PAS JETÉ WITH A TURN

This movement is done with a 1/4 circle turn and a throw of the leg to the side in Second Position. The turning push is done with both legs with an active participation of the entire body, arms, and head as in the movement without the turn.

Example: To a measure of 2/4, beginning in Fifth Position, épaulement croisé, a pas jeté is done to the side onto the leg standing in back in the Fifth Position. It is done as a 1/4 circle turn as the other leg, having done the push off the floor, ends in sur le cou-de-pied behind the supporting leg. The turn was en dehors. The leg which was thrown is the leg on which the jump ends. All this is repeated from the beginning with stops in demi-plié on each second 1/4 of the measure. Then the exercise is repeated without stops and each jump to 1/4 of the measure. This is followed by a full measure for a pas de bourrée en tournant with a change of legs and ending in Fifth, and an entrechat quatre the last 1/4. This is then done from the other leg. The arms at first are kept in Preparatory Position and later are used as in small poses. All the rules for the pas jeté are strictly kept and lightness and clearness in the turn itself should be practiced.

PAS EMBOÎTÉ WITH A TURN

This movement is done with a 1/2 circle turn. Beginning in Fifth Position, en face, a demi-plié is made on the back leg, as the other leg, at the same time, moves to sur le cou-de-pied front. From here, a small jump is made during which both legs stretch out into a minimum Second; then the leg that made the jumping push (the back foot) moves into sur le cou-de-pied in front as the other does a demi-plié at the same time. All this is done with a turn of 1/2 circle, en dedans and with a very small advance in the direction of the leg in sur le cou-de-pied. The first turn ends with the student's back to the mirror (facing upstage) and is then repeated with the next turn en dehors, ending facing the mirror (or downstage). This movement may be done four to eight times in a row and in a diagonal line as well as parallel to the mirror. If the movement is done in reverse, the sur le cou-de-pied is placed in back every time and the first half turn is done en dehors.

The arms in demi-plié are in Preparatory Position. The arm corresponding to the direction of the turn is in First, and the other is in Second. During the jump and turn, the arm in First goes into Second and the other moves from Second into First, etc. The body is turned to the front if the pas emboîté is done in a parallel line to the mirror. If the movement is done diagonally, the body moves in épaulement.

The head, before the first jump, is turned toward the advance. At the first emboîté, it keeps this position; at the second, it turns a little faster than the body in the same direction. If the movement is done in reverse, the arms and body reverse their movements as well. The head, before the final jump, is turned in the direction of the advance. At the first emboîté, it turns a little faster than the body in the same direction. At the second emboîté, it keeps the position, etc. It should be studied in a quiet tempo, in not too great a number. To a measure of 2/4, six emboîtés should be performed to each 1/4 of the measure. At the first 1/4 of the measure, a pas glissade with a change of legs into Fifth Position is done, and to the second 1/4 of the same measure, the forward leg rises into sur le cou-de-pied front. Then the exercise is ready to be performed on the other leg once more from the beginning, and in reverse. Later, the emboîté may be done at a normal tempo to 1/8 of a measure. In this case, the speed of the movement is increased and each full turn requires three emboîtés.

For example: Two emboîtés with a turn of 1/2 circle to each 1/4 of the measure is performed. Then three emboîtés of 1/3 of a circle to each 1/8 of the measure follows, with a demi-plié on 1/8 ending the exercise. All is repeated to the other side; to each side again, and then reversed.

In this movement, a light push must be practiced and a clear stretching of the leg in flight, with an exact transfer to sur le cou-de-pied in its diminished form. The demi-plié must be elastic and a true line of advance with equal distances between each jump observed. There must be the proper action in the arms, head and body.

The entire movement must be compact, very clear in design and without any disheveled action in the upper or lower portion of the body. (Notice the small minimum movement to Second between jumps for added brilliance in this method.)

PAS JETÉ WITH AN ADVANCE TO THE SIDE OF 1/2 CIRCLE

This movement is done with an advance parallel to the mirror or diagonally, following the rules of the petit jeté.

Beginning in Fifth Position en face in a 2/4 measure, a pas jeté is done with the front leg with an advance toward the same side and an en dedans turn of 1/2 circle. The other leg, having made the push, is transferred at the end of the jump into sur le cou-de-pied in back. The same jeté is then done with the back leg en dehors of 1/2 circle en face. The arms in the starting demi-plié in Fifth are in Preparatory Position. They rise with the arm corresponding to the advance into First Position, as the other arm moves to Second Position. During the flight, the arm in First opens into Second. At the end of the jump the arm in Second moves into First, etc. The body is straight and shapely. During the push and the flight, and at its end, it is trajected onto the supporting leg. The head at the start of the movement is turned toward the forthcoming jump. During the flight and at its end it is kept in the same position. Only the entire body turns. At the next jump, the head turns back to the starting position. Each jump is done to the first 1/4 of the measure and the second 1/4 is for the demi-plié.

In this manner, four pas jetés are performed and, at the last 1/4 of the fourth measure, the exercise is ended with a pas glissade to the side without a change of legs to Fifth Position. The exercise is then ready to be repeated to the other side and to be reversed. The turn is then en dehors with the student's back to the mirror, and the second jump is en dedans, facing the mirror or en face.

Then the movement is done without interruption with each jump on 1/4. Finally, it is done on a diagonal and introduced into other combinations.

In this movement, there must be a wide and vigorous advance with stretched legs in flight and a clear turn performed at the last instant. The entire jump must be exact, elastic, without flabbiness and no untimely bending of the leg for the sur le cou-de-pied position and no sharpness at the landing of the jump.

SAUT DE BASQUE

This movement is a development of the previous pas jeté and is divided into a small, large and double form.

PETIT SAUT DE BASQUE

Beginning in Fifth Position, en face, a demi-plié is made on the back leg as the other leg, at the same time, rises into a somewhat elevated sur le cou-de-pied in front. That leg then opens to the side to 45 degrees in Second and at once moves into demi-plié with a jumping push and turning sendoff of the entire body en dedans. The other leg at this moment glides lightly along the floor through First and is thrown into Second Position at 45 degrees. The leg that performed the push in flight *is fixed in a perpendicular position*. In this way, the body turns 1/2 circle in flight, ending with the student's back to the mirror. Immediately upon landing, the perpendicular leg clearly bends into an elevated sur le cou-de-pied front. The other leg descends from its 45 degrees into a finishing demi-plié. All this is repeated in a 1/2 circle which places the end of the jump in the same starting position, en face.

At the start of the demi-plié, the arms follow this pattern: The corresponding arm to the direction of the turn is in First Position, the other is in Second. During the transfer onto the open leg, the arm moves from First clearly into Second. The other arm, during the jumping push, is sent from Second energetically into First. This is the position in which they are fixed as seen from the student's position with his back to the mirror in the jump. At the landing or the second half of the turn, the arms move into the starting position and remain there during the finishing demi-plié. The body is straight throughout the movement but follows the side movement and the turning movement together with the legs. The head at the starting demi-plié is en face. Together with the leg opening to the side, it turns in the same direction. In flight, it does not change. At the end of the jump it returns en face. (See illustration #152.)

---

152   Petit saut de basque

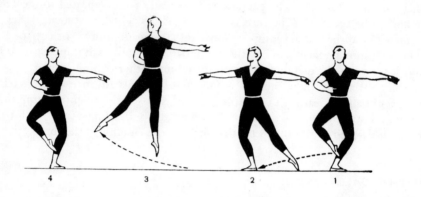

4   3   2   1

The petit saut de basque is done with a small advance and minus the pas chassé Second approach. When the movement is done diagonally, then placement of the body before and after the jump is in épaulement.

In practice, the student should strive for the proper opening to 45 degrees with a sufficiently broad transfer from toe to heel and an elastic demi-plié. The push should be vigorous, and the throw of the leg exact and light through First into 45 degrees. The fixing of the outstretched legs at the culmination of the jump should be clear and a soft, light, and elastic demi-plié should finish a light flight.

A slack turnout, unclear sur le cou-de-pied, or overly high throw of the leg should not be permitted. A weak demi-plié before and after the jump or a blunt ending and a sendoff by the body that is too big or too small are equally undesirable. The advance, as well, must be neither too big nor too small in flight.

The arm must move in a clear pattern somewhat lowered in its positions, but not in a sharp manner. The body is pulled up, and the shoulders open and easy. The weight of the body must be exactly and in proper time over the supporting leg. The head is straight and the look directly in the line of the turn.

The study of this movement begins en face, and there are stops on each finishing demi-plié. The measure is 2/4, with the opening of the leg to 45 degrees before the measure; 1/4 is for the push and flight; 1/4 for the finish of the jump; 1/4 for the stop in demi-plié; 1/4 for the free leg to open again to the side, etc. All is repeated four times but, instead of a final pause in demi-plié, a small assemblé is done into Fifth Position closing in back. The last 1/4 finds the leg in front opening to the side through sur le cou-de-pied. Then the exercise is ready to be repeated on the other leg.

In reverse, the exercise is as follows: The starting position is the same but the demi-plié is on the forward leg in Fifth Position as the other leg, through sur le cou-de-pied, opens from the back to 45 degrees. Then there is a transfer onto the leg from a push with the turn of the body en dehors. The other leg, at the same time, lightly glides along the floor through First and is thrown into Second at 45 degrees. The leg, having done the push, is perpendicular. In this way, the movement of flight with the turn of the body of 1/2 circle, is fixed with the back of the student to the mirror. Then, the pushing leg bends into sur le cou-de-pied in back. Finally, the demi-plié is done on the other leg. The second half ends en face. The arms, head and body follow the pattern described above. Later, the pauses or stops are omitted and the movement is used in combinations.

GRAND SAUT DE BASQUE

This movement is done like the small form, but all the movements in this larger form are intensified. The jump is big, the leg is thrown to 90 degrees, and the arms are thrown at flight into Third Position. The body and head actively participate, the advance is increased, and the start and finish in sur le cou-de-pied are even more elevated. The movement has pas chassé as an approach into Second to achieve a higher and more soaring flight.

The approach may start from a small arabesque pose as in the performance of the revoltade or other big jumps.

The arms in pas chassé open into Second and, during the jumping push, are sent through Preparatory Position and First into Third, where they stay during the flight. At the final demi-plié, they may remain or change into Second. The head and body act as in previously described patterns. The study must be done at first with stops, then without the stops. In reverse, the movement is done like the grand assemblé en tournant or the revoltade.

DOUBLE SAUT DE BASQUE

This movement is done with the highest possible jump and with a double turn of the body. The leg is thrown to 45 degrees, as the other leg in flight maintains the elevated sur le cou-de-pied front position.

As an approach, the pas chassé in Second is used with an accent for a maximum push, not for an advance. The arms in the pas chassé are in Second. During the saut de basque they are, as a rule, in Third Position or the arm corresponding to the direction of the turn goes into First as the other goes into Third. They might also be fixed in a rounded and lowered First Position, but this would be an exception.

The body actively participates by being straight and shapely. The transfer to the supporting leg must be sure and on time. The head turns twice as for the

usual saut de basque pattern. In the jump, the entire body must be strictly perpendicular, not leaning to either side in the final demi-plié.

The jump may be finished in sur le cou-de-pied with an exit into a pas tombé
in Second, or with an exit into first arabesque, attitude or to the floor on one
knee. In all cases, the transfer must be very elastic, flowing and stable with no
excessive force. Therefore, there must be practice for a suitable turning sendoff.
Students sometimes produce only a medium high jump with excessive sendoff
which results in an unstable finish of the jump and a fast, hasty tempo for the
two turns.

In the double saut de basque, the practice must be for a light approach, good
force for the jumping push, with an elastic transfer to the heel, a free and high
flight and a clear and resolute fixing of the body as it turns. There must be an
elastic and stable transfer into the final demi-plié and into the following movement.
In flight the arms must be directed vigorously, with free and stable positions.
The body must be stable, collected and not weakened at the final demi-plié. The
arms must act, like the body, with plasticity and with aplomb.

The body must be pulled up, shoulders open and lowered. The body must be
carried lightly and transferred exactly over the supporting leg. Boldness and exactness are demanded from the actions of the head, especially in the second turn.
There must be a sure and direct look to the proper point in space. The loss of
orientation here is inadmissible. The exact and proper tempo of both head turns,
together with the action of the arms, add considerably to the stability of the
performance. The flight and both turns must be technically exact, high and forceful. They both must have élan, inner dance; and the sendoff must be strict and
masculine in character with no fluttering lightness or acrobatics.

Before the study, the pupil must have mastered the tours en l'air from Fifth
into Fifth Position; then from Fifth into Fourth Position. He must have mastered
the pas chassé as an approach and such movements as the grand pas assemblé
with one turn and the revoltade, a grande cabriole derrière with a fouetté turn,
etc. The double saut de basque is different and complex and its study must be
given only to the pupils who may be able to master its technique. (This movement
as a single full turn movement is similar to the Cecchetti grand jeté en tournant
en avant except that the movement contains a rond de jambe and bent knee instead
of a perpendicular, and a leg in 45 degrees to the side.)

An exercise for the study of the movement is as follows: In a starting position
of second arabesque in profile, with the leg, toes to the floor and parallel to the
mirror, the arabesque leg moves back into a pas chassé along Second and steps
into a demi-plié with sufficient force to push off for a double saut de basque en
dedans, ending in sur le cou-de-pied. Then a 1/4 turn into the starting pose is
made onto the sur le cou-de-pied leg and the exercise is ready to be repeated
from side to side, four times. The arms in the pas chassé open into Second; at
the saut (jump), open into Third and, later, opening through Second, assume the
second arabesque position. The body, in chassé, turns en face and at the push
increases this turn to the jump, turning twice. At the end, it is still en face, and
at the transfer into second arabesque, it turns in profile. The head fixes en face.

At the final demi-plié, it turns in the direction of the advance. At the change into the starting pose, it smoothly assumes the second arabesque pose.

As an exercise: To a measure of 2/4, a pas chassé is performed before the measure; 1/4 is used for the jumping push; 1/4 for the flight and the end of the jump; 1/4 for the transfer into second arabesque; 1/4 for the demi-plié and transfer to the back leg to begin the combination again. At first the double saut de basque must be done only to one side, then to the other side with only one turn. Later, both sides may be done with a double turn.

This movement may then be incorporated into other combinations, first in its simple, then its more complicated form. After that, the study of the transfer into arabesque and on one knee should begin.

The double saut de basque may be done with a sur le cou-de-pied in back. This introduces variety and allows for an exit into Fourth Position back into small poses or to one knee.

This form is studied in the same pattern, but it is not performed on a straight line from side to side but on a diagonal upstage (toward the upper corners of the room, #4 and #6).

In the same pattern, the study may end in Fourth on one knee. In general, the saut de basque is combined in exercises done en face, parallel to the mirror, diagonally up or down and in a circle. In addition, the double saut de basque must be studied with an exit through pas tombé and tours chaînés. In the practice of the saut de basque simple combinations should progressively give way to more complicated forms. They should be practiced with the obligatory repetitions to fortify the qualities necessary for their execution. Only then should they be placed in more complicated combinations.

PAS CHASSÉ WITH A TURN (OR EN TOURNANT)

In this movement, the 1/4, 1/2 or full turn is done in flight. An example of a 1/4 turn: Beginning in third arabesque, a demi-plié and pas chassé is done toward the opposite lower corner of the room ending in attitude effacée. An example of a 1/2 turn: Beginning in second arabesque along a diagonal line in a lower corner, a pas chassé is done to the opposite upper corner of the room, with a turn toward the side of the supporting leg, ending in a fourth arabesque sauté. (The back of the pupil is toward the mirror.)

As an example of a full turn: Beginning in a first arabesque in a diagonal from a lower corner, a pas chassé is done into the same lower corner of the room with the turn to the side of the supporting leg and ending in the same pose. Or: Starting in écarté front, with the arms open into Second allongé, pas chassé into the upper corner of the room with a turn toward the side of the supporting leg, which, in flight, is led back into Fifth Position and ends in the starting pose.

The arms in the last two examples, as a rule, move energetically and with roundness, joining in a lowered First. They end opening to the starting pose. But they may open into Second allongé, or rise to Third Position. The body is straight in the air, and the head at the start of the turn is held back a little; then, before the body, it takes the starting pose. It must be added that if the turn is done *toward* the side of the supporting leg, the turn is en dedans.

If the turn is done away from the supporting leg, the turn is en dehors. In addition, all the examples may be done in reverse, with the turn reversed as well. The larger the degree of the turn, the stronger the turning sendoff must be and the higher the jump required to complete the turn.

These movements, if practiced in all their forms, teach a sense of space and give the pupil the ability to turn and be steady.

The qualities for which to strive are: elasticity at the starting and the finishing demi-plié; a sufficiently energetic advance in flight; a shapely and free plasticity in the turn; clear and coordinated movement of the arms, body and head. Special attention should be paid to the end of the jump, which should be done with a light, gliding movement of the opening leg, as it is required for the pas chassé without the turn.

The study of the turn with 1/4 or 1/2 circle turns should be practiced as given or in combinations. The full circle pas chassé may be done separately as follows: For instance, beginning in Fifth Position épaulement croisé, sissonne tombeé forward is done into third arabesque; two pas chassés in the same direction follow into the same third arabesque pose, each with a full turn en dedans; and assemblé en arrière into Fifth Position (closing back). All this is done along Second, en face, in the direction of the forward leg. Then the combination is ready to be repeated on the other leg in the opposite direction and then in reverse on both sides.

The arms in each pas chassé join in a lowered First and at the pas assemblé move into Preparatory Position. At the sissonne tombée along Second, the arms open through First into Second and at each pas chassé they join in First and at the pas assemblé they move into Preparatory Position. The body and head act as described above.

When the combination is reversed, the first sissonne tombée is done to the back; the two pas chassés are done in the direction of the leg in back in Fifth; both turns are en dehors, both assemblés are done to the front or en devant into Fifth Position. The arms, body and head act as described above. Each jump in these combinations may be done to 1/4 of a 2/4 tempo or to one 3/4 measure in a fast tempo.

The turn of a full circle may be used in combinations and as an approach to such movements as the grand assemblé en tournant, the revoltade, the grand and double saut de basque. It may also be performed as an independent movement in an accelerated tempo along a straight or diagonal line or combined with tours chaînés, etc. The movement of the arms may vary in the starting pose and in their pose during the turns.

GRAND PAS JETÉ EN TOURNANT

This movement is done in an attitude or arabesque with a turn of 1/2 circle. The jeté and the attitude are usually done from an approach such as the sissonne tombée, the temps levé tombé, and the pas failli. These approaches are tied with the pas jeté by means of the pas coupé en tournant en dehors in a 1/2 circle.

If, for instance, the grand jeté is preceded by a sissonne tombée in croisé forward, then the free leg, by doing a pas coupé, is able to push off the body by replacing the supporting leg in back in demi-plié, enabling the body at the time of the pushoff to make a 1/2 en dehors circle. In this way, with the pushing help of the pas coupé, the body may turn to the upper corner of the room for the grand jeté of a 1/2 circle and land toward the opposite lower corner of the room. If a pas failli precedes the grand jeté, then the free leg is also exchanged from a pas coupé with the supporting leg into an en dehors turn of 1/2 circle. (See illustration #153.)

---

153   Grand jeté into attitude croisée derrière from a turn in pas coupé

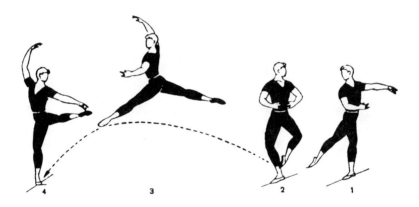

This coupé is done in the form of an elastic pushoff by the supporting leg, which, without losing the tempo of the movement, is thrown forward by means of a grand battement jeté. The other leg, after making the jumping push, is thrown in the same tempo to 90 degrees. The arms, before the coupé, in both cases are in the following position: The arm corresponding to the direction of the turn is in First, the other is in Second Position.

At the moment of the coupé, the arm from Second is forcefully moved through First into Third, and the other arm moved from First into Second. The body, at the approach, gives a slightly forward lean but straightens out at the coupé and, during the flight, rushes diagonally forward. The head, at the approach and at the coupé, is turned toward the advanced shoulder. In flight, it clearly turns along the direction of the movement. All actions during the flight are done in one tempo.

In the performance of the coupé, the pupil may sometimes try to turn and advance more than needed by putting the pushing leg not in back of the supporting leg, but in the direction of the performance of the jeté. This, of course, introduces incorrectness and carelessness into the movement. The grand jeté into first arabesque is usually done as a series in a lengthened jump with an advance diagonally or in a circle. Each of these jetés is tied with the aid of the pas coupé. At the finish of the jump, the leg that opens forward moves into a demi-plié with a turn of the body of a 1/2 circle en dedans. The leg which opens in back, in tempo, is led to the supporting leg and performs a forceful push. The free leg dashes immediately forward into the next jeté with a turn en dehors of 1/2 circle.

The arms during the demi-plié join in a lowered First Position. During the coupé, they open into first arabesque and stay to the end of the flight. The body is pulled up with a proper sendoff in the direction of the jump and the turn. The head, in flight, keeps in first arabesque position, and at the pas coupé, it clearly turns as for a small pirouette. The look is in the direction of the movement.

---

154 Grand jeté en tournant ending in first arabesque

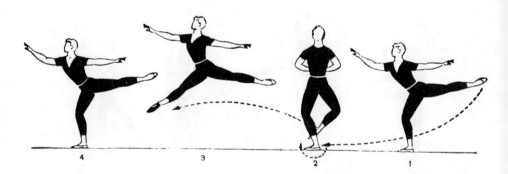

In doing this jeté, the step into Fourth must be clearly fixed, with no diminishing opening of the leg, especially in back. Otherwise, the lightness and impetus of the flight is lost. (See illustration #154.) The transfer into demi-plié and coupé must be elastic in order not to break the progressive inertia of the jump and the turn. The arms in flight must speed resolutely and exactly in their movements. The coupé must be performed energetically so the turning sendoff with the exit into the next jump may be stable and secure.

The body and its center of gravity are sent boldly but with calculation. An overly strong or too weak calculation will break the design and tempo of the movement. In performing this jeté on the diagonal or in a circle, the accent is on the jump, not the coupé. Any evenness in the tempo here would be out of place and would lead to monotony and a heavy flight. (When this step is performed in a circle leaning back at an acute angle, the step is called tour de reins—turn of the back.)

The leg in coupé must join as clearly and closely as possible to the supporting leg and make a short, light push with the supporting heel on the floor. The shoulders must be kept open, not squeezed together, especially when the jeté is done in a circle.

At times, when the pupil turns his back to the center of the circle, the shapeliness of the arabesque is marred. It is true that the performance of the jeté in a circle is based upon the mirage of a lean by the entire body away from a straight line. But it must not lean to the extent that it destroys the harmoniousness of the construction of the pose. Each jeté must be done as the continuation of the other along an uninterrupted flying line, like a spreading jump. The pas coupé should be short, fast and performed with an elastic push.

The jump is always done before the measure: Beginning in Fifth, épaulement croisé, sissonne tombée croisée and coupé-jeté with a turn into attitude croisée; end with pas assemblé croisé back. The arms and body perform as usual. The sissonne tombée starts before the 2/4 measure; 1/4 coupé; on the second 1/4 of the first measure, the jeté; on the third 1/4, pas assemblé; stop, on the fourth measure. It is repeated from the other leg. Then repeated once more.

In the following examples more complicated approaches and combinations of jumps may be used.

The study of jeté into first arabesque begins as follows: From Fifth Position, épaulement croisé, jeté is done into first arabesque onto the front leg; coupé; repeat all four times with a diagonal advance into the lower corner of the room (the starting place should be an upper corner of the room, #6); but instead of a last coupé, the series is finished with an assemblé forward into Fifth Position. This series is repeated from the other leg.

Each movement is done, at first, evenly to each first 1/4 of the measure. Later, the jeté is done with an accent on the crest of the jump. Still later, this movement may be combined in other jumps and joined with tours chaînés after the coupé.

The jeté in a circle is also studied at first with even accents, with no accent on the jump. It is performed in a series of twelve turning jumps and ends with tours chaînés and a final step into a small pose—second arabesque. It must begin in a lower corner of the room and keep to a well-defined circle ending in the opposite corner from its start.

Later, this movement may be done with the accent on the flight in a circle (en manège), then changes, after the third quarter of the circle, into a diagonal line into the lower corner of the room. This change is difficult and demands meticulous practice. (Beginning in corner #8 and traveling straight across the front or mirror of the room, the circle continues to corner #2, 3, 4, 5 and at corner #6 a sharp turn is necessary to focus on corner #2, which is the goal of the diagonal line's ending. This turn is seldom reversed on stage, although it must be practiced in the opposite direction, unless the dancer turns exceptionally well to the left.)

Mastery of this form permits a more complex form: Jeté into first arabesque on the diagonal is done with the opening of the arms into Second allongé; or the one that is contrary to the direction of the turn may be raised, while the other is in a lowered position.

The jeté in a circle (en manège), in first arabesque as described above, may be performed with an attitude instead of the arabesque. It should be high but not a drifting flight, with a smaller advance. This form requires a more energetic accent in the jump. The entire body must seem to float in air, clearly moving in a circle in a shapely yet supple series of attitudes.

GRAND JETÉ FOUETTÉ

This jump is performed from one pose into another through a fouetté movement. The pose remains in flight and changes into another with the turn of 1/4 or 1/2 of a circle.

Usually, it begins in first arabesque and ends in effacé forward in a 1/4 turn, or backward into an upper corner of the room in a 1/2 circle. (See illustration #155.)

This jeté is usually begun with an approach which makes a high jump possible in order to have an exact turn. A sissonne tombée, pas glissade, pas failli or pas de bourrée are the usual approaches.

---

155   Grand jeté in fouetté from first arabesque en l'air into effacé devant

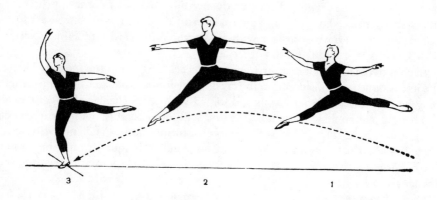

The method of performance is as follows: After one of these approaches mentioned above, such as the sissonne tombée croisée forward, the leg behind, together with a jumping push, is thrown forward to 90 degrees in a jeté that takes the first arabesque pose. At the crest or apex of the jump, the body clearly and energetically turns en dehors from the forward leg in a 1/4 circle, taking the pose effacée forward; the landing is on the leg that has done the throw.

The special feature of this jump is that the turn in the hip joint into another pose occurs at the apex of the flight with both legs and the body, instead of being a fouetté on the floor.

The arms, at the approach, move forcefully from Preparatory Position to First in flight or the pose required. During the fouetté, they immediately transfer into the final pose but without passing through First. The body, in flight, gives a bit forward and, at the ending, leans a bit to the back in accordance with the pose. The head stays turned toward the direction of the flight throughout.

In performing this jeté, all the rules for the jump and the fouetté must be observed. On the whole, the jump must flow, be light and clear during the turn, have lightness in the advance. There must be no dragging in the first pose, nor roughness in the final demi-plié. All must flow from one pose into the other freely, but with a dynamic quality.

The study, at first, is without an approach but from a pose. From a croisé forward, a jeté is done into first arabesque and back into the same pose. Then an approach is practiced: From Fifth Position, épaulement croisé, sissonne tombée forward in croisé and grand jeté into first arabesque diagonally toward a lower corner; ending in a fouetté turn of a 1/4 circle effacé forward; temps levé tombé forward in the same pose effacée and assemblé forward into Fifth Position.

In sissonne tombée, the arms move from Preparatory to First. During the flight, they assume the pose for first arabesque. At the end of the jump, the arm in first arabesque rises to Third as the other stays in Second. During the temps levé tombé, the arm in Third opens into Second and, at the assemblé, both arms descend into Preparatory Position.

The body at the sissonne and during the jeté is pulled up with a little push forward. At the end of the jump, it turns and leans a bit backward. On the temps levé it keeps leaning and, at the assemblé, straightens into the starting pose.

The head, at the approach, turns toward the hands in First and, at the jeté, is in the position for first arabesque. At the end of the jump, it is kept toward the advanced shoulder, where it remains until the end.

Then the exercise is done from the other leg and repeated on each side. Each jump is done to 1/4 of the measure.

Another example: From Fifth Position, a pas failli forward is done with a jeté into first arabesque diagonally to a lower corner, with a fouetté of 1/2 circle ending effacé forward with the student's back to the lower corner. This exercise is ended with a sontenu en tournant en dehors of a 1/2 circle and is ready to be repeated on the other leg. It is repeated on both sides. Both jumps are done to 1/4 of a 2/4 measure and the soutenu is done in one measure.

Later, a more forceful approach may be used such as the pas glissade, or pas de bourrée and combined in more complicated combinations.

GRAND JETÉ EN TOURNANT (GRAND JETÉ ENTRELACÉ)

(This movement has a variety of names, the "tour jeté" being the most frequently used misnomer. It is also called the grand jeté dessus en tournant or, in the pre-Soviet terminology, the grand jeté entrelacé—interlaced.)

This movement is done with an en dedans turn of 1/2 circle and, as a rule, into an arabesque ending. It requires maximum height in the air and therefore usually starts from a vigorous approach, such as the pas chassé in Second. In order to master the technique of this movement the components must be understood very well. First, the flight during which one leg (let us say the right leg) is thrown to a height of 90 degrees forward, as a result of the 1/2 circle fouetté, is then in back of the body. Second, the other leg (the left leg), at the same time, after doing the push, is thrown up to the right leg at 90 degrees and passes it at the point of the fouetté. Third, the leg in the back fouetté descends, having achieved at the apex of the jump the first arabesque pose. (Hence the word entrelacé. When a battu is added, the interlacing is more apparent.) (See illustration #156.)

---

156 Preparation and grand jeté en tournant ending in first arabesque

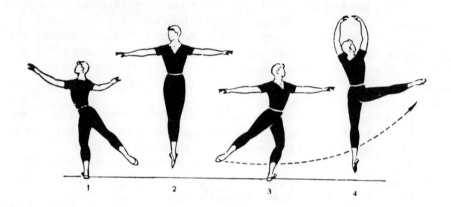

It should be clear from this explanation that the first element to master is the fouetté with the jump 1/2 circle and the jeté passé. Then the study of the grand jeté en tournant, a complex movement which needs much practice, may begin.

In the performance of this jeté the following rules must be strictly observed: The approach, pas chassé, may start from a small arabesque pose or a jump, but it must always be energetic with a strong sendoff into a large jump without an advance. The pas chassé form, along Second, must be very exact. It must not become a stocky, squat backward run, which has no place in classical dance. During the performance of the pas chassé, the legs in flight must be well stretched and joined in Fifth Position, with the leg that does the push in back. At the moment of ending the pas chassé, the body makes a clear turn of 1/4 circle. The leg which moves forward from the pas chassé elastically transfers the weight from the toes through the foot to the heel to perform the jumping push. In the performance of the jeté itself, the first throw of the leg must be done forcefully and exactly *through First and not in Second Position*. During the flight, the pushing leg must be just as forcefully thrown back in the fouetté. At the crest of the jump, the legs must meet, pass closely but not touch. Both throws of the legs must be strong, light, and clear, but not rough. The final pose in arabesque must be achieved in the air before landing. The leg must not be lowered from 90 degrees in the arabesque ending. The landing leg must not be thrown forward but must descend vertically into demi-plié. And, finally, the legs during this movement must be turned out, straight in flight and elastic in demi-plié.

The legs must move freely and clearly, keeping the accent at the crest of the jump. The arms in pas chassé, as a rule, open to Second. In the jeté, together with the first throw of the leg, they move forcefully through Preparatory and up through First into Third so that, together with the turn in the air and the end of the second throw of the leg, they may lower into a first arabesque position.

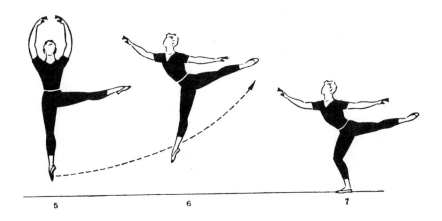

5   6   7

If the jeté ends effacé, then the pose is first or second arabesque. If the ending is in croisé, then third or fourth arabesque arms end the movement. On the whole, the arms must act with pliability, exactly accenting the moment of the flight, then transfer into arabesque position.

The body, during the pas chassé, is totally straight. At the push and jeté, it gives exactly onto the supporting leg and participates actively in the jumping and turning sendoff.

The head, during the chassé, is turned toward the advanced shoulder and at the first throw clearly moves in the same direction.

On the whole, this jeté must be done in a crisp tempo and with a soaring flight. If, after this jeté, a jump with an advance backward or forward is required, then the final demi-plié landing must be considered an approach for the next movement, such as a pas de bourrée en tournant, etc.

The choreographer, in staging this jeté, may give this movement, as well as the others, a most varied tempo and plastic character. But in the school, this movement must be studied in its fullness and in high flight. Then its technique may become a forceful and vivid means of expression for the acting powers of the dancer.

The study must begin in first arabesque, from pas tombé. The place is a lower corner of the room with a starting pose of second arabesque, as a small pose with the toes on the floor. From this position, a fouetté en dehors of 1/2 circle is done at the same time as the supporting leg does a relevé to demi-pointe and the fouetté leg opens to 45 degrees. Then a pas tombé forward is done and a jumping push as described above. All is repeated four times from one leg and four times from the other. The tempo is 4/4: 1/4 for the fouetté; 1/4 for the pas tombé; 1/4 for the jeté; 1/4 for the rest.

After this exercise has been well learned, the study may begin from pas chassé, at first with a stop after the jeté, then without the stop. For instance: Starting from the same position, a pas chassé is done diagonally to an upper corner; followed by the jeté into first arabesque and a relevé onto demi-pointe in the same pose; a passing demi-plié prepares the way to continue the movement four times in the same direction. It should then be repeated from the other leg. The tempo is the same: pas chassé to 1/4; jeté to 1/4; relevé and demi-plié to 2/4.

Later, it may be performed in a circle pattern keeping strictly to the rules.

In the male graduating class, this jeté may be done in a 3/4 circle which demands more force in the turning sendoff. Beginning in an upper corner of the room in a starting pose of second arabesque facing back to the mirror and on demi-pointe, a pas chassé is done along Second diagonally from the upper back corner.

The first throw is not forward but to the side along Second Position. The rest of the movement is the same and ends after a 3/4 circle in first arabesque on a diagonal facing downstage.

The movement of the arms, head and body are the same as for the jeté with the 1/2 circle turn. The first throw of the leg is done here to the side in regard to the body, in order to shorten the fouetté to a 1/4 circle and, in this way, make the turn more freely. This method somewhat breaks the plastic character of this movement, but it allows an increase in the degree of the turn of the body in the jump and, therefore, increases virtuosity.

In addition, it is useful, in the graduating class, to perform the usual 1/2 circle jeté from the same big jump ending in first arabesque, as, for instance, from a grand pas jeté in a rebounding form. The first throw is done forward without delay directly from a demi-plié ending the preceding movement. In this way, the end of the grand jeté is at the same time the beginning of the next thrown jeté.

By the use of the same method, a thrown jeté may be done side to side from a preceding grand temps levé into a first arabesque. This demands great force and exact calculation since the directions of the turns do not coincide. However, in practice, this exercise is very useful. It develops the ability to switch from a complicated approach to a turn in the opposite direction.

The jeté with the pas chassé approach and with the 1/2 turn may be done a few times in succession along a diagonal or in a circle, but the exactness of the movements must be strictly maintained.

In the male classes, this movement may end with a turn from pose into pose through a fouetté. (See illustration #157.) In that case, the pose in arabesque must be fixed at 90 degrees in flight, but at the moment of the close to the ending of the jump, a turn en dehors of a 1/2 circle is done through a fouetté into the pose effacée forward at 90 degrees. The final end of the jump is done in this pose or with a transfer from it into pas tombé, if the following movement requires such a beginning. Usually, this jeté is done on a diagonal line from an upper to a lower corner of the room, or the opposite, from a lower to an upper corner.

For instance: Beginning in the upper corner of the room, in a starting pose of second arabesque, the leg is slightly raised; a pas chassé along Second is done into the lower corner of the room, followed by a grand jeté en tournant, in which both throws are done in the same direction and the last ends, through a fouetté, en dehors of 1/2 circle.

In this way, a turn from pose into pose culminates at the moment the body lowers from the crest of the jump.

---

157 Change from first arabesque through fouetté en l'air into ending in effacé in demi-plié

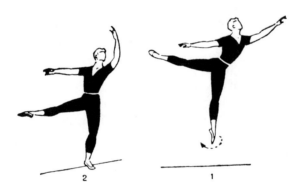

The approach to this jeté must always be as energetic as the jumping push and the turning sendoff. The entire body turns in a full circle, which requires a corresponding effort and resolve.

All the rules pertaining to the jeté to 1/2 circle and the fouetté to 1/2 circle must be observed. The flow of the movement must be free and clear.

The arms, head and body follow the positions required and accepted for the grand jeté with a turn and for a pose to another pose, by means of a fouetté.

The study includes stops, then without. The movement is then incorporated into simple and, later, into more complicated combinations, with an exit into pas tombé. The study of this movement is done only in the graduating class.

TEMPS LEVÉ SIMPLE EN TOURNANT

This step may be done in 1/4, 1/2 or 3/4 circles. For instance: Beginning with a sur le cou-de-pied front, épaulement croisé, a demi-plié is done and a jump with a turn en dehors to 1/4 circle; ending in a demi-plié, épaulement effacé.

Before the jump, the arm corresponding to the supporting leg is in a lowered First and the other in Second. In flight, both arms exchange positions at the same time and remain in that position until the final demi-plié. The body is held straight with a hardly visible bend toward the shoulder opposite the supporting leg. In the jump, the body straightens and turns toward the shoulder *corresponding* to the supporting leg.

The head, during the first demi-plié, is turned toward the advanced shoulder and in flight turns toward the other shoulder, where it stays until the final demi-plié.

Another example: Starting in sur le cou-de-pied back, épaulement croisé, a demi-plié is done and a jump en dehors to 1/2 circle. During this movement, the free leg stays as close as possible to the other leg, but not touching it, and moves into sur le cou-de-pied front. This makes it easier to turn the half circle. The jump ends with the student's back to the mirror.

Before the jump, the arm opposite the supporting leg is in a lowered First and the other in Second. In the jump, they exchange places at the same time and remain in the same position through the final demi-plié. The body is straight with a very slight lean toward the shoulder corresponding to the supporting leg. In flight, it straightens, turns and, on the final demi-plié, leans slightly toward the shoulder corresponding to the supporting leg. The head, before the jump, is turned toward the back shoulder. In flight, it turns to the opposite shoulder and stays in that position until the end of the jump.

At the same time, according to the given directions, the leanings of the body and the head may be reversed, or combined. Additionally, the turn of a 1/2 circle may be done en dedans starting from sur le cou-de-pied front and ending in back.

Like the turn of a 1/4 circle, the 1/2 circle turn may end in a small pose depending upon the preceding and its following movement. The temps levé simple with a 3/4 circle turn is done in the same manner as the turn of 1/2 circle, except that the degree and force of the turning push must be correspondingly increased. The actions of the head and body are the same as for the previous patterns.

In this jump to 1/4, 1/2 and 3/4 circles, there must be lightness and an elastic turning push by the supporting leg from demi-plié as well as a fully stretched leg in flight—the one that is not in sur le cou-de-pied. The sur le cou-de-pied foot must be kept exactly and without rigidity, in a high sur le cou-de-pied position that is turned out throughout the movement. The arms must move with exactness, but freely with no extra pressure. The center of gravity must be kept exactly over the supporting leg without a belated or anticipated sendoff for the flight. The lean of the body is done lightly, with a feeling of plasticity. The head turns clearly and freely, as do the arms and body. The eyes look forward in the same direction as the head. In performing this movement, the entire body must participate actively in the turning sendoff, but it should be done with freedom and stability. The greater the degree of the turn, the higher the jump required. The final demi-plié must be done in coordination with the tempo of the measure and in the character of the movement that is to follow.

The study of the turn to 1/4 and 1/2 circle may be done as follows: Starting in sur le cou-de-pied back, épaulement croisé, three temps levés simples are done with a turn en dedans of 1/4 circle followed by a pas emboîté sauté with a turn in the same direction of 1/2 circle. It is then repeated from the other leg; once more to the first side and reversed to the other side. All the jumps are to an even 1/4 or a 2/4 measure.

The arms, head and body follow the previous pattern. The study of turns to 1/2 and 3/4 of a circle may be joined with a petit jeté, petit ballonné, etc.

Examples like these are countless, but all must be repeatable, logical in development and done with stability.

TEMPS LEVÉ TOMBÉ EN TOURNANT

This movement is a development of the preceding temps levé and is done in a 1/4, 1/2 or 3/4 circle. For instance, starting in a sur le cou-de-pied front, épaulement croisé, a demi-plié is done and a flight with a turn en dehors in 1/4 circle with an advance toward a lower corner of the room. The jump ends on the leg which did the pushoff and the demi-plié, as the other leg, with a light, gliding movement along the floor, opens into effacé front into a tombé.

The movement ends in first arabesque to 45 degrees, followed by an assemblé derrière into Fifth Position, or another ending. The arms, during the first demi-plié, are in Preparatory Position. In flight, the arms rise into a lowered First. In the tombé, they assume the position for second arabesque. The body, during the flight, is straight. During the tombé, it lightly leans forward. The head, in the demi-plié, is turned toward the advanced shoulder, and in flight turns toward the other shoulder, where it remains to the tombé. The movement must flow and be elastic with a clear advance and a soft fixing of the final pose.

The turn of a 1/2 circle is the same but the push for the jump and the turn must be stronger. The start and final position of the arms may vary depending upon the given instructions. The turn to 1/2 of a circle is done at the crest of the jump. The change of sur le cou-de-pied is done as in the temps levé simple.

The study of this movement with turns of 1/4 and 1/2 circle may be separate or in a combination, to a slow 3/4 tempo in the following exercise: Starting in Fifth Position, épaulement croisé, a sissonne simple is done to the back without a turn; temps levé tombé with a 3/4 circle turn en dehors changing to sur le cou-de-pied into croisé front; end with a petit assemblé derrière into Fifth Position. The same exercise is done along Second, repeated and reversed. Each jump is done to each 1/4 of the measure. The head, arms and body conform to various small poses to make the turn easier to perform.

TEMPS LEVÉ IN POSES WITH A TURN

This jump is performed with large poses and a turn of 1/4, 1/2 or a full circle. It usually begins from a movement that enables an energetic turning, trajecting the entire body with a flow in the direction of the turn. The movement may be a pas tombé, sissonne tombée, temps levé tombé, sissonne ouverte, pas failli, etc.

For instance, a sissonne tombée in first arabesque is performed, followed by a jump with a turn en dedans of 1/4 or 1/2 circle in the same pose.

In doing sissonne ouverte in pose écartée to the back, one may go into a temps levé in the same pose, with a turn en dehors of 1/4 or 1/2 circle. Or, after a pas chassé along Second diagonally to an upper corner of the room, move into temps levé in à la seconde at 90 degrees in the jump.

The turn here would be en dedans in a full circle. The arms are usually fixed in Third and the pas chassé requires a vigorous and calculated approach as for the grand saut de basque.

Independent of the pose, the direction or the degree of the turn, the jumping push must be done by the supporting leg with a short demi-plié that is supple and with the active participation of the entire body. But all this must be done lightly and with no extra effort and according to the rules of the pose performed. Each jump must be soft with the pose kept exactly.

The study may begin as follows: Starting in Fifth Position, épaulement croisé, a sissonne tombée forward in effacé, ending in first arabesque, is performed, followed by three temps levé in the same pose, each with a turn of 1/4 circle en dedans. Then a bourrée en tournant with a change of legs into Fifth Position follows and three small entrechats quatre end the combination.

All is done from the other leg, repeated again and reversed.

The head, arms and body follow the rules for each movement to a measure of 2/4. The first four jumps are done on each 1/4 of the measure; the pas de bourrée en tournant to one measure; the three entrechats, to 1/8 each.

To compose an exercise for the study of this movement with a turn of 1/4 circle in poses along Second, the suggestions for the exercises with a jump with a 1/2 circle turn may be followed.

The first exercise for the turn of a full circle may be as follows: Beginning in a small second arabesque pose facing an upper corner of the room, a pas chassé along Second en face is performed; in the same direction a temps levé with a throw of the free leg through First into Second to 90 degrees and a turn en dedans of a full circle follows. This movement is fixed during the jump and at the end in an à la seconde.

The arms in pas chassé open into Second and at the push and jump are thrown through Preparatory Position into Third, where they remain. The body is straight and exactly over the supporting leg. The head during the pas chassé stays en face but in flight turns toward the thrown leg and remains there until the final demi-plié. The look is in the direction of the turn of the head. (It prevents eyes wandering to the mirror to see how the jump is progressing!)

After the pas chassé is repeated, followed by a relevé to demi-pointe into second arabesque, the exercise may be repeated on the other side. The tempo may be 3/4. All the elements are performed in an even tempo with an accent on the temps levé in the first part of the first measure. (The pas chassé begins before the measure.)

A pliable yet strong sendoff of the body must be practiced without an advance for this movement. It requires a free and exact fixing of the pose and a supple, stable end to the jump. Later, the movement may be done in a full circle turn from a pas chassé on the diagonal combined with other large jumps.

TEMPS LEVÉ FROM ONE POSE INTO ANOTHER

This movement may be done through a développé, a grand rond de jambe en l'air or a fouetté. They will be examined in that order.

TEMPS LEVÉ DÉVELOPPÉ

This movement is done in a 1/4 circle with a starting pose, écarté to an upper corner on the diagonal. The jump, during which the free leg passes at the knee into a croisé forward, turns en dedans in 1/4 of a circle.

The arms during the jump change positions. The arm corresponding to the supporting leg rises from Second into Third, and the other, from Third moves into Second. The body is kept straight and exactly over the supporting leg. The head, in the jump, turns toward the advanced shoulder.

This jump may be done in reverse with a turn of en dehors of 1/4 of a circle ending in third arabesque or attitude croisée back.

Another example: Starting in croisé forward, the jump and turn en dedans of 1/4 circle transfer the leg through passé at the knee into third arabesque. The arms in the jump move through First into third arabesque. The body, in the jump, is straight, and at the end leans a bit forward but exactly over the supporting leg. The head turns to face the lower corner of the room.

These jumps must flow, be clear and high, and observe all the rules in order to create a suppleness in the movement of the head, arms and body. The legs must at all times be turned out. The pushing leg must stretch fully from the hip to the toes as the free leg bends in the passé position and moves through it into the final pose. All the rules for a pliable and unhindered développé at 90 degrees must be followed. The arms move in time with the leg, the design at the start and the finish of the movement. The body is kept gracefully collected and pulled up, with only the slightest bend required for the given pose.

The performance of jumps demands active participation in the entire figure for a calculated, forceful and stable descent.

The study must join these jumps with sissonne ouverte and other movements involved with the performance of big poses, as in the following exercise: Sissonne ouverte into écarté to an upper corner on the diagonal; a temps levé is performed with a turn en dedans to 1/4 of a circle into écarté forward; followed by a grand jeté into third arabesque and a petit assemblé derrière. The same may be repeated from the other leg, repeated and reversed once more. The tempo is 2/4 or 3/4. In the 2/4 measure, each jump is to 1/4 of the measure. In the 3/4 tempo, each jump is done to each measure.

This jump may begin from the sur le cou-de-pied position and end in a big pose at 90 degrees. All the rules are to be observed, but the free leg in the jump from sur le cou-de-pied rises to the knee and opens through développé at the *start of the final demi-plié* in the proper direction with a turn of the body of 1/4 circle.

The arms, head and body act according to the given pose. For instance, beginning with the supporting leg in demi-plié, the other in sur le cou-de-pied back, épaulement croisé, a temps levé with a turn en dedans in 1/4 circle is made into first arabesque. The arm corresponding to the supporting leg is in First, the other is in Second. The body is straight and the head turned toward the advanced shoulder.

It is a possibility that should not be excluded, to use this jump with the leg opening to 45 degrees, in combinations.

TEMPS LEVÉ—GRAND ROND DE JAMBE EN L'AIR

This jump is done with a turn of 1/4, 1/2 or a full circle. The energetic transfer of the open leg permits a forceful resilience for the performance of the turn which adds an element of virtuosity.

The turn of 1/4 circle is done through the transfer of the open leg from a pose along Second into a pose along Fourth en arrière (to the back).

The turn of 1/2 circle is done through the transfer of the open leg from Fourth devant into a pose along Fourth en arrière. For instance: From écarté front, a turn of 1/4 en dehors into third arabesque accomplishes the transfer in grand rond de jambe en l'air. Another example: From croisé forward, a turn of 1/2 circle en dehors into third arabesque.

The arms, body and head act according to their rules as in temps levé, the starting pose, the jumping push, the rond de jambe with a change of arms, the finish of the jump and final pose.

The body must participate with vigor in all the turns which must be done from the most convenient position from which to rebound in the jump. The arms must be in a comfortable position especially in the 1/2 circle turns. The legs, from a preceding jump such as the sissonne ouverte, must have a forceful and elastic push. The body aids in the ease of performing movement of the legs. The arm movements contribute to the turn of the body which, at the crest of the jump, is a speedy dash in the proper direction kept in the required form.

The head, during the jump, turns surely and together with the body, and keeps its position in space at the time of the turn.

On the whole, the movement must flow, balloon with lightness and descend with softness.

To a measure of 3/4 and from a pose of Fifth Position épaulement croisé, the study may begin with a sissonne ouverte in écarté to an upper corner. A temps levé with a turn en dehors of 1/4 circle into third arabesque and a petit assemblé into Fifth derrière complete the exercise. This is performed on the other leg, repeated and reversed. Each jump is done to one measure with a stop on the fourth measure.

The jump of 1/2 circle may be studied with a grande sissonne in a simple combination: sissonne ouverte in croisé devant; temps levé with a 1/2 circle turn en dehors into third arabesque; two pas emboîtés with a 1/2 circle turn in the same direction, petit assemblé en arrière into Fifth Position ending in épaulement croisé. Repeat this combination on the other leg, begin again and reverse.

The tempo is 2/4. The first two jumps are on each 1/4 note, and the following three jumps are on 1/8 notes each.

Later, the jump of 1/2 circle may be introduced into more complicated goals.

There is another form of temps levé with a turn en dehors of a full circle, which is done as a series in a diagonal from an upper to a lower corner of the room. This diagonal begins with a sissonne tombée in effacé devant; followed by a pas coupé behind the supporting leg; a temps levé with a rond de jambe jeté into third arabesque at 90 degrees; a pas de bourrée en tournant with a transfer into Fourth effacé devant where it begins again with the pas coupé, etc.

The arms during the sissonne tombée move from Preparatory Position into First for the arm corresponding to the direction of the turn, and into Second through First for the other arm. In the pas coupé, they remain in the same position, but on the temps levé they open with energy into third arabesque position and remain there until the final demi-plié. During the pas de bourrée, they join in a lowered First and, in the jump, open again into third arabesque. The body, during the pas tombé, leans forward toward the leg and in flight, and in the final demi-plié, remains in the same position. During the pas de bourrée, it straightens again, etc.

The head during the sissonne tombée is turned with the face in the direction of the advance. At the pas coupé, in the jump and at the finish, it turns with the body. During the pas de bourrée, it lags behind a bit, then returns to the starting position before the body arrives to its position (as in a pirouette).

On the whole, these turns must be performed in a solid tempo, with an uninterrupted and clear change from one jump to another.

The study of this movement on the diagonal should be performed in a somewhat slowed tempo and number four to six turns, ending each pas de bourrée in a Fifth Position followed by a clear movement into effacé for the sissonne tombée devant. The measure for this study may be 2/4 with the sissonne tombée done before the measure, the pas coupé and temps levé on 1/8 of the measure and the pas de bourrée en tournant in 2/4.

When the turn has strengthened, the movement may be done in a quick waltz, 3/4 tempo. At this point, the study may exclude the sissonne tombée on the diagonal and end with the pas de bourrée into a Fourth Position which prepares for the next turn. In this case, the pas coupé, temps levé and pas de bourrée are done in one measure of 2/4. In this movement, if a 3/4 tempo is used in a quick tempo, the pas coupé is done in 1/4 of the measure, the temps levé and its end in 2/4, and the pas de bourrée to a whole measure.

TEMPS LEVÉ—FOUETTÉ

This jump is done with a 1/4, 1/2 and full circle turn. It has the characteristics examined previously in the chapter on turns and spins on the floor (par terre).

Here, they are described only as a jump, and in conjunction with the fouetté and its study.

This jump may begin from any large pose. The fouetté portion of this movement is done in the second pose, which is fixed at the finishing demi-plié. For instance, if the jump is begun in a pose écartée to a back corner of the room and must turn 1/4 of a circle into first arabesque, it changes into this pose in the fouetté performed at the crest of the jump. Or, beginning from a second arabesque from an upper corner of the room on the diagonal, a turn en dehors of 1/2 circle through the fouetté movement will end the movement in an effacé devant.

The arms, head and body, which are in the pose of the Preparatory Position for the jump, change in flight into the pose for the given final position following all the rules for port de bras, etc. The supporting leg must perform the jumping push with resilience, be stretched fully during the turn, and the working leg held in an exact 90-degree position, stretched especially at the end of the jump. A strict turnout must be kept, and the usual soft ending is obligatory.

The turn in the air must be light, with no obvious strain in the body or, especially, in the arms. The beginning and ending poses must be clear in design and the body in the air must be pulled up, collected, and otherwise correctly placed with its center of gravity over the supporting leg in the air as well as in the descent.

In the study of this movement, it is advisable to permit the student to sense the characteristics of movement through a form already known to him, the battement divisé en quarts. This exercise is complicated by the addition of the jump and the following rise to demi-pointe with the simultaneous fixing of the open leg at 90 degrees. The jump here takes the place of the relevé to demi-pointe, with a turn en dehors or en dedans of 1/4 circle.

The working leg bends into the passé knee position and the supporting leg remains on demi-pointe. All is repeated again. The arms, head and body follow the performance for the movement as done on the floor (par terre).

The jumps in temps levé with a turn en dedans of 1/2 circle may be done from any approach along Fourth forward, like the sissonne tombée, the pas chassé, pas glissade or the pas failli. If such an approach is used, the jump is performed with the aid of a grand battement jeté forward through First into Fourth. The glide of the leg through First in this case must coincide with the resilient demi-plié of the supporting leg and the turning sendoff of the entire body.

The arms move with the energy previously described for jumps in the air and perform at the same time as the throw of the leg. They rise through First into Third and open into the final pose. The head and body perform as usual but with a stronger accent in the flight. The grand fouetté, discussed in the turns-on-the-floor section of this book, applies here with the reminder that the rules for temps levé must be applied as well. The rules for the performance on demi-pointe and for a jump with a turn must be observed as well.

The grand fouetté, different from the performance on demi-pointe, may begin with a petit jeté or a pas coupé, instead of the demi-pointe movement.

ROND DE JAMBE EN L'AIR EN TOURNANT

This movement is based upon the temps levé and is performed with a turn en dehors or en dedans in 1/4 circle.

For instance, beginning in a Fifth Position, épaulement croisé, simultaneously a throw of the front leg to the side at 45 degrees is done with a jump en dehors with a 1/4 circle turn. At the crest of the jump, the thrown leg executes a small rond de jambe en dehors and ends together with the demi-plié of the supporting leg. All is repeated three times in a row, not from Fifth Position, but from the open position at 45 degrees. Then a pas de bourrée en tournant is done with a turn in the same direction, ending in Fifth Position, from where two small pirouettes en dehors may be done, ending in a Fifth Position front in the first turn, and in Fifth Position in back on the second turn. This enables the exercise to be repeated on the other side, and reversed.

The arms move from Preparatory and into Second through First at the first jump, and remain in this position for the next three jumps. During the pas de bourrée they lower into Preparatory Position once more and, at the end, the arm coinciding with the direction of the turn goes into First, as the other arm goes into Second. At the pirouette, the arms are in a lowered First Position.

The body is kept straight and exactly over the supporting leg, lightly corresponding to the plastic movement of the head.

The head, during the rond de jambe en dehors, is turned toward the open leg and is slightly bent forward. In performing the rond de jambe en dedans, the head leans slightly backward. During the pas de bourrée, and the two pirouettes, it is straight and performs according to the rules for turns.

All this must be done with a flow, a clear and stable design. The turning and jumping pushes must collect and pull up the body.

The study of this movement should begin with the simple form from Fifth Position, then be studied from the open position ending in a petit assemblé in both cases. The preliminary exercises may be done to 2/4 with no stops. Later, a 3/4 measure may be used. This jump is combined into the enchaînement of the more advanced and graduating classes, as a double rond de jambe, after it is mastered in its simple form.

PAS BALLONNÉ EN TOURNANT

This movement is also based upon the temps levé and is divided into petit and grand forms.

PETIT PAS BALLONNÉ

The jump is done in various poses with the leg opening to 45 degrees devant, à la seconde and en arrière (front, side and back). The turn is 1/4 circle en dehors and en dedans. For instance, beginning in Fifth Position épaulement croisé, four pas ballonnés forward are done each with a 1/4 circle turn en dehors, followed by a grand jeté into first arabesque. This is followed by pas ballonné devant through First Position in croisé devant; a grand jeté en avant into attitude croisée with an ending of assemblé derrière into Fifth Position.

The arms on the first ballonné move from Preparatory Position to Second for the one corresponding to the direction of the turn, and First for the other. They remain in this position for the three following ballonnés. During the first grand jeté, the arms rush into first arabesque position and, during the following ballonnés, return to the former position. During the second grand jeté they move into Second and, at the assemblé, move into Preparatory Position.

The body, during the four ballonnés, leans slightly backward. During the jeté into first arabesque, it leans slightly forward. During the second ballonné and second jeté, it straightens.

The head, during the four ballonnés, leans very slightly in the direction of the body's movement, turning toward the advanced shoulder. During the first jeté, it turns in profile and, at the pas ballonné, it assumes the position as in the beginning and remains there during the second jeté and pas assemblé.

The exercise must be done lightly, clearly and with a gradual strengthening of the second part in the force and height of the jump. This is except for the pas assemblé, which must be small and an ending movement.

Another example: Beginning in Fifth, épaulement croisé, four ballonnés are performed to the side, each with a turn en dehors of 1/4 circle; followed by two jetés with an advance to the side and in 1/2 circle; followed by a grand jeté opening into écarté to an upper corner of the room on the diagonal and ending with a petit assemblé front into Fifth Position.

The arms, during the first ballonné, open from Preparatory through First into Second Position and remain there for the next three jumps. During the first jeté with an advance to the side, the arms are in an allongé position during the jump, and at the end of the jump the arm opposite the direction of the turn goes into First as the other stays in Second.

During the second jeté the arms, by the same means, change positions. At the grand jeté and écarté movement, they open through allongé into Second and at the assemblé return to the Preparatory Position.

The body, during all the jumps, is straight but leans with a slight nuance according to the rules of the performance of each movement.

The head, in all the ballonnés, is turned toward the working leg and, during the two jetés, with the advance, moves according to the rules of that movement. During the grand jeté into écarté, it turns toward the advanced shoulder and remains there at the final assemblé.

The exercise is repeated from the other leg and is reversed. The tempo is 2/4; all jumps are done to each 1/4 of the measure with lightness and flexibility and a gradual increase in the size of the jump in the second half of the exercise.

This pas ballonné may be done alternating from the right to the left leg using a pas coupé approach and turning in the same 1/4 circles. In this case, the tempo is better at 3/4 so the push, jump and ending demi-plié may be done on each 1/4 of the measure.

In general, the petit pas ballonné with a 1/4 circle turn may be done in various rhythms but it must always be fluid and in character with the other movements in the combination.

The study should be simple with no further complications needed. As an example: The first part of the given exercise may be done within any combination and the second part may be structured from simple small jumps or simple entrechats.

Later the movement must be gradually complicated. Still later, it may be performed with a fouetté turn of 1/4 or 1/2 circle in this manner: The jump may start from an open leg in a small pose or in effacé forward and end with a turn en dedans of 1/4 circle in sur le cou-de-pied back. The same may be done in reverse or with a turn of 1/2 circle ending the jump back into a lower corner of the room.

The study should begin for pas ballonné without the turns, then be combined with other small jumps according to the rules for the fouetté.

GRAND PAS BALLONNÉ

This movement is done with a turn of 1/2, full or double circle. As an example: Beginning in first arabesque in profile on a high demi-pointe, a pas chassé is done en face along Second with a grand pas ballonné in Second Position turning en dedans in a 1/2 circle. (The stop is with the back to the mirror in a heightened sur le cou-de-pied front position.) From this position, a temps levé simple is performed with a turn en dedans of a 1/2 circle with a transfer of the free leg into sur le cou-de-pied back, ending the exercise with a grande cabriole into second arabesque.

The arms in the pas chassé are opened to Second, and at the pas ballonné move through Preparatory and First into Third. During the temps levé simple, they are fixed in this position, and at the cabriole, they open into second arabesque.

The body is always straight except in the second arabesque, where it leans a bit forward.

The head, during the pas chassé, turns en face, and at the ballonné turns in the direction of the throw of the free leg and remains there during the temps levé simple.

All is repeated from the other leg and repeated again on both sides.

This jump is not done in reverse. The tempo may be 2/4 or 3/4. In the 2/4 tempo, each jump is done to 1/4 of the measure, and, in the 3/4 tempo, the whole measure is used.

This pas ballonné may be done a full turn in the same direction, but it continues differently. In its performance, the pose in the jump in à la seconde position at 90 degrees must be firmly fixed and lowered into a heightened sur le cou-de-pied position only at the end of the descent in demi-plié. An elastic and resilient push is required for the jump, and a stable finishing demi-plié.

This movement is done by the graduating class with double turns, but only by the pupils who have an excellent technique. In this case, the throw of the leg from the same approach is done into Second, not to 90 degrees but to 45 degrees, and it is led at once into the heightened sur le cou-de-pied forward position. This method is very much like the performance of the grand assemblé with a double turn, only in this case the moment of flight is fixed, not in the Fifth Position, but in sur le cou-de-pied front, and it ends on one leg instead of two legs.

The finish of the double turn may be done fermé (closed) into Fifth Position or ended in pas tombé forward.

The study of pas ballonné may start after grand assemblé and the grand saut de basque with a double turn has been mastered.

An example: Beginning in second arabesque, a pas chassé along Second is performed, followed by a pas ballonné with a double turn en dedans; and a temps levé tombé croisé devant follows with a jeté back into second arabesque. Then the position is ready to begin the movement from the other leg and to be repeated on each leg again.

After this, the pas ballonné may be executed, ending with a closed Fifth Position front and a tombé into Fourth. It is then introduced into other complex combinations.

The arms and body, in the pas ballonné with a double turn, act as described above, although there might be some deviation. For instance, in the jump, the arm corresponding to the opening leg may be moved into First instead of Third, or both arms may join, rounded, in a lowered First.

The head, in the jump, acts as for the grand assemblé or the grand saut de basque with a double turn.

In performing the grand pas ballonné with a double turn, the push must be stronger, more rebounding and be collected into a clear, short and powerful thrust. This applies in particular to the movement of the arms.

Finally, the grand pas ballonné may be done through a fouetté movement in a 1/4 or 1/2 circle in the pattern of the small, or petit pas ballonné. For instance, in Fifth Position, a pas failli is done followed by a grand pas ballonné through First devant in 90 degrees into effacé with a turn en dedans of 1/4 circle ending in a pose écartée toward the lower corner of the room. This jump ends in sur le cou-de-pied back, épaulement effacé. From this position, further in the study, a grand jeté en tournant may be done.

The arms in the failli perform as usual and at the grand pas ballonné in flight, the arm opposite to the thrown leg moves through Preparatory Position into First as the other remains in Second.

At the moment of the turn in écarté, the arm in the First Position opens into Second, and the other stays in Second. At the end of the jump, the arm corresponding to the bending leg moves from Second into First, and the other stays in Second.

The body, in the pas failli, performs as usual, but in the pas ballonné it leans slightly backward in flight. During the fouetté turn, it straightens, and at the end of the jump, leans slightly backward.

The head, at the pas failli and pas ballonné, during the flight, is turned toward the advanced shoulder. During the fouetté, it turns toward the other shoulder and remains there until the end of the jump.

The same pas ballonné may start in a croisé forward position from a sissonne tombée approach in effacé forward, or it may be done with a fouetté turn of 1/2 circle. Then the jump will end in the lower corner of the room, where it started. This jump is never reversed since it would be a very awkward movement in the learning progression of this movement and would answer no purpose.

In performing this grand pas ballonné by means of a fouetté, the look must always be a flying design, culminating in a fixed and clear pose. The open leg must never descend into the sur le cou-de-pied position ahead of time, but be closed with energy into the heightened sur le cou-de-pied and joined into the supple finishing demi-plié.

The arms, head and body must participate totally in the turning push with a feeling for the plasticity of the jump, but showing no extra effort.

The study of pas ballonné with a fouetté turn should be combined with petit ballonné without the turn and then studied from the approach of a big jump.

CABRIOLE EN TOURNANT

This movement is done with a turn of 1/4, or 1/2 circle in 45-degree and 90-degree poses, turning en dehors and en dedans.

The performance of temps levé with a turn and cabriole has already been described. Here is a description only of two contributory elements.

The cabriole without a change of pose may be done in a 45- or 90-degree pose with an en dedans or en dehors turn. As in: Beginning in Fifth Position, épaulement croisé, with a sissonne tombée into first arabesque at 45 degrees. This is followed by three cabrioles in the same pose, each with a turn en dedans of 1/4 circle, followed by a jeté passé into third arabesque to 90 degrees and two cabrioles in that pose with a turn en dedans of 1/2 circle and an assemblé derrière into Fifth Position.

The arms in sissonne tombée from Preparatory Position rise through First into first arabesque and remain through all the cabrioles until the final assemblé, when they lower into Preparatory Position.

The body, during the sissonne tombée, leans a bit forward toward the supporting leg and remains there for all the cabrioles in strict coordination with the arabesque pose. At the final assemblé, it assumes the starting position. The head in all the cabrioles turns with the body, keeping all the rules of the arabesque. In the final assemblé, it turns toward the advanced shoulder, assuming the starting pose.

It is all repeated from the other leg and reversed. The tempo is 2/4 with each jump on 1/4 of the measure.

Of course, the study of the cabriole en tournant cannot begin with such a complicated exercise, but its description gives a clear idea of the basic characteristics of this movement. This cabriole may begin from the same position and approaches as were described for the cabriole without a turn. Naturally, the same rules apply.

The study should begin with a simple exercise. Sissonne ouverte is done into third arabesque at 45 degrees, followed by two cabrioles in the same pose with a turn en dehors of 1/4 circle and an assemblé derrière into Fifth Position ending with the student's back to the mirror.

This exercise is repeated four times, then practiced separately in reverse to a 2/4 measure, 1/4 for each jump.

More difficult exercises follow this example and include small jumps or sissonne simple, temps levé simple or a petit pas jeté, etc.

Then the cabriole is performed at 90 degrees in the same tempo and, to add to the complexity, the cabriole at 45 degrees is included with small beats, other small jumps and turns. Finally, these cabrioles may be done in combinations closing into Fifth Position or in tombé into Fourth.

CABRIOLE WITH A CHANGE OF POSE

This cabriole is done through a fouetté only in a pose of 90 degrees and only with an en dedans turn. For instance, beginning in Fifth Position, épaulement croisé, a pas failli is performed followed by a temps levé with a throw of the free leg into a big effacé forward. At the crest of a fouetté jump from this position, an en dedans turn of 1/2 circle is done into first arabesque. At the end of this turn, a cabriole with the supporting leg pushing off to perform a beat on the open leg ends the exercise. The jump ends on the same pushing leg fixed in the first arabesque pose.

The arms in pas failli open from Preparatory Position into a lowered Second and descend again into the Preparatory Position. At the moment of the next push to temps levé, they are strongly thrown through First into Third. During the fouetté, they open into first arabesque and remain there until the end of the jump.

The body in pas failli bends as it turns a bit toward the leg moving through First into Fourth Position, and on the temps levé, leans a bit backward. It thus assumes the pose for first arabesque.

The head in pas failli turns toward the advanced shoulder and, at the crest of the jump in the temps levé, keeps that position. During the fouetté it turns into the first arabesque position.

This is all repeated from the other leg with the pas failli starting not from the Fifth Position, but directly from the first arabesque.

Therefore, the body does not turn as in the first pas failli, and the arms do not open into Second. The head and body follow the same movements.

This kind of exercise is usually repeated four to eight times in a series to a 2/4 or 3/4 tempo. In the 2/4 tempo each jump is done to 1/4 of the measure, and in the 3/4 tempo it is done to a full measure.

This cabriole may also be performed from other approaches, such as the sissonne tombée, the pas glissade, pas chassé and from the third arabesque. In this case, the approach is the pas chassé along Second into the upper corner of the room.

Finally, the cabriole may be done in the form of a grand fouetté with a turn en dedans into third arabesque in this manner: Starting en face, Fifth Position, a sissonne ouverte into à la seconde to 90 degrees is done, and a temps levé into a pose écartée en dedans of 1/8 of a circle. Then the open leg is thrown through First Position into Fourth devant and a temps levé with a turn en dedans of 1/2 circle becomes a third arabesque. This turn ends with a cabriole from the supporting leg beating the raised leg. For a finale, a petit assemblé back into Fifth Position may be chosen.

The arms in sissonne ouverte open from Preparatory Position through First into Second. During the jump of the temps levé, they turn palms down into allongé. In the second temps levé, at the moment of the transfer into flight, the arms vigorously and together with the movement of the open leg go into Preparatory Position and rise to Third through First Position. At the fouetté, they open into third arabesque and remain there to the end of the jump. At the assemblé, they return to the Preparatory Position.

The body is straight and exactly placed over the supporting leg. At the turn into third arabesque, it leans forward and remains there until the finishing demi-plié.

The head, during the sissonne, is en face; at the jump into écarté, turned toward the advanced shoulder; at the throw of the leg through First, turned toward the upper corner of the room and, together with the body, turned into the proper third arabesque position. During the assemblé, the head is turned toward the advanced shoulder.

Then this exercise is done from the other leg and repeated twice more in a 2/4 or 3/4 tempo. In the first case, each jump is done to a 1/4 beat, and in the 3/4 tempo, a full measure is used for each jump.

This same cabriole may be done in a slightly more complicated form, repeated from one leg a few times in a series. This version is done with the use of the temps levé and a throw of the leg from third arabesque through first into écarté forward. From here, a grand fouetté with the cabriole may be performed, etc. The measure is 2/4 and the temps levé is done before the measure into écarté; 1/4 is used for the jump into cabriole and 1/4 to end the jump. The arms, head and body perform as previously described.

The cabriole with a turn, except for the last form described with the grand fouetté, may be done at the beginning, not at the end of a turn. In such a case, the cabriole must be done devant with clarity and a flowing movement and turning into the final pose, which is usually an arabesque through a fouetté movement.

For instance, from a pas chassé along Second into an upper corner of the room, a cabriole forward is done in the same direction with a fouetté into arabesque. Or the movement may begin with a pas failli into a cabriole effacée forward with a fouetté ending in first arabesque, etc.

CABRIOLE WITH A DOUBLE BEAT

This same cabriole may be done with a double beat by two means: 1. Both beats may be done derrière at the end of the fouetté into arabesque, or 2. The first beat may be done forward and the second in back of the pushing leg at the end of the fouetté.

Finally, ordinary cabrioles with a fouetté may end in a tombé into Fourth or close into Fifth. The double cabriole is done only by means of the tombé approach. All these cabrioles with a turn must be performed clearly, in a pliant descent, with lightness and in one tempo. It is not permissible to break the pose, its rush into flight or its ending.

Neither should there be a weak or unclear beat of the legs, especially in the double cabriole. A harsh or unstable demi-plié ending is undesirable. The body should appear relaxed without raised shoulders and there should be no overcharged acts or reflexes, from the movements of the body, in the arms.

It is advisable to keep to the order of the description in the study of this movement, starting with simple exercises and comfortable approaches like the sissonne tombée, the pas failli, pas glissade and pas chassé. It may be joined in combinations only after a very thorough study of these movements in the elementary exercises.

In the cabriole without a turn, it is mentioned that it could be done through a soubresaut. The cabriole with a fouetté may also be done through a soubresaut, but only to the back in this manner: into a first arabesque from a pas failli, or into a third arabesque from a pas chassé along Second.

CABRIOLE WITH ONE BENT LEG

The same cabriole may be done with a bend of the pushing leg to the knee of the raised leg, remaining in that position for the culmination of the jump.

The arms in the cabriole, with the outstretched legs, act as previously described, but in the cabriole with the bent leg, they remain in Third and, at the end of the jump, open into arabesque or in the third arabesque position.

The body and head act as usual for the cabrioles with the fouetté.

In both cases, the student must practice the technique for ballon—that strong resilient push and a clear fixing of the pose in the air with lightness maintained throughout the entire movement.

In the study, the approach of the pas failli and the simplest construction of the exercise should be used. In the practice of the cabriole in the passé position, the pushing leg must work with great resilience and force, bending to the knee of the raised leg without the slightest delay and must maintain this position during the jump. It must straighten just as energetically and descend through the toes to the heels, into a soft demi-plié.

It is obvious that the work of the supporting leg demands a very detailed study. The open leg in the jump and after the jump must be exactly fixed at 90 degrees. It must make not the least movement toward the pushing leg and must keep its point in space.

The study of this cabriole must begin with the stretched legs, then the passé position. As strength and technique develop, the time for the holding of this position in the air may be gradually increased to its utmost limit.

RENVERSÉ

In the chapter on turns and spins on the floor, this movement was examined in the attitude position in relevé. It may be done as well with a jump, by means of the temps levé. This movement with a jump fully follows the description of the movement par terre, except that the jump replaces the relevé on demi-pointe.

Beginning in attitude croisée, together with a demi-plié, and a slight bend of the body forward, including the head and arms, and with no delay, a jumping push is done. The flight finds the body straight and the jump ends in attitude croisée in demi-plié and transfers to a pas de bourrée with a slight and flexible bend of the spine to the back as described in the renversé on demi-pointe. The movement ends in Fifth Position in demi-plié, a total of three demi-pliés: one energetic demi-plié at the moment of the slight lean forward, one that is softer after the jump, and the third, a soft demi-plié after the pas de bourrée.

On the whole, this movement must be done yieldingly, lightly, but with a high flight and a fluid movement of the body.

The study begins in simple combinations at once, but with the attitude croisée derrière and the pas de bourrée en dedans. Then the study may be in the attitude croisée forward pose with the pas de bourrée en dehors. Beforehand, the renversé en attitude on demi-pointe and the temps levé in the corresponding poses must be well learned.

REVOLTADE (OR RIVOLTADE, TURNING OVER)

This form of jump is done in the first or third arabesque pose with an en dehors turn of a full circle.

The jump, as a rule, is done from an approach such as the sissonne tombée, temps levé tombé, pas chassé or pas failli. Beginning in Fifth Position with the right leg forward, épaulement croisé, a sissonne tombée forward en croisé is done and a pas coupé with the left leg in back of the right. Then without delay, through First, the flight with a turn en dedans (to the right) of 1/2 circle is done at the same time the right leg is thrown forward.

The left leg joins and passes the right leg front in Fifth Position in the air and, as the left lowers into demi-plié, the right rises slightly higher than 90 degrees in back to end the movement.

The arms rise at the sissonne from Preparatory, the right in First and the left through First into Second. At the pas coupé and the flight, both rise into Third, then together at the end of the jump, they open into first arabesque.

The body, at the sissonne, leans a bit forward and, on the pas coupé, straightens out. In flight, it leans a bit backward and at the moment the jump ends in first arabesque, it assumes that position.

The head, during the sissonne, leans a bit forward; at the pas coupé, straightens; in flight, leans back, and at the end is in the first arabesque position. The head is turned toward the right shoulder in the sissonne and, at the pas coupé and jump, turns with the body and ends with the jump in the first arabesque position.

The entire body of the dancer in the flight takes on an almost horizontal position and, at the end of the jump, descends into the first arabesque.

The revoltade is done with a big jump, in a dynamic tempo with a clear and light turn of the entire body, strictly in the character of classical dance, and without acrobatics. (See illustration #158.)

---

158   Revoltade

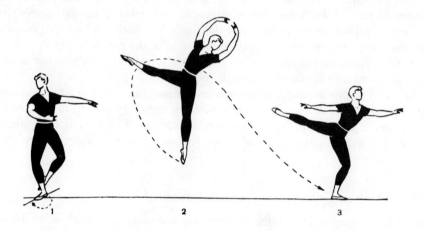

The pas coupé must be done with pliability, strength and exactly through Fifth Position. The throw of the free leg is done with just as much vigor and strength and must be placed in alignment to the body. The pushing leg also must be vigorous and, with no delay, follow the thrown leg; both, in flight, must stretch out fully at the knees, insteps and toes.

The joining and the separation of the legs must be done lightly with a clear passing movement through Fifth Position. The end is a soft demi-plié. The leg must be fixed in back in a clear and light 90 degrees. The turnout must be preserved throughout.

The arms act throughout with vitality and in one tempo with the other elements. The body is collected, pulled up and harmonious, actively participating in the turning and jumping push. The head moves surely and clearly, supplementing the action of the body and arms.

The study of the revoltade should be at first in first arabesque, with a stop, and should be studied separately from a combination. For instance, in a 2/4 measure, a sissonne tombée is done on the first 1/4 of the measure, the pas coupé and revoltade on the second 1/4. Pause on the first 1/4 of the second measure in demi-plié. On the next 1/4, the leg is placed in Fifth Position forward and the exercise is ready to be repeated four times from one leg. It is then repeated from the other leg.

After it is learned, the basic revoltade may be used in simple combinations. At the same time, it may be practiced in third arabesque. Here, the sissonne tombée is done effacé forward. Then both revoltades may be used in complex combinations.

REVOLTADE WITH A DOUBLE TOUR

Some performers of great virtuosity are able to do the revoltade with a double turn. This, of course, is very difficult.

The students of the graduation classes may be allowed to try this revoltade with the double turn only if they possess special gifts and are excellently trained. The most difficult, and even dangerous, is the final jump. Here, the least miscalculation or inexactness may harm the ligaments of the legs. Therefore, before permitting a student to attempt the double revoltade, his abilities must be carefully assessed. It must be remembered that the movement is performed in strict classical style and without tricks.

BEATS WITH TURNS

Beats, incorporated into a turn or jump, as in the grand jeté en tournant, introduce dynamics into classical dance and give the technique a virtuosic character.

At the same time, beats look better without the turn, and performed en face. The beat, done in profile, hides from the spectator the clear movement of the legs. If, however, the entrechat quatre is done with a full turn, then the movement of the legs is partially shadowed, but there appears a new element of dynamics which may be used by the choreographer as a vivid and expressive addition. Therefore, the student must master to perfection all the forms of beats with a turn from the smallest to the most complex.

Beats are examined in this portion in the same groupings as those without the turn which were previously described. The technique for the performance of these beats will not be discussed unless the turn introduces a new factor or unless the beat changes the turn in some way. And yet, it should be remembered here that the study of beats with a turn may, in the beginning, contain certain faults: a lack of coordination in the pushing sendoff and the beginning of the beat; insufficient clarity and force for a big movement; separation of the legs before the beat in an arc instead of in a Second Position; an overly strong push with a harsh, unstable ending to the jump; reflex movements in the arms; lack of harmoniousness in the use of the body; lack of free head movements; inexact rhythms, etc.

These faults must be eradicated, but, most important, mechanical joining of the turns and beats must not be allowed. There must be a constant striving for the plasticity of dance.

ENTRECHATS EN TOURNANT

ROYALE

This beat is done with a 1/4 or 1/2 turn and begins, as a study, with a 2/4 measure: Fifth Position, right leg forward, épaulement croisé. Four royales are performed, each in 1/4 circle to the right; three quick entrechats quatre without a turn; one royale with a 1/4 circle turn with a change of épaulement. All the royales are done to each 1/4 of the measure and the entrechats quatre to 1/8 of the measure.

The arms in all the beats and jumps are held in Preparatory Position. The body is straight and the head in the starting pose is turned toward the advanced shoulder. At the last royale, it turns toward the other shoulder.

The exercise is repeated on the other side and the turn is in the opposite direction and repeated once more on both sides. The performance of this exercise should at first be in a moderate tempo to perfect the exactness of the turn and the beats. Then the study or royale may proceed to include a 1/2 circle turn.

As an example: Beginning in Fifth Position with the right leg forward, épaulement croisé, four royales are done each in 1/2 circle to the right; three quick entrechats quatre without the turn; one changement de pied with a full turn to the right.

The arms during all the jumps are in Preparatory Position except for the last entrechat quatre when the arm corresponding to the direction of the turn rises to First and the other into Second Position. At the last changement de pied, they join in a rounded and lowered First Position and on the final demi-plié open slightly.

The body is straight and the head at the start of the exercise is turned toward the advanced shoulder. During the four royales, it is straight in respect to the body and turns with it.

At the entrechat quatre, the head turns toward the advanced shoulder. At the changement de pied, the head follows the pattern for the tour en l'air. Then all is repeated in the opposite direction and repeated on both sides once more.

The tempo is 2/4 and each royale is done to 1/4 of the measure and the changement de pied is done to 1/8, with the last changement de pied to 1/4 of the measure. There is a rest of 1/4.

Each exercise may be constructed as a more simple or more complicated combination but only in accord with the pupil's ability to perform the exercise correctly. If the pupil does not master the beats and the turning movements separately, he will only learn the general shape of the movement without working out the elements in order to perform them as dance.

ENTRECHAT TROIS

This beat is done in a 1/4 and 1/2 circle with its study beginning as follows: To a 2/4 tempo, in Fifth Position, épaulement croisé, one entrechat trois is performed with the sur le cou-de-pied ending in back in a 1/4 turn en dehors. It is followed by a petit assemblé derrière into Fifth Position.

This is then reversed with a turn en dedans of 1/4 circle assemblé en arrière. This is followed by three petit changements de pieds with a full turn in the same direction and an ending of an entrechat quatre without a turn and an advance forward in croisé.

The arms at the first entrechat trois move from Preparatory Position to First for the arm corresponding to the direction of the turn, and Second for the other arm. On the assemblé, the arms do not change. At the second entrechat trois, they change positions. During the three petit changements de pieds, they move back into Preparatory Position and remain there until the end of the exercise.

The body is straight during all the jumps. At the end of the second entrechat trois, it leans a bit forward. The head, during both entrechats trois, turns toward the arm in First and on the assemblé croisé forward, it straightens out and turns toward the advanced shoulder. During the three petit changements de pieds, it gradually turns toward the opposite shoulder and stays until the end of the exercise.

The exercise is then repeated from the other leg and both sides once again. After a little rest, it is reversed. Each petit changement is done to 1/8 of a measure and all the other jumps to 1/4 of the measure.

An example with a turn of 1/2: To the same tempo and starting pose of the previous exercise, two entrechats trois are performed in sur le cou-de-pied back, with a turn en dehors of 1/2 circle each and a petit assemblé à la seconde ending in Fifth Position forward. This is followed by three rather low entrechats quatre without a turn and one changement de pied with a full turn in the same direction.

The arms are in Preparatory Position during the first four jumps and at the third entrechat quatre the arm corresponding to the direction of the turn rises into First as the other rises into Second. At the changement de pied, they join in a rounded and lowered First and at the final demi-plié are opened slightly.

The body is straight throughout the exercise. The head at first turns toward the advanced shoulder and, at the first entrechat trois, turns toward the other shoulder. At the second entrechat trois, it returns to the starting position and remains there during the three small entrechats quatre. During the changement de pied, the head turns as for a tour en l'air.

The exercise is repeated on the other side, repeated again and then done in reverse. Each entrechat quatre is done to 1/8 of the measure and all other jumps to 1/4 of the measure each.

ENTRECHAT QUATRE

This beat is done with a turn of 1/4 and 1/2 circle. As an example: To a 2/4 tempo, beginning in Fifth Position, right leg front, épaulement croisé, four entrechats quatre are done each with a turn of 1/4 circle to the right. This is followed by three small entrechats quatre without turns; one jeté fermé to the right with a change of Fifth Position and one entrechat quatre without a turn.

The arms during all the jumps are in Preparatory Position except at the jeté, during which they rise slightly in the direction of Second Position and lower again.

The body is straight, but on the jeté it leans a little in the direction of the advance. At the last jump, it straightens once more.

The head, during all the jumps, is turned toward the right shoulder and, at the jeté, turns toward the other shoulder.

The exercise is repeated from the other leg and once more from the beginning on both sides. The three small entrechats are done to 1/8 of each measure and the rest, to 1/4 of the measure.

An example for an exercise with the entrechat quatre in a 1/2 circle turn begins in the same tempo and starting position: One entrechat quatre is done, followed by two more entrechats quatre each with a 1/2 circle turn to the right; followed by two more entrechats quatre, each with a 1/2 circle turn in the same direction and a changement de pied with a full turn to end the exercise.

The arms during the jumps are in Preparatory Position except for the last two. At the jump before the last, the arm corresponding to the direction of the turn rises into First and the other into Second. At the last jump, the arms are rounded and join in a lowered First. At the final demi-plié, they open slightly.

The body is straight. The head at the start is turned toward the advanced shoulder. At the first six jumps, it remains in the same position. At the first entrechat quatre of 1/2 circle, it delays a bit, but at the second 1/2 circle, it turns to the starting position.

During the changement de pied, the head turns as for a tour en l'air. Then the exercise is done from the other leg and repeated once more on both sides.

The first entrechat is done to 1/4 of the measure; the two following, to 1/8; the same is repeated; then each jump is done to 1/4 of the measure.

These examples may be structured differently but should always be within the ability of the students and hold to the elements under study.

ENTRECHAT CINQ

This beat is also done with a turn of 1/4 and 1/2 circle. For example: To a measure of 2/4 beginning in épaulement croisé, entrechat cinq ending sur le cou-de-pied back is done in a 1/4 circle followed by an assemblé back into Fifth; repeated twice more; ending with three small royales with a 1/4 turn.

At the first entrechat cinq, the arms move from Preparatory Position to First—for the arm corresponding to the direction of the turn—and Second for the other arm. During the assemblé to the back they remain in these positions. During the second entrechat, they change positions and remain the same at the assemblé. At the third entrechat, the arms again change positions and stay the same for the assemblé. At the three small royales, they return to the Preparatory Position.

The body at the first entrechat cinq leans slightly away from the perpendicular toward the free leg and remains there for the assemblé. In flight, during the next entrechat cinq, it straightens and, at the end of the movement, leans slightly toward the supporting leg, etc. During the three small royales, the body is straight.

The head, before the start of the exercise, is turned toward the advanced shoulder. During the first entrechat it turns toward the opposite shoulder and remains there during the assemblé. During the third entrechat, it turns again toward the advanced shoulder and remains there until the end of the exercise. The entire combination is repeated on the other leg and once more on each side, then reversed.

Each small royale is done to 1/8 of the measure while all the other jumps are done to 1/4 of the measure.

An example of an exercise with a turn of 1/2 circle would be: In the same measure and starting position; three entrechat cinq to the sur le cou-de-pied position in back with a turn en dehors of 1/2 circle followed by the assemblé back into Fifth Position. Then the exercise ends with a grand changement de pied de volée (flying) forward with a turn en dehors of 1/2 circle.

The actions of the arms, body and head are the same as for the other exercises. During the changement de pied, the arms lower into Preparatory Position and the body straightens out. The head is turned toward the advanced shoulder.

The entire exercise is done from the other leg, repeated on both sides once more and then reversed. Each jump is done to 1/4 of a measure.

ENTRECHAT SIX

This beat is done with no more than a 1/4 or 1/2 circle turn. The study is helped by this exercise: To a 2/4 tempo, beginning with Fifth Position right leg front, épaulement croisé; three entrechats six are done each with a 1/4 turn to the right.

The arms at the third entrechat six are thrown into Third, and during the rest afterward, the arms lower through Second into Preparatory Position.

The body is straight and the head, at the third jump, turns toward the other shoulder. The exercise is repeated three times, then performed in the opposite direction.

Each jump is done to 1/4 of the measure with a rest after the third entrechat six of 1/4 measure.

As an example for a 1/2 circle turn: To a 2/4 measure and from the same starting position, two entrechats six with a 1/2 circle turn to the right on each six; grande sissonne ouverte par développé into à la seconde and a petit assemblé to the back, end the exercise.

The arms during the first two jumps are in Preparatory Position. At the sissonne ouverte, they open through First into Second and at the assemblé return to Preparatory.

The body during the entrechat six is straight. At the end of the sissonne, it leans a little away from the leg, which opens to 90 degrees. At the assemblé, it straightens.

The head during the two entrechats remains in the starting position. At the sissonne, it turns to the other shoulder and remains there until the end of the assemblé. Then all is done on the other leg and reversed.

All the jumps are to 1/4 of a measure each. Later the entrechat six with a turn must be introduced into combinations where there are big jumps with an advance.

ENTRECHAT SEPT

This is usually performed in no more than a 1/4 circle. The reason is the difficulty of the movement in finishing on one leg while the other is in sur le cou-de-pied front or back following a complicated beat and a high jump.

An example: Beginning in Fifth Position, épaulement croisé, one entrechat sept with the sur le cou-de-pied position in back and a turn of 1/4 circle ends with a pas coupé and a small assemblé croisé forward. These movements are repeated twice more and the end of the exercise is two sissonnes fermées in écarté forward.

The arms during the first entrechat sept rise from Preparatory Position with the arm corresponding to the direction of the turn in First, the other through First into Second. At the pas coupé and the petit assemblé, there is no change. During the second entrechat sept, they change positions, etc.

The body, during the jump, is straight. At the end of each entrechat, the body leans a little away from the free leg and remains in that position during the pas coupé and assemblé. This is repeated and the exercise repeats. During the two sissonnes fermées, the body leans slightly in the direction of the advance.

The head, during each entrechat, turns to the opposite shoulder and remains there during the pas coupé and the petit assemblé. During the sissonnes fermées, the head is turned toward the advanced shoulder. All is done from the other leg and reversed. Each pas coupé and each petit assemblé is done to 1/8 of the measure while all the other jumps are to 1/4 of the measure.

In this beat, the arms must remain free with no apparent strain. The movements must be clear and elastic.

The entrechat huit is not described here because it is not done with a turn.

PAS BATTU EN TOURNANT
(STEPS WITH A BEAT AND A TURN)

PAS ÉCHAPPÉ BATTU

Example: In a 2/4 measure in Fifth Position with the right leg forward, épaulement croisé, the jump is done from Fifth Position into Second with a small beat and a right turn of 1/4 circle. The second jump from Second into Fifth is with a small beat, but without the turn. Both beats are done with the right leg beating back, left front. These jumps are repeated three more times with turns, in the same direction, but the last beat is done with the right leg beating front. Then the exercise is ready to begin with the turn in the other direction.

The arms, head and body act as usual for a petit échappé battu. All the jumps are done exactly to a 1/4 count. The same exercise may be performed with a turn at each jump, repeating two full turns to the right and the same to the left.

Later, this exercise must be done with the second jump ending in sur le cou-de-pied in front and ending in back. When this is the case, the first beat is not done and the second beat starts with the right leg in front for the beat and ending sur le cou-de-pied back. The second pas échappé begins from this position and ends with the left leg in sur le cou-de-pied back, etc. The last jump is ended by a beat of the right leg in front of the left leg, into Fifth Position, left foot front. Then the exercise is ready to be repeated from the other leg and reversed with the transfer of the free leg into sur le cou-de-pied front.

The arms, head and body act as in a petit échappé battu with the sur le cou-de-pied ending.

GRAND PAS ÉCHAPPÉ BATTU

This beat may be done in a 1/4 or 1/2 circle. Example: With the starting pose the same as for the petit échappé, the first jump from Fifth into Second with a big double beat and a turn to the right is done in a 1/4 circle. Then the second jump from Second into Fifth with a big beat and a right turn of 1/4 circle follows. The first beat is done with the right leg beating behind the left leg. Then the legs exchange position and from there open into Second in demi-plié. At the second half, the first beat is done with the right leg exchanged in Fifth in the air behind the left, opens again and ends in Fifth right leg front. This grand échappé is repeated once more and the exercise ends with three small entrechats quatre and two tours en l'air in the same direction. The entire exercise is repeated four times. The arms, head and body act as in échappé battu with double beats.

Each small entrechat is done to 1/8 of the measure while all the other jumps are to 1/4 of the measure.

In the same exercise, both grands échappés may be done with two full turns. Each jump is 1/2 circle and, performing two échappés, there will be four turns.

Then the study of this échappé may begin ending on one leg, the other in sur le cou-de-pied front or ending in back. The tempo is 2/4 with the same starting pose. The first jump in grand échappé battu is done with a turn of 1/2 circle. Then the second jump in grand échappé battu with a turn is in the same direction and also with a 1/2 turn, but the ending is on the right leg with the other in sur le cou-de-pied back. Then a pas coupé and a small assemblé in Second, closing in back in Fifth and two small entrechats quatre end the exercise. The position is ready for the exercise to be repeated from the other leg, repeated once more on both sides. In reverse, it is done ending in échappé in cou-de-pied front, etc. The arms, head and body act as in the movement without the turns. Each échappé is done to 2/4 of the measure and all other turns to 1/8 of the measure.

SISSONNE OUVERTE BATTUE EN TOURNANT

The petite sissonne ouverte battue turn is executed in 1/4 and 1/2 circles. To a 2/4 measure in Fifth, right leg front, épaulement croisé, a petite sissonne battue is done with the opening of the left leg in écarté and an advance in flight into the right upper corner of the room, en dedans, in a 1/4 turn to the right. The beat is executed by the left leg striking the right leg in front and then opening to 45 degrees into a small écarté front, followed by a petit assemblé into Fifth back. All is repeated three more times, but the last and fourth assemblé ends in front in Fifth so that the entire exercise may be repeated on the other leg.

Each sissonne has an advance in flight in the direction of the diagonal corners of the room (#4, #6).

The arms, head and body act as in the movement without the turns.

In the performance of the reverse sissonne, the right leg opens to écarté to the back and the advance in flight is into the left lower corner of the room. At the same time, the turn is en dehors in a 1/4 circle. The beat is with the right leg behind the left followed by a throw of the right leg to 45 degrees écarté.

The arms, body and head follow the pattern for the movement without a turn.

It is useful to do the exercise with a turn of 1/2 circle en dedans and en dehors, with the beat in each sissonne as in the 1/4 circle exercise.

If the sissonne is done en dedans, then the advance in the flight is toward the upper left corner of the room of the performer, and the écarté is with the left leg opening toward the lower corner of the room.

The following sissonne is with a turn in the same direction but the advance in flight is into the opposite lower corner of the room. Both petits assemblés after the sissonnes are into Fifth Position in back. Then three petits changements de pied and one entrechat quatre de volée forward end the exercise. Then all is ready for the other leg. If the movement is in reverse, the first sissonne is done with a turn en dehors and the advance is to the right lower corner of the room. The jump ends with the throw of the right leg to 45 degrees into a small écarté from the back.

The second sissonne is with a turn in the same direction but the advance is in the opposite, upper corner of the room. The jump ends with a throw of the same leg into écarté front. Both petits assemblés are into Fifth forward; the petits changements de pied and the last entrechats quatre de volée go to the back.

The arms, head and body act as for the jumps without the turns.

In all the exercises described above, each jump is done to 1/4 of the measure except the petits changements de pied, which are done to 1/8 of the measure each.

This sissonne is just as useful to do in small poses with the leg opening to 45 degrees backward or forward in croisé or effacé. The procedure is the same as in the preceding exercises with turns of 1/4 or 1/2 circle.

For instance, to a 2/4 measure, starting in Fifth Position, right leg front, épaulement croisé, a petite sissonne battue with the leg opening backward is done in a turn en dedans of 1/4 circle to the right. The advance is toward the lower corner of the room. The beat here is the ordinary one, with the left leg beating front followed by an opening to the back into a small pose. Then a petit assemblé follows to the back in Fifth and the exercise is repeated three more times with the turns in the same direction. The last and fourth assemblé, however, is done forward into Fifth with an en dedans turn of 1/4 circle. Then the exercise is done from the other leg.

The arms at the first sissonne rise from Preparatory with the left in First and the right through First into Second. They remain there until the last assemblé, then return to Preparatory Position.

The body, at each sissonne, is in a slight lean forward and, at the assemblé, straightens. The head at the start is turned to the right shoulder. At the first jump, it turns toward the other shoulder and stays there until the last assemblé. In the performance of this exercise from the other leg, the head turns toward the opposite shoulder.

Reverse of this exercise begins in the position as the pose for petite sissonne battue with the opening of the right leg forward into effacé. At the same time, a turn is made en dehors to the right, and the advance to the lower corner of the room.

The beat is made by the right leg in back and opening to 45 degrees into a small pose effacé forward. Finally, the petit assemblé is in Fifth Position forward. All this is repeated three more times with a turn in the same direction, but the last and fourth assemblé is done into Fifth in back with a 1/4 circle turn.

Then the entire exercise is done from the other leg. The head, arms and body follow the same pattern.

This exercise may be done into other small poses—arabesque, for instance, or alternating poses.

This exercise develops the ability to perform simultaneously a jump, a beat, a turn and an advance which prepares the student for the study of more complex and bigger beats with turns.

The study may begin only after all the elements have been well absorbed.

GRANDE SISSONNE OUVERTE BATTUE

This movement is done with a turn of 1/4, 1/2 and 3/4. It may be studied after the procedure for the petite sissonne battue with a turn of 1/4 circle. But added to this movement is a larger jump, a double beat, an enlarged advance and a big pose in écarté.

If a grande sissonne is done with a turn en dedans, the left leg beats the right one first in front, then in back and is thrown to 90 degrees into a big pose écartée. All the petits assemblés are the same as in the exercise for the petite sissonne ouverte battue.

For the study of the sissonne battue with a 1/2 circle turn, with poses in Fourth, the procedure for the petite sissonne battue may be used.

For grande sissonne battue with a turn of 3/4 circle, start in Fifth Position, right leg in front, épaulement croisé. A grande sissonne ouverte battue is done into third arabesque with an advance into the right lower corner of the hall (corner #2). The jump starts from the spine with a turn of the left shoulder and ends on a diagonal in the third arabesque. The beat is a double one: right leg in back of the left leg, then in front, and then it is thrown back to 90 degrees for the arabesque. This is followed by a petit pas coupé and a petit assemblé forward into Fifth Position.

The arms at the sissonne move from Preparatory Position into First and open into the third arabesque, or through First move into Third. At the pas coupé and the petit assemblé, they move back into Preparatory Position.

The body's center of gravity during the sissonne must energetically give in the direction to the final point of the jump and, while still in demi-plié, lean away from the perpendicular axis in the direction of the advance.

In flight, the body rushes along the trajectory into the right lower corner of the room and, at the end of the jump, returns exactly to the supporting leg, which is lowering into a supple demi-plié.

At the pas coupé the body straightens out, and at the assemblé it rushes toward the other lower corner of the room.

The head, before the sissonne, is turned toward the advanced shoulder. In flight it, together with the body, turns freely to the right lower corner of the room and remains there in third arabesque. At the pas coupé and the petit assemblé, it turns toward the other shoulder.

Then the entire movement is done with an en dedans turn to a 3/4 circle in the other direction, and once again from the beginning. After a rest, it is done from the other leg.

Each sissonne is performed to 1/4 of a measure, each pas coupé and petit assemblé to 1/8 of the measure. Each rest falls on the fourth and eighth measure.

In reverse, the grande sissonne ouverte battue is done in a large pose with the leg opening forward in croisé and the advance toward the upper corner of the room.

This jump starts from the chest with a turn of the left shoulder and ends along a diagonal to the pose croisée. The beat is a double one, the left leg hits the right in front, then back and is then thrown forward to 90 degrees. The pas coupé and the petit assemblé backward into Fifth end the exercise.

The arms in the sissonne move from Preparatory into First but may open differently as well: The left moves into Second, the right into Third; or both into Third; or the left into Second and the right into First. Both arms transfer through allongé into the given poses. At the pas coupé and petit assemblé, the arms return to Preparatory Position.

The body, during the sissonne, leans toward the final point of the jump and, while still in demi-plié, leans away from the perpendicular in the direction of the advance. In the flight, it points along the trajectory toward the upper corner of the room, and at the end of the jump transfers exactly onto the supporting leg, which is descending into a supple demi-plié. At the pas coupé, the body is straight again and, at the assemblé, points toward the other upper corner of the room.

The head, before the sissonne, is turned toward the advanced shoulder. In flight and at its end, it turns together with the body to face the lower left corner of the room and keeps this position in the big pose croisée forward. At the pas coupé and petit assemblé, the head turns toward the other shoulder. Then all is repeated with the turn en dehors of 3/4 circle in the opposite direction and then repeated once more.

All grandes sissonnes with turns, especially of 1/2 and 3/4 circles, may be studied in the last two years.

PETIT ASSEMBLÉ BATTU

This movement is done with a 1/4 circle turn. To a 2/4 measure, Fifth Position right foot front, épaulement croisé, a petit assemblé with the left leg along Second is done with the turn en dedans and a single beat, left, beats the right leg in back. The jump ends with the left foot front in Fifth Position.

Then a petit assemblé is done with the right leg performing the battu, with the turn in the same direction of 1/4 circle. These two movements are repeated and the circle is complete. In all, four assemblés have been performed, two with the right leg, two with the left in a series in a full circle. The first and third turns were en dedans; the second and fourth, en dehors.

Then three petits changements de pied with a turn in a full circle in the same direction end the exercise, along with two final entrechats six.

The arms during the first assemblé move from Preparatory in the direction of Second and, at the end, the left is moved into a lowered First, while the right stays in a lowered Second. The arms correspond to the successive assemblés but move each time from the ending positions, not from Preparatory Position.

During the three petits changements de pied, the arms lower into Preparatory smoothly and remain there for the two entrechats six.

The body is held straight. The head during each assemblé turns a bit toward the opening leg. During the three changements it turns smoothly toward the other shoulder and remains there. Then the entire exercise is repeated from the other leg and reversed.

The petits changements are done to 1/8 of a measure while all other jumps are 1/4 to the measure.

When the exercise is done in reverse, all assemblés are begun with the leg moving from the front Fifth Position with the turn to the right. Then the exercise is repeated to the left. The beat is a single one, with the front leg beating front after it is thrown into 45 degrees side and closes into Fifth Position in back.

At the end of each assemblé, the arm opposite to the thrown leg moves from Second into First as the other stays in Second. All other movements are the same.

(The assemblé in the French and Cecchetti systems has gathered a great many adjectives in addition to petit and grand: dessus, dessous, devant, derrière, en avant, en arrière, en tournant, battu, coupé, coupé derrière, coupé devant, de suite [continuously], élancé [darting], porté [carried in the air], en descendant [downstage], en remontant or en reculant [upstage], soutenu [with straightened knees after the descent], not to mention all the assemblés described for pointe work. The major difference, however, is in the execution of the pas itself. In the Cecchetti assemblé, both knees are bent after the battement so that the flat of the toes of both feet meet in the crest of the jump.)

GRAND ASSEMBLÉ BATTU

This beat is done only with an en dedans turn in a 1/2 or full circle. As an example:

Beginning in the left lower corner of the room (#8), in third arabesque on a high demi-pointe, the left leg raised to 45 degrees, a pas chassé along Second is done with a turn of 1/4 circle to the left. The back is toward the mirror or spectator. Then a grand assemblé battu with the right leg thrown into écarté into the upper corner of the room opposite the starting point (#4) is done in an en dedans 1/2 circle. The beat is a double one—right leg beats the left in front, then in back and is transferred front into the closing Fifth Position. Then a pas glissade along Second to the upper diagonal corner is done (same direction as the assemblé) and a sissonne ouverte into third arabesque completes the combination. (The third arabesque is in the starting pose once more.)

The arms in the pas chassé open from third arabesque into Second and, during the grand assemblé, are thrown energetically through Preparatory and First, and in allongé (palms down) the right arm moves into Third and the left into Second. During the pas glissade, the arms return to Preparatory Position and, at the sissonne ouverte, rise through First into third arabesque. The body, at the chassé from third arabesque, straightens out, remains straight during the assemblé but at the pas glissade leans slightly in the direction of the advance. At the sissonne, it leans a bit forward for the third arabesque which follows.

The head, during the pas chassé, is delayed at the starting position and at the pas glissade turns toward the other shoulder. At the sissonne ouverte, it takes the pose for the third arabesque.

All this is done from the other leg and repeated once more.

Each jump is to 1/4 of a measure but later must be done more energetically to a 3/4 tempo performing each jump in one measure.

This exercise is not done in reverse, but the assemblé with a full turn may be done as follows: Beginning in the right lower corner of the room (#2) in a first arabesque pose on a high demi-pointe, with the left leg at 45 degrees, a pas chassé is done diagonally, followed by a grand assemblé battu with a throw of the right leg to écarté into the opposite upper corner (#6) and a turn en dedans of a full circle. The beat is a double one as described in the previous exercise. Then a sissonne tombée croisée forward and a jeté passé into first arabesque complete the combination.

The arms in the chassé are in Second; at the assemblé they are thrown through Preparatory and First into Third; at the sissonne tombée they lower into First, and at the jeté passé, open into first arabesque.

The body at the pas chassé straightens and remains straight during the assemblé and sissonne tombée. At the pas jeté, it leans a bit forward.

The head during the pas chassé is delayed a bit in the starting position, but at the assemblé, clearly turns in the direction of the advance. At the end, it remains turned toward the advanced shoulder. At the sissonne tombée, the head turns toward the hands, which are moving through First and at the jeté passé move into the first arabesque position.

This exercise is repeated from the other leg and twice more. All jumps are made evenly in 2/4 or 3/4 tempo. Later this movement must be incorporated with other big jumps in combinations.

PAS JETÉ BATTU EN TOURNANT

PETIT PAS JETÉ BATTU

The petit pas jeté battu is done with a turn of 1/4 and 1/2 circle. An example: Beginning with the right front in Fifth Position, épaulement croisé, a petit jeté by the left leg is done along Second with an en dedans turn of 1/4 circle. The beat is a single one—left beats behind the right. The jump ends in a transfer of the right leg sur le cou-de-pied back together with a demi-plié on the left leg. Then a jeté is done with the right leg and a turn in the same direction of 1/4 circle. All together, there are four jetés battus in the exercise in the same pattern as described in the petit assemblé battu. Then three petit emboîtés sur le cou-de-pied back are performed with a full turn en dedans and one cabriole in third arabesque and a petit assemblé croisé back into Fifth Position complete the exercise. Instead of the cabriole, the last assemblé may be done dessus-dessous.

The arms, head and body perform as for the petit assemblé battu. At the three emboîtés, they descend smoothly into Preparatory Position and, during the cabriole, open through First into third arabesque. During the final assemblé, they return to Preparatory Position.

The body is straight and leans only on the cabriole, slightly forward. The head during each assemblé turns a bit in the direction of the thrown leg. During the three petits emboîtés, it turns smoothly toward the other shoulder. At the cabriole it assumes the position for the third arabesque and, at the assemblé, turns toward the advanced shoulder.

Then all is done on the other leg and reversed. The petits emboîtés are done to 1/8 of the measure and all other jumps to 1/4 of the measure.

When the combination is reversed, all the jetés begin with the front leg, first with a 1/4 circle turn to the right, then to the left. The beat is made with the thrown leg beating front and the sur le cou-de-pied ending with the other leg in front. The three petits emboîtés and the final assemblé are performed devant (forward).

The arms at the end of each jeté perform as for a petit assemblé battu reversed. During the three emboîtés, they lower into Preparatory Position and, at the cabriole, rise into First. Then the arm corresponding to the pushing leg is transferred in allongé into Second; the other moves into First. At the final assemblé, both are in Preparatory Position.

JETÉ BATTU WITH AN ADVANCE TO THE SIDE IN A 1/2 CIRCLE

Example: In a measure of 2/4, en face as a starting position, the front leg performs a jeté with an advance to the right in an en dedans 1/2 circle turn in the same direction. Before the descent, the left leg, which made the pushing jump from the floor, does a single beat in front of the right leg and transfers into sur le cou-de-pied back. (The student's back is to the mirror.) Then the left leg does the next jeté with an advance and a 1/2 circle turn en dehors in the same direction. Before the descent, the right leg, which has done the pushing jump, does a single beat in back of the left leg en face, and transfers into sur le cou-de-pied front. This is followed by two temps levés simples sur le cou-de-pied front and a jeté battu with an advance to the side in a 1/2 circle, etc., and is repeated twice more. To end this exercise or combination, a petit assemblé back into Fifth Position permits the combination to be performed on the other side. Then it is all reversed. The jumps are on an even 1/4 of the measure.

JETÉ PASSÉ BATTU EN TOURNANT

This movement is done in a 1/4 circle turn to a 2/4 measure. Beginning in Fifth Position, right leg front, épaulement croisé, a sissonne ouverte in third arabesque; a jeté passé battu is also done in third arabesque with a turn en dehors—right— in 1/4 circle turn; a grande cabriole follows in the same pose and a petit assemblé back into Fifth Position finishes the exercise. The beat is a single one—the right leg beats the left at the crest of the jump. The beat is done as a brisé from the Fourth not the Second Position, when the leg is almost in a horizontal position. After the beat, the legs pass one another and the left leg descends into a demi-plié as the right rises a bit.

The arms during the jeté rise through First and the body leans a bit forward. The head turns to face the right corner (#2). All the movements follow the pattern for the beat without a turn.

The exercise is repeated four times, practiced on the other leg and reversed. Each movement is performed to 1/4 of the measure in an energetic and assertive manner in a clear rhythm.

JETÉ BATTU FOUETTÉ EN TOURNANT

An example of this movement begins in the lower right corner (#2) and is performed in a 2/4 tempo. The starting position is a first arabesque on a high demi-pointe. A pas chassé along Second is followed by a thrown jeté toward the opposite corner of the room (#6) by the right leg devant, followed by a throw of the left leg in the same direction. At the crest of the jump, the first beat is done by the right leg front and the left back; and in the continuation of the turn, the second beat is done by the right leg back and the left, front. The legs then separate, pass each other and the right descends into demi-plié and the left rises a bit. The movement ends in first arabesque and is done impetuously and clearly, preserving all the rules for the thrown jeté and a double beat.

This is followed by a relevé to a high demi-pointe in first arabesque and the entire movement is repeated in the same direction. The second thrown jeté (a fouetté movement) ends with a temps levé tombé with an en dehors (left) 1/4 circle turn and a petite cabriole in first arabesque.

The temps levé is done through the shin position with an advance toward the lower left corner of the room (#8). The movement is repeated on the other leg and again from the beginning.

The arms, head and body perform as for the movement without the beats. All the jumps are on 1/4 of the measure.

Attention must be called to the jeté passé battu since the legs are in a horizontal position. This adds to the difficulty of the movement but it introduces the effect of high flight. The legs must move freely and forcefully. The body must show no strain or stress as a reflex to the beating.

Before the study of this movement, the double beat with a turn and the fouetté with beats must be mastered.

When this throw (grand battement) is well learned with the double beat as well as other big jumps, it may be performed with a double cabriole beat. This should only be attempted in the graduating class by students who have an excellent preparation and a big jump. This double cabriole is done at the crest of the jump in back by the leg that descends.

The double beat in the cabriole replaces the double beat in the jeté and is performed backward at the crest of the jump but at the end of the fouetté. This small but most difficult detail must be studied well and practiced as a double cabriole with fouettés into the third and first arabesques.

This thrown jeté with the double cabriole must be performed even more assertively and with a quicker throw of the first and second leg to gain even fractions of a second in order to give more time to the double beat.

This movement with the double cabriole is examined here in a general context since it is impossible to explain, in a short, clear description, this rarely performed and highly virtuosic movement.

PAS BALLONNÉ BATTU EN TOURNANT

This movement is only performed in its small form with a 1/4 turn. The study may begin in a 2/4 tempo, Fifth Position, right leg front, épaulement croisé. The exercise consists of three pas coupés and a petit pas ballonné battu along Second with a turn to the right of a 1/4 circle at the same time. At the beginning a demi-plié is done on the front leg as the other rises to sur le cou-de-pied in back. All the pas coupés are in back of the supporting leg and each beat is in front with a transfer of the closing leg into sur le cou-de-pied back. The first and third ballonnés are performed with the right leg; the second, with the left leg. At the end of the three coupé-ballonné repetitions, two pas emboîtés in sur le cou-de-pied back, each with a 1/4 turn in the same direction, end the exercise. Then all is repeated on the other leg.

The arms at the starting demi-plié rise from Preparatory Position into First. During the pas coupé, and the pas ballonné, the right arm opens into Second and the left remains in First. At each repetition of the coupé-ballonné, the arms change but remain fixed in the last position for the emboîtés.

During the starting demi-plié and at the end of each ballonné, the body leans slightly toward the supporting leg and remains there during the emboîtés.

The head, during each coupé, turns away from the leg opening into the ballonné and remains in that last position for the two emboîtés.

The exercise is then performed on the other leg and reversed. In the case of reversing the ballonné, if the right arm moved to Second in regard to the right leg performing the ballonné, then in this case, it is moved into First and the left moves into Second. The body leans slightly toward the leg performing the ballonné and remains there during the two emboîtés.

The head at each ballonné turns in the direction of the lean of the body. Each movement is done to 1/4 of the measure.

Another example: In 2/4 tempo, Fifth Position, right leg front, épaulement croisé, a petit pas ballonné battu with the right leg to the side is done simultaneously with a turn en dehors (right) of 1/4 circle.

The beats are done with the right leg in front and its transfer is to the back in sur le cou-de-pied. Then the movement is repeated by the same leg in reverse with the turn of 1/4 circle in the same direction. The first ballonné battu of a 1/4 circle to the right is repeated, followed by a temps levé simple and a final petit pas emboîté back in a 1/4 turn in the same direction, with a final assemblé to the front.

The arm, head and body basically perform as described earlier but with the following changes: 1. The arms at the temps levé simple are fixed at the previous position and the emboîté arms open into a lowered Second while the last assemblé finds the arms lowered into the Preparatory Position; 2. The body during the pas emboîté and the assemblé is straight; 3. The head during the emboîté turns en face and, during the assemblé, turns toward the advanced shoulder.

Then the entire exercise is done on the other leg and is reversed with the arms, head and body performing in the same manner, including the last two jumps.

Each movement is done to 1/4 of a measure. All the rules for the performance of ballonné battu must be strictly observed.

GRAND FOUETTÉ BATTU

In this movement the beat is done in a fouetté and a 1/2 circle turn. As a study: To a 2/4 measure and beginning in the lower right corner of the room (#2) from a first arabesque in a high demi-pointe, a pas chassé along Second is done to the upper corner (#6). This is followed by a grand fouetté with a double beat; the right leg is thrown forward into the upper corner (#6), with the pushing left leg following in the same direction. At the crest of the jump, the left leg beats back with the right in front. As the fouetté continues in the air, the second beat—right leg back, left front—takes place. The left descends into a supple demi-plié as the right leg rises a bit into third arabesque.

The exercise continues with a pas chassé along Fourth into the lower left corner (#8), with a 1/4 circle turn en dehors and a petite cabriole into first arabesque. All is repeated from the other leg and performed once more from the beginning.

The entire movement is done impetuously, clearly and strictly according to the rules of fouetté and double beats.

The actions of the arms, head and body are as in the movement without the beats. The jump is done to 1/4 of the measure.

Later, the movement must be studied from other approaches such as the pas failli and the sissonne tombée, ending in first arabesque.

BRISÉ EN TOURNANT

The movement example starts in Fifth Position, with a 1/4 circle turn in 2/4 measure, right leg front, épaulement croisé. The brisé is forward with an en dedans 1/4 turn. The left leg, which is in back, is thrown in space starting in Second and ending in Fourth, actually like a hardly noticeable fouetté. The pupil must be made aware of this movement and perform it exactly.

This is followed by two petits changements de pied and all the movements are repeated three more times with turns in the same direction. However, after the fourth brisé, the exercise ends with, instead of the two changements, a pas glissade to the right and a change of legs into Fifth Position. Then the exercise is done on the other leg and, after a rest, is reversed.

When the brisé is reversed or done backward, with the turn en dehors of 1/4 circle, the leg is thrown from the Fifth Position with the advance to the point the toe leads (#6 or #4).

If this movement were pictured in a pattern on the floor, it would look like a square. And both movements would look like two squares.

The arms, head and body perform as they would in the brisé movement without a turn.

Each brisé with a turn and the pas glissade are done to 1/4 of a measure and each petit changement de pied is done to 1/8 of a measure.

As a second example: Beginning in the same position as the last exercise, a brisé forward is done with a turn to the left, en dehors of 1/4 circle followed by an entrechat quatre; then the brisé is done backward turning in the same direction in 1/4 of a circle, followed by an entrechat quatre. All this is repeated except for the last entrechat quatre, which is replaced by a royale. Then the exercise is ready to be repeated on the other leg.

Later, the brisé with a turn may be joined to other, more complicated beats with or without a turn.

In this kind of brisé with a turn, the thrown leg must move from Fifth into Fourth with a fully turned-out position and along an exact straight line. It is inadmissible to move the supporting leg or to shorten the length of the advance. The turning sendoff from the supporting leg must be sufficiently powerful and exact. The center of gravity is sent toward the same point in space as the thrown leg. The slightest mistake will result in an incorrect advance, turn and even an incorrect beat. The arms and head must participate actively and rush toward the same point in space. And, of course, all the rules for the jump, beat and turn, must be scrupulously observed.

BRISÉ DESSUS-DESSOUS EN TOURNANT

This brisé is done with a 1/4 turn. As an example: Beginning in Fifth Position, right leg front, épaulement croisé to a 2/4 measure, a brisé dessus forward with a 1/4 turn en dedans is executed. The jump ends on the leg that made the throw; the other, after the beat, transfers into sur le cou-de-pied front. This is followed by a temps levé simple. Both these movements are done in reverse with the turn in the same direction and the jump ending on the leg that made the throw with the other in sur le cou-de-pied back.

The movements are repeated from the beginning, except for the ending after the fourth brisé, which is a petit pas ballonné battu to the side ending in sur le cou-de-pied back instead of the temps levé simple.

Then all is ready to be repeated on the other leg. In doing the brisé, dessus or dessous, the leg must be thrown into the same point in space, a corner of the room beginning in Second and ending through a fouetté into Fourth.

Each jump is to 1/4 of the measure.

As another example: Beginning in the same starting pose and with the same pattern of movement, brisé dessus-dessous with a turn of 1/4 to the left. All together, there are four brisés, two dessus and two dessous. This is followed by three petits emboîtés with a 3/4 turn in the same direction and a brisé dessus-dessous without the turn. The entire movement is ready to be performed on the other leg and reversed. In that case, the first brisé dessous is with a turn to the left.

Each petit emboîté is done to 1/8 of a measure and all other to 1/4 of the measure.

When the pupil has performed this exercise correctly, he has learned to orient himself in space and is ready to perform more exercises of virtuoso quality. But it must be remembered that if he has merely learned to perform only the turns and the beats and has not mastered the artistry, then he is not ready for the creativity of the stage. He has only exercised the technique of movement.

TOURS EN L'AIR

This group of movements consists of big jumps which are done with double turns in the air and are named, in a general sense, tours en l'air.

In the performance of these movements one may find the changement de pied, the temps sauté and various sissonnes. The double turn in space contributes a new dimension, a new quality to these movements. These jumps, done with a partial or full turn, hardly change qualitatively and in a considerable measure preserve the plastic structure of the jump. But the addition of two quick turns seems to change the image of these movements and the turning becomes the leading basis for them.

Therefore, these movements are discussed here as tours en l'air—turnings in the air—and not as jumps complicated by double turns.

The tour en l'air as a means of expression is widely used in many ways in the art of classical ballet. But exactness and stability in performance alone, as well as in other movements of classical ballet, cannot disclose the character and imagery of the dance action. What is needed is mastery of expression.

The tours en l'air done in the role of Albrecht in *Giselle*, Danilo in *The Stone*

Flower or Basil in *Don Quixote* may be the same in method of execution, but they are very different in character and style.

The task for the pupil in learning the tours en l'air is to gradually learn to express the plastic character of the movement by increasing or softening the jump, by shortening or deepening the demi-plié, by adding impetuosity or restraint to the movement of the arms, head and body. In time, of course, each pupil will develop his own style and tempo of performance for the tours en l'air, but still, the stability in the performance of these tours must gradually obtain ever increasing and refined musicality.

Moreover, the tours en l'air are not merely effective jumps. They are dance gestures which may be inspired, full of the feelings of inner action or demonstrative. And all these things must be considered in teaching the exercises, as well as later on stage.

In short, tours en l'air must be prepared for the future dancer in a way that will enable him to give them live nuances and virtuosity. These preparations must be exercised during the lessons.

There are some dancers of the past and present who are able to perform the tour en l'air with three turns! This, of course, is the highest form of virtuosity, but only if the turns incorporate artistry.

The study of these turns must not start until small and large jumps have been well learned, as well as the turns of a 1/4, 1/2 and full circle. Like the study of the pirouette, which should not begin until the elements are mastered—stability on demi-pointe, a strengthened spine, and mastery of exercises with turns—the study of the tour en l'air begins when the force for a jump, stability and turnability have been mastered.

In addition, all tours en l'air must be practiced on both sides, including "one's own" and the "alien" side. This develops the technique of turning in general. But if the pupil, because of limited gifts, cannot perform a double tour on the "alien" side, and is in danger of incurring a serious injury to the legs, he must perform only one turn on the weaker side and be given help in overcoming this weakness in order to assist him in performing a double turn on this side.

TOURS EN L'AIR FROM FIFTH POSITION TO FIFTH POSITION

These tours are done with the assistance of the grand changement de pied. Beginning in Fifth Position, right foot forward, épaulement croisé, a demi-plié is made with an elastic and even pressure on the heels for a forceful, strictly perpendicular and trampoline-like turning push to the right. At the moment of the flight, the legs next to one another (in First Position), clearly exchange places during the turn in the air and remain tightly joined until the final demi-plié landing, which is soft and exactly into a Fifth Position onto both heels with an even pressure.

The arms at the start move from a Preparatory Position, the left through First into Second and the right into First Position. At the moment of the turning push, the left arm is sent forcefully from Second into First and, without delay, both energetically join in a rounded and lowered First Position or are thrown into Third Position. In the jump and during the turn, they are kept in one of these positions, and at the final demi-plié they clearly and freely open into a lowered Second Position.

The body actively participates in the turning sendoff by remaining straight as well as being collected throughout the spine, with open, free and lowered shoulders.

The head, at the beginning of each turn, is slightly delayed. Then, ahead of the body, it clearly fixes its position. The eyes look straight front as in small pirouettes. The neck must not be strained, nor the facial muscles.

The tours en l'air require a high and light jump in a definite and vigorous tempo and a soft, free and stable finish. To accomplish this, the student must learn to compute the force needed for the turning push and the height required for the jump. If, for instance, the jump is not high enough but the push forceful, the tours will become too fast and fuzzy and the finish, rough and sharp. With too forceful a push, the pupil, as a rule, performs a less high jump with less strength. This must be eliminated from the performance. If the push is too weak, the tours become unstable, muddied and inexact at the finish. The tour must be practiced with moderate force for the spinning push but be sufficient for two full, clear and high turns which will allow a free finish descending into a soft demi-plié as one would end in a simple grand changement de pied.

The legs, in their clear and active change, turn themselves. If the change is flabby or the legs are not joined in Fifth Position, they will become a brake in the spin of the body.

The arms, like the legs, turn themselves, when joined vigorously into a close and lowered First Position. If this movement is done weakly, or too quickly and forcefully, the spinning in the air will be made more difficult.

The body, incorporating the turning effort of the legs and arms, must itself rush impetuously in the same direction. But if the sendoff is too weak or too rough, the tempo and balance of the body will be destroyed.

The head turns itself as well, with the aid of a clear and separate movement of the neck. But if that is too forceful, or in a weak tempo, it as well will interfere unfavorably with the spin of the body.

Consequently, the movement of the arms, legs, head and body, during the turning push, cooperate. They must be in one tempo and be commensurate in effort for a correct, virtuoso performance. Inadmissible in the performance are:

1. a disturbance in the turnout; a delay in the joining of the heels during the turning push; a wide, flabby exchange of the legs during the jump; a failure to keep the legs in Fifth Position during the jump; a weakening in the knees, instep or toes during the jump; a rough or inexact ending of the jump in Fifth Position;

2. a violation of the plasticity of the arms by moving them to the side opposite the direction of the turn at the moment of taking force for the turn; overstraining or breaking the rounded line of the lowered First Position by raising or lowering too much; weakly or deliberately opening the arms into lowered Second Position at the end of the jump;

3. the overstraining or weakening of the body; a lean away from the perpen-

dicular; a turn before the spin to the opposite direction; an inexact alignment of the center of gravity over the legs in the turning push and the final demi-plié;

4. a lean by the head away from the perpendicular; a turn in the same tempo as the body; a pressure of the chin into the sternum; a focus downward, failing to look directly front.

The general style and character of the tour en l'air must be strict, restrained, free of artifice and emotionally sure and masculine. Any casual, colorless or mechanical performance of this movement has no place in classical dance.

An example of an exercise: To a 2/4 measure, Fifth Position, right foot front, en face, three petits changements de pieds are performed followed by two tours en l'air. The third changement ends with a stronger and deeper trampoline-like demi-plié which becomes the spinning push and tosses the body from the floor to the required height.

Tours en l'air end in a soft and stable demi-plié and a pause. The exercise is repeated three more times in full and then is done in reverse.

Each petit changement group is done to 1/4 of the measure; the tours to 1/4 each and the pause in the final demi-plié, 1/4 of the measure. The changement de pied is useful to the performance of the tours en l'air. The repetition of these jumps, which distribute the weight of the body on freely springing legs, prepares for a stable and correct performance of the tours.

These complications are useful in further study:

1. omitting an approach, a spot or place, but including a rest or pause after the spin;
2. omitting an approach and adding the performance of small jumps after the spin;
3. performing the tours from petit assemblé along Second and Fourth with a stop after the spin;
4. performing the tours from pas glissade from Fifth into Fifth;
5. performing the tours from a pas de bourrée simple or en tournant;
6. performing the tours with a transfer into a big jump such as the sissonne ouverte and into big poses.

The exercises for tours may be constructed in a great many ways and many degrees of difficulty, but they must gradually and progressively lead to the mastery of an exact, stable and artistically dynamic spin during the jump.

The tours en l'air may be usefully introduced into the middle or end of combinations with big jumps. When the technique for spinning strengthens, the tours may be introduced into adagio movements and into exercises consisting of grand battement jeté, etc. This is done so that the student will perform the tours as a usual component in a combination, not as something special or a movement that has a specific or familiar approach.

Finally, the raising of the arms into Third during the tours may be incorporated into the exercises when there appears to be a free tempo to the spin, a high flight and a stable ending. The arms must not be held in front of the body, but in Third Position directly above the head in one perpendicular axis with the body in order not to interfere with the spinning process.

Another approach for the tours is the relevé onto a high demi-pointe in Fifth

Position. This is a traditional approach and merits every attention, but it seems to me that if the student has learned well the diverse turns and spins on the floor as well as in the air, which have been part of the teaching, then the usefulness of the relevé onto demi-pointe is not very great.

This approach should be used, and rightly so, but it is more in the style of historic choreography than a contemporary method for the development of difficult and complicated technique.

TOUR EN L'AIR IN TEMPO (IN SUCCESSION)

This tour en l'air is performed as a jump from two legs onto two legs for a successive tour. The two tours are called tours en l'air in tempo. Their peculiarity is in the fact that the first jump is done as a temps sauté without the changement de pied in Fifth, and the second jump with a changement de pied with a change of legs. The leg which ends in back corresponds to the direction of the turn.

The transfer from one jump to another must be done in a trampoline-like rebound, and from a short, fast, passing demi-plié, so that the spinning is not interrupted and the ending of the first jump serves as the beginning of the next.

The arms must take force as described previously, but in one tempo with the turning push of the body.

Total perpendicularity, a totally collected body and evenness in the push by both legs are of decided importance. Additionally, these tours must be done strictly in one place, with no jumps to the side.

These tours are studied last, in the graduating classes and only by the students who have sufficient gifts. If the method is well learned, it may be repeated three or even four times in succession. In such a case, the last tour is performed as described, with the change of legs.

An exercise for the beginning of the study: In a measure of 2/4, Fifth Position, right foot front, en face, the tours à tempo is performed (two successive turns en l'air). This is followed by three changements de pied and all is repeated three more times. These tours are practiced only on one's own (preferred) side, which can support such a complicated spinning sequence.

The first tour begins before the measure and ends on the first 1/4 of the first measure. The second tour is done on the second 1/4 of the first measure. Each petit changement de pied is done to 1/8 of the second measure.

The following exercises must take into consideration the gradual increase in complexity of the approaches and the performance of these tours.

TOUR EN L'AIR PAR SISSONNE SIMPLE

The performance of sissonne simple with one tour has already been described. The tour en l'air by way of the sissonne simple is constructed in the same way except for a correspondingly increased height in the jump and a greater force for the turning push.

The legs during the jump might be used in two ways: 1. They may remain joined in Fifth Position during the jump, opening just before the descent, into sur le cou-de-pied by the front leg. (The turn is en dehors. If done in reverse, it is en dedans.) 2. They may exchange places at once as in the basic tour en l'air except with a transfer to the back into sur le cou-de-pied by the front leg. (The turn is en dehors. If, however, the transfer is forward, the spinning is en dedans.)

Each method has its difficulties. The first form is difficult because it does not contribute to a free spin of the body in air. Therefore, the spinning push must be taken with more force than for the basic tour from Fifth Position. And yet all the rules must be observed for its correct execution. On the other hand, a push that is too forceful is not suitable since it may easily disturb the stability of the ending of the turn, which is on one leg with the other in sur le cou-de-pied. The force must be carefully estimated to permit a soft and stable ending to the jump.

The second method is difficult because the foot in flight moves into the sur le cou-de-pied position front or back. On the other hand, the exchange of legs in the air permits this tour to be done with less force and it, therefore, has a softer and freer ending which is more stable as well. The change of legs in the air must be done clearly into a heightened position of the sur le cou-de-pied position. In this push and flight, both legs must work with equal force while one leg remains perpendicular and the other, passing as close as possible, with a strongly held thigh, fixes a somewhat heightened position in sur le cou-de-pied back for the en dehors turn, or front for the en dedans turn.

The arms and head as well as the body follow the pattern for the previously described tours en l'air. As a first exercise: In a 2/4 tempo, Fifth Position, right foot front, épaulement croisé, two tours en l'air are performed with the right foot bending into sur le cou-de-pied front; followed by a petit assemblé along Second ending in Fifth Position back; and three petits changements de pieds.

The arms, during the tours, remain in a lowered First until the changements, when the left arm, through First Position, rises to Second and the right arm rises to First Position.

The body is straight, pulled up and harmonious. At the final demi-plié, the center of gravity must be correctly over the supporting leg. This is a very important element and if not mastered the study will be unsuccessful.

In the assemblé, as well as in the changements, the body changes épaulement in turns of 1/4 circle. The head, during all the tours and in all the other movements, performs in the usual pattern.

The exercise is repeated four times to the right side, and separately on the left. Then it is reversed.

The tours and the petit assemblé are performed each to 1/4 of the measure and each petit changement to 1/8 of the measure.

Later, the petit assemblé may be replaced by a pas glissade to the side, and the petits changements replaced by entrechats quatre.

The first example for study: Two tours en l'air en dehors are performed with a transfer of the right leg into sur le cou-de-pied back; petit assemblé to the back into croisé in Fifth follows; three petits changements end the exercise. The arms and body perform as in the previous exercise.

This is repeated four times to the right with a rest instead of the changements.

(The assemblé ends with the left shoulder advanced.) It is then repeated to the other side. After a short rest, the exercise is reversed. The first two turns are done to 1/4 of the measure, the next to 1/8, followed by a rest of a full measure.

Later, instead of performing the petit assemblé, a pas glissade en croisé to the back and to the front may be substituted. Or a pas de bourrée simple with a full turn in the same direction may be the substitution with more complicated jumps instead of the petits changements.

There exists still another accepted form of joining these tours without an exchange of legs—by a renversé en attitude. At the moment of the end of the tours, the leg in sur le cou-de-pied in front, together with the performance of the second jump, is thrown by means of a rond de jambe jeté through Second, into attitude croisée back. This is done with an even raise of the leg to 90 degrees from the rond de jambe to the attitude, which must be completed together with the final demi-plié on the supporting leg. Then, a pas de bourrée with a full turn is done into Fifth Position.

Together with this movement, the arms move from a lowered First into Second Position. At the moment of the transfer of the leg into attitude croisée back, the arms move into the position for renversé en attitude. The body and head perform in the usual pattern.

Both jumps must flow and be plastic.

As an exercise: To a 2/4 tempo, from Fifth Position, right foot front, épaulement croisé, two tours en l'air en dehors without a change of legs are performed, the last tour becoming a renversé en attitude croisée back; pas de bourrée into Fourth Position follows; a petit assemblé to the back into Fifth Position ends the exercise. The head, arms and body perform in the usual manner for this movement. The tours are performed before the count; and all the rest of the exercise, evenly. The exercise is done on a diagonal downstage (#6 to #2 or #4 to #8 on the left side) and then practiced on the other leg. These two joined jumps may later be introduced into more complicated exercises.

TOURS EN L'AIR PAR SISSONNE TOMBÉE

These tours are a development of the preceding form. They are performed by means of a tombé opening the leg from sur le cou-de-pied followed by a "fall" into Fourth or Second Position. This must be a supple flow at the final demi-plié.

The characteristic of this movement is an advance during the tombé which must be estimated carefully and move into a final demi-plié with a sendoff of the entire body in the direction of the opening leg.

In these tours, both forms of spinning and both forms of leg movements—changing and not changing—are used.

The tombé in these tours is done by leading the free leg, toes along the floor. The arms, head and body at this moment assume the position for a small pose, effacé, croisé devant or en arrière, à la seconde or écarté.

As a first exercise for tours without a change of leg: To a 2/4 measure, beginning in Fifth Position, right foot front, épaulement croisé, two tours en dehors are done by means of a tombé devant into a third arabesque by leading the toes of the free leg along the floor; a petit assemblé into Fifth back follows. The head, arms and body perform as usual for the tours. During the assemblé, the arms move from third arabesque, the left First into Second and the right, from Second into First to prepare for the next repeat of the exercise—a total of four times except for the last tour, which is done from Fifth into Fifth Position. Then the exercise is done on the other leg. Each jump is to 1/4 of a measure.

Later, this tour may be studied with a tombé into a small pose with the toes moving along the floor à la seconde. The exercise is in the same form.

Finally, these tours may be done with a tombé into third arabesque and followed by petit assemblé to the back into Fifth Position eight times in a row. The eight tours are done into Fifth Position.

Then, the tombé may be alternated in direction: to the front, to the side or joined with other, more complicated exercises.

As an example of these tours *with a change of legs*: In the same measure and beginning position, two tours en dehors are performed by means of a tombé to the back into croisé, with the free leg leading backward, toes along the floor; a petit assemblé into Fifth devant; an ending with three petits changements de pieds.

The arms, head and body perform as usual for the tours. On the tombé, the right arm opens into Second and the left stays in First. At the assemblé, the left arm opens into Second but the right does not move. During the petits changements, the right arm moves into First.

The exercise is repeated four times with the last tour ending in Fifth and an entrechat quatre added. Then the exercise is repeated on the other leg and reversed with the tours en dedans, and the tombé forward. Each tour and petit assemblé is done to 1/4 of a measure. Each changement is to 1/8 of a measure; the entrechat quatre to 1/4; and a rest for one full 2/4 measure.

Later, the same tours may be studied with a tombé onto Second in this same form, alternated, then joined into more complicated jumps with a raising of the arms into Third Position.

TOURS EN L'AIR PAR SISSONNE OUVERTE

These tours may be done with a change of legs in the air, as in the previously described turns, with an en dehors direction, but only with an opening of the leg to the back into Fourth with the whole foot on the floor; onto one knee; into 90 degrees into third arabesque or attitude croisée derrière.

TOUR EN L'AIR INTO FOURTH POSITION

In this movement the leg in front, at the crest of the jumping turn, quickly and exactly moves into an elevated sur le cou-de-pied in back. This transfer must be done as close to the other leg as possible and immediately after the turning push. The leg on which the jump ends is kept perpendicular. Both legs are turned out and fully stretched at the knees, insteps and toes. At the end of the jump, the leg which is bent stretches at the knee, is led back in croisé and is put on the floor with flexibility—the entire foot in Fourth Position. This occurs at the same time as the demi-plié on the supporting leg. The arms, head and body are in third arabesque position. The first exercise: In 2/4, Fifth Position, right foot forward, épaulement croisé, two tours are done into Fourth Position back in croisé. The supporting leg straightens from demi-plié as the back leg is pulled into a Fifth Position and a demi-plié on both legs. The arms, head and body at the end of the tours are in third arabesque.

During the demi-plié into Fifth, the arms move into the pose required for the next tours in the other direction. All is repeated four times. The tours are done before the count with a stop on the first 1/4 of the measure in third arabesque par terre; 1/4 for the stretch of the supporting leg from demi-plié; 1/4 for the following demi-plié into Fifth.

The third arabesque position is only the first form of the study. It may later include arms opened into a lowered Second; into an attitude through the usual positions; or in allongé.

The tours as well may end differently in Fourth: in effacé, first arabesque and other poses. The head and body always suit the pose. The study of this movement must be gradual and joined in combined exercises.

TOURS EN L'AIR TO THE KNEE

These tours are done in the same manner as those in Fourth described above, but only en dehors with a change of legs and an elevated sur le cou-de-pied back.

At the moment the turn ends, the leg that was led to the back position must clearly and elastically descend onto its knee. The leg must not be straightened and the toes, which are stretched, must touch the floor, cushioning the knee from the tips of the toes to the knee. The knee must not hit the floor but descend softly and exactly into Fourth Position in its relationship to the supporting leg.

Inadmissible to this movement is a leading of the knee too near to the supporting leg or too far from it in back. Nor would it be acceptable to have the knee end to the side along Second, since those directions would not observe the characteristic of this turn. The supporting leg, together with the leading of the other leg, does a demi-plié exactly that accepts the weight of the body with suppleness. The demi-plié must not be weak, rough or prolonged. It must be soft, light, clear. On the whole, the work of the legs must be free, in one tempo, turned out and pliable.

The arms during the turns are kept in a lowered First or Third Position. At the moment of the transfer to the knee, they may open into Second; into an attitude pose with rounded arms; into an attitude with arms allongé. The body during the turn must be straight and collected. At the moment of the descent to the knee, it leans slightly back in order to be supported evenly on both legs. This must be done with a correct estimate and not too forcefully or the body will be forced to "sit down" on the back leg. If this lean backward is not done, the body is pulled forward, which interferes with the work of the supporting front leg and causes a loss of balance. The head performs as usual and, at the end, takes the position suitable to the pose. On the whole, the arms, head and body act strictly and clearly, with aplomb but without any underscoring for effect.

As an example for study: To a measure of 2/4 in Fifth Position, right leg forward, épaulement croisé, two tours are performed to the back knee. Then simultaneously with the straightening of both legs with a transfer of weight to the forward leg, the right leg remains in croisé back and closes back into Fifth in demi-plié.

The arms, during the tours, act as previously described, and, at the descent to the knee, open into First. Upon rising from the knee, the arms remain in the same position, but when the leg closes into Fifth Position in back, the arms move into Preparatory Position.

The body is straight. The head, during the tours, acts as usual. During the descent to the knee, it turns toward the advanced shoulder and stays until the end of the movement.

These tours are done before the measure; the descent to the knee uses 1/4; a rest is 1/4; the rising from the knee is 1/4 and the closing into Fifth, 1/4.

Then the movement is done on the other leg and repeated once more on both. Later, the tours to one knee may be joined with other combinations of big jumps and different positions given to the arms. The rise from the knee must be free, light and a continuation of the dancing. It is not an ordinary, everyday movement.

TOUR EN L'AIR IN ARABESQUE AND ATTITUDE AT 90 DEGREES

This form of tour is performed in the same method as the tour to Fourth, in the direction en dehors, with a change of legs in air and the raised position of the sur le cou-de-pied in back opening at the end of the spin clearly into 90 degrees in back.

The opening of the leg must end fully stretched if the tour ends in arabesque, and somewhat bent, if the tour ends in attitude croisée derrière.

In both cases, the leg opens together with the final demi-plié and opens without delay or increased speed into its final position. Both legs at this moment act in one tempo with suppleness and are turned out so that the final point of the tour is at one with it and actively a part of it.

Inadmissible to the performance of this movement is a flabby or rough demi-plié, the slightest lowering of the thigh of the open leg or breaking of any of the rules for the execution of the grande sissonne ouverte, into a given pose.

The arms in the performance of the tours into first arabesque rise energetically into Third and open in one tempo with the final demi-plié into first arabesque. This must not be done with too feeble or loose a movement or one that is too aggressive or too bold. Strictness and measure are necessary here as in all other movements of classical dance.

If the tours are performed ending in attitude croisée, the arms rise into Third and, on the demi-plié, the arm corresponding to the rising leg in back remains in Third and the other opens into Second.

The body during the tours into first arabesque remains upright, collected and, at the transfer to the supporting leg in demi-plié, leans slightly forward. These movements must be done very softly and quietly so as not to lose balance in the placement of the body, and the leg opening back at 90 degrees.

The body, after the tour into attitude croisée, leans slightly forward to a lesser degree since the leg in back is half bent, and therefore needs less counterbalancing. The head during the spinning performs as usual and at the final demi-plié is turned in the direction for the first arabesque of the attitude croisée derrière. The eyes look straight and with sureness in the same direction—a rule in the performance of these tours. On the whole, all the forms of these tours must end in a light and soft demi-plié, free of inertia, from the proper taking of force and in a single tempo to the final pose.

An example for the study to "one's own side" would be to a measure of 2/4, from Fifth Position, épaulement croisé. A double tour en l'air is done into first arabesque from the preferred side. Then a pas chassé in effacé forward and a petit assemblé devant into Fifth ends the exercise. The arms during the tour rise with vigor into Third and, at the end of the tour, lower into first arabesque. During the pas chassé, the arm in First transfers into Second and the other arm moves from Second into First and remains there during the petit assemblé. The body during the tour is straight, harmonious and, at the end, leans slightly forward. At the pas chassé, the body straightens and remains straight for the assemblé.

The head, before the spin, is turned in the direction for the first arabesque—downstage on the diagonal (#2 or #8). It moves as usual during the tours and into the pose for the first arabesque, and at the pas chassé is turned toward the advanced shoulder. At the assemblé it returns to the starting pose.

This exercise is repeated three times on the diagonal, downstage, ending in a small pirouette en dehors from Second Position.

Double turns are done before the measure and end on the first quarter of the measure. A rest of 1/4 follows in first arabesque; 1/4 is used for the pas chassé; 1/4 for the petit assemblé. The last two measures are used for a small pirouette en dehors from Second in the same direction as the exercise.

When these tours are performed on the preferred side, the rest may be omitted but must be practiced on the "alien" side as well. Then they are incorporated into exercises with big jumps.

The tours into attitude are studied somewhat later in an exercise like this: To the same measure and same starting pose, a double tour en l'air to attitude croisée back is performed on the preferred side; then a temps levé tombé in effacé forward through the calf position is done; a petit assemblé back into Fifth Position keeping the épaulement effacé position ends the exercise.

The arms during the tour rise energetically into Third. At the final demi-plié, the arm corresponding to the supporting leg opens into Second, the other remains in Third. During the temps levé tombé, the arm in Third goes into Second and at the petit assemblé moves into First as the other stays in Second.

The body, during the turning, is straight and pulled up. At the end it leans somewhat forward but at the temps levé tombé, it straightens and remains straight until the end.

The head, before the spin, is turned in the direction of the final attitude, diagonally downstage. During the tour, the head acts as usual, but at the end of the spin it turns toward the advanced shoulder. At the temps levé tombé, it returns to the starting position.

All of this exercise is repeated three times with an advance diagonally downstage (to corner #2 or #8) and ends in a small pirouette en dehors in the same direction.

The double tour is done before the measure, and ends on the first 1/4 of the measure; followed by 1/4 for a rest in attitude; 1/4 for the temps levé tombé; 1/4 for the petit assemblé to the back. The last two measures at the end of the exercise are used for small pirouettes.

When this has been well learned on the preferred side, it may later be combined with other exercises.

When both forms, the arabesque and the attitude ending, have been mastered, the student may attempt to end in a third arabesque or an attitude effacée derrière. But it must be attempted with care in order not to distract the student from the correct method or to shake his self-confidence.

If this should happen, the attempt should immediately be stopped and the attempt made again at a later time in combination with other jumps. In other words, one should search for another approach for the mastery of this difficult movement.

Finally, when all these tours have been learned, they may be approached from a small pirouette. This is done during the course of the turning of a pirouette by means of a quick lowering of the foot from sur le cou-de-pied into Fifth Position front in demi-plié. This lowering must be done en face from the toe through the heel with a flexible movement and exactly in Fifth Position, not an approximate position. Both feet at this moment, and in a trampoline-like manner, with equal force, press on both heels and, vigorously maintaining the spin of the pirouette, continue its force into a jumping push.

The arms at the moment of the passing demi-plié assume the position used for taking force for a tour en l'air. It must be done quickly and at the correct time, so that when the body reaches the en face position, they are already in place. Then they perform as usual.

The body is kept straight, harmonious and collected. During the passing demi-plié, it presses evenly on both legs and, continuing the spin, strengthens it for the jumping push.

The head moves in the manner for a pirouette and for a tour. But it must not lose tempo during the performance of the demi-plié. This slowing up for the demi-plié into the tour must be gradually overcome so that it is at its minimum but not to the extent that the movements lose plasticity.

There must be a constant effort to preserve the general perpendicularity of the axis during the small pirouettes and until the end of the tour. Then the spinning will get stronger and acquire the free and virtuoso character required for this movement.

Petites pirouettes into tours en l'air are usually done from a second, en dehors beginning of no more than three or four turns. The double tour ends in Fifth Position.

Later, after this has been well learned, the number of pirouettes may be increased and ended in different poses.

An example: To a measure of 2/4, Fifth Position with the right foot in front, body en face, three petites pirouettes en dehors in Fifth are done. A double tour is followed by three petits changements de pieds and another double tour in the same direction from Fifth into Fifth Position.

The arms, during the last tours, rise into Third but the rest of the movement follows the usual pattern. The approach to the petite pirouette is made before the measure; each pirouette is to 1/8 of the measure, the passing demi-plié with an accent is on the first 1/4 of the second measure; the tour to 1/4; petits changements to 1/8 of the second measure; the next tour to 1/4 and a rest of 1/4 of the measure.

Then all is done on the other leg and repeated two more times. To perform this exercise only on the preferred side is not advisable. It is necessary to "unravel" oneself, although the pirouettes may start on the preferred side.

Later, this method of transferring from petites pirouettes into tours en l'air may be used in more complicated combinations with more complex endings.

A progression for the study would be: 1. performing the study from Fifth into Fifth Position; 2. performing the tours by means of the sissonne simple; 3. performing the tours by means of the sissonne in tombée; 4. performing the tours by means of the sissonne ouverte; 5. in combination with the small pirouette; 6. "in tempo" (successive tours).

FROM THE AUTHOR

All of the material in this book is but a small part of the variety at the disposal of the teaching system in the Soviet School of classical dance. Therefore my recommendations may not coincide in every way with the training received in the school for teachers.

Many of the best teachers of classical dance, who prepare dancers in the choreographic schools throughout our country, use various methods of teaching and educating. One hopes that these masters, and their pupils, will in time compile their knowledge and put their ideas and experience into printed form. Nothing so enriches and sustains a teacher as a knowledge of individual methods that will help him deal with troublesome worries in his profession.

Like the whole of Soviet choreographic art, the Soviet School of classical dance has preserved its traditions in order to perfect and develop itself creatively. Though the school is sometimes berated for not giving the future artist enough practice in new styles of dance—the grotesque, eccentric and acrobatic—one may answer that if the teacher has mastered well the teaching of the school of classical dance, and is talented, he will have at his disposal all the necessary resources to formulate original and contemporary designs.

The choreographers of various styles prefer to work with performers who have finished the academic school of classical dance. Experience has shown that these performers, during rehearsals and stagings, can master roles in the various dance styles.

The school of classical dance is not for the memorizing of complex movements. With the aid of its exercises, it teaches the body and educates the mind of the performer so that he may act as freely and with as much variety and expressiveness as his choreographer needs for his creations.

Of course, next to the creativity of the theater the school takes a very modest position, but as its teaching melts into the mastery of the choreographer and the performer, it carries weight. The school is a near, true and useful creative friend of the choreographer of any specialty if its teaching is understood and mastered by him.

Having freed itself from mannerisms, especially in the teaching of male dancers, the Soviet School became more purposeful in its reach for ideas, more virtuosic in its technique and more nearly perfect in its methods and forms. It has enjoyed constant success here and abroad. Its choreographers, performers and teachers are welcome specialists everywhere, and it has made a rich contribution to the development of dance throughout the world.

To preserve a high academic style, to develop and perfect virtuoso mastery and culture—this is the task of the teacher.